PHYSIOLOGY OF MAMMARY GLANDS

PHYSIOLOGY OF MAMMARY GLANDS

Edited by
AKIRA YOKOYAMA, HIDEO MIZUNO, and HIROSHI NAGASAWA

JAPAN SCIENTIFIC SOCIETIES PRESS, Tokyo
UNIVERSITY PARK PRESS, Baltimore

JSSP No. 01412-1104
Printed in Japan

Published jointly by
JAPAN SCIENTIFIC SOCIETIES PRESS
Tokyo
and
UNIVERSITY PARK PRESS
Baltimore

Library of Congress Cataloging in Publication Data

Main entry under title:

Physiology of the mammary gland.

Bibliography: p.
Includes index.
1. Mammary glands. I. Yokoyama, Akira. II. Mizuno, Hideo. III. Nagasawa, Hiroshi.
QP188.M3P47 599′.01′6 78-7191
ISBN 0-8391-1303-X

PREFACE

We have organized a physiology of lactation research group in Japan, and have had workshops once or twice a year since 1962. For 3 years from 1972, the studies of our group were supported partly by cooperative research grants from the Ministry of Education, Science and Culture, Japan, and our experiments progressed greatly during those years. We thought, therefore, that it would be worthwhile publishing our experimental results in the form of a book.

This book is composed of two sections, a retrospective part and prospective part. In the latter part, recent advances in the various aspects of the physiology of lactation are reviewed not only by members of our group but also by Dr. J. S. Tindal, England. A general survey of the literature is not intended in this part, but the prospective view of specific aspects, based on each contributor's work, is presented. Although many books extensively reviewing the physiology of lactation have been published in the last decade, these books deal mainly with present knowledge. In the quest for truth, we need first to look backward and then to follow the paths of thought of senior scientists in either the same or different research fields. From this point of view, it is edifying, in the first part of this book, to study papers that have been contributed by distinguished scientists in the field of lactation regarding the retrospective, as well as philosophical views of their research.

We believe this book will be of great benefit not only to students, but also to the younger scientists working on the physiology of the mammary glands in understanding and searching for ways to solve the problems with which they are confronted.

This book is dedicated to Dr. K. Fujii, Professor of Emeritus, Tokyo Medical and Dental College, Dr. T. Hosi, Professor of Emeritus, University of Tokyo, and Dr. M. Naito, Professor of Emeritus, University of Tokyo, who were pioneers in lactation studies in Japan.

We thank Mrs. Y. Niwa and Mr. K. Ito for preparing the typescript and bibliography. The help given by Mr. T. Miyazaki, Japan Scientific Societies Press, Tokyo, in the preparation of the book is most gratefully acknowledged. For permission to reproduce various figures, we are much indepted to the editors of the following journals: *Anatomical Record*, *Development, Growth & Differentiation*, *Journal of National Cancer Institute*, *Endocrinologia Japonica*, *Endocrinology*, *Nature*, *Proceedings of National Academy of Science*, *Science*, *Zeitschrift für Anatomie und Entwicklungsgeschichte*, and to the following publishers: American Association for the Advancement of Science, J.B. Lippincott Company, Japan Endocrinological Society, Japanese Society of Developmental Biologists, MacMillan Journals Ltd., Springer-Verlag, The National Academy of Science, The Wistar Institute Press, U.S. Department of Health, Education and Welfare.

June 1978

A. Yokoyama
H. Mizuno
H. Nagasawa

CONTENTS

Preface v

I. RETROSPECTIVE OF THE STUDY ON THE PHYSIOLOGY OF MAMARY GLANDS

THE INITIATION AND MAINTENANCE OF LACTATION .... R. L. Baldwin, Jr. 5

MILK EJECTION AND SYNTHESIS OF MILK IN RUMINANTS .... G. Peeters 23

BACKWARD GLANCES .... A. T. Cowie 43

STUDIES IN SUCKLING .... B. A. Cross 59

LACTATION INHIBITION BY ERGOT DRUGS .... E. W. Flückiger 71

HOW I BECAME A NEUROENDOCRINOLOGIST .... M. Kawakami 85

EARLY STUDIES ON CONTROL OF INITIATION OF LACTATION AND PROLACTIN SECRETION .... J. Meites 107

II. RECENT ADVANCE IN THE PHYSIOLOGY OF MAMMARY GLANDS

NORMAL AND ABNORMAL GROWTH OF THE MAMMARY GLAND .... H. Nagasawa and R. Yanai 121

1. Methods for Evaluating Mammary Growth 121
2. Normal Mammary Growth 123
3. Abnormal (Preneoplastic and Neoplastic) Mammary Growth 129
4. Longterm Effects of Perinatal Treatments with Hormones and Drugs on Normal and Abnormal Mammary Growth 141

5. Mammary DNA Synthesis as an Important Factor for Mammary Tumorigenesis 143
Summary 147

MAMMARY TRANSPLANTATION AND ITS HISTOGENESIS IN MICE .... K. Hoshino 163
1. Genetic Donor-host Relationships 164
2. Methods of Mammary Transplantation in Mice 171
3. The Quantitative Transplantation of Mammary Ducts 171
4. Site of Transplantation 173
5. Transplantability in Relation to the Origin Duct-segments 186
6. Directional Preference of Mammary Duct-segments in Regeneration 190
7. Sexual Differences in Mammary Transplantability 190
8. Heterochronic Donor-host Relationship 193
9. Life Span of Mammary Parenchyma 195
10. Pretreatment of Donor Mice 199
11. Parenchymal-stromal Interactions in Mammary Grafts 200
Conclusion 221

PROLACTIN RECEPTORS IN THE MAMMARY GLAND .... K. Kohmoto and S. Sakai 231
1. Iodination of Prolactin 232
2. The Existence and Characterization of a Prolactin Receptor in the Mouse Mammary Gland 233
3. Development of the Binding Site for Prolactin during Pregnancy and in Lactogenesis 239
Summary 245

SOME ASPECTS OF CASEIN BIOSYNTHESIS IN THE MAMMARY GLAND .... S. Komine 251
1. Effects of Hormones 252
2. Locality of Casein Biosynthesis, Change of Ribosomes, Casein Phosphorylation, and Secretory Mechanism 255
3. Messenger RNA for Casein 256
4. Precursors of Casein 257
5. Energy Source for Casein Biosynthesis 257
Summary 259

HORMONAL CONTROL OF THE INDUCTION OF LACTOSE SYNTHESIS IN THE RAT .... A. Yokoyama and K. Ôta 265
1. Plasma Concentration of Corticosterone during Pregnancy and Daily Fluctuation of the Concentration in the Rat 267

2. Induction of Lactose Synthesis in the Mammary Glands of Pregnant and Pseudopregnant Rats by Ovariectomy 272

EFFECTS OF CONCURRENT PREGNANCY AND CONTINUOUS SUCKLING ON TWO CONSECUTIVE LACTATIONS
.... H. Mizuno and N. Sensui 287
1. Concurrent Pregnancy and Lactation 288
2. Continuous Suckling and Subsequent Lactation 295
Summary 299

CENTRAL PATHWAYS IN OXYTOCIN AND PROLACTIN RELEASE
.... J. S. Tindal 305
1. Brainstem Pathways Involved in Oxytocin Release 305
2. Brainstem Pathways Involved in Prolactin Release 311
Summary 317

HORMONE SECRETION AT LACTOGENESIS AND DURING LACTATION IN DAIRY FARM ANIMALS ....T. Johke 325
1. Methods of Radioimmunoassay 325
2. Serum Hormone Levels during Late Pregnancy and Early Lactation in Dairy Cows and Goats 327
3. Effect of 2-Br-α-Ergocryptine on Serum Hormone Concentration and Lactogenesis in Cows and Goats 329
4. Milking Stimulus and Release of the Hormones 333
5. Effects of 2-Br-α-Ergocryptine on Hormone Secretion and Lactation 336
Summary 337

ROLE OF MILKING IN INITIATION AND MAINTENANCE OF LACTATION IN THE DAIRY ANIMALS ....Y. Shinde 347
1. The Effects of Milk Removal on the Mammary Function and Induction of Lactation in the Goat 347
2. The Effect of Milk Removal from the Udder of the Dairy Cow upon Milk Secretion 352
Summary 358

PHYSIOLOGICAL SIGNIFICANCE OF VARIATION IN THE ELECTROLYTE CONCENTRATION IN COW'S MILK ......M. Oshima 363
1. Variation in the Electrolytes in Milk due to Non-physiological Causes 364
2. Variation in Milk Composition and Osmotic Pressure of Milk 369
3. Inverse Relationship between Electrolytes and Organic Constituents in Normal Milk of Different Cows 373

Summary 380

SUBJECT INDEX 383

I. RETROSPECTIVE OF THE STUDY ON THE PHYSIOLOGY OF MAMMARY GLANDS

I-1

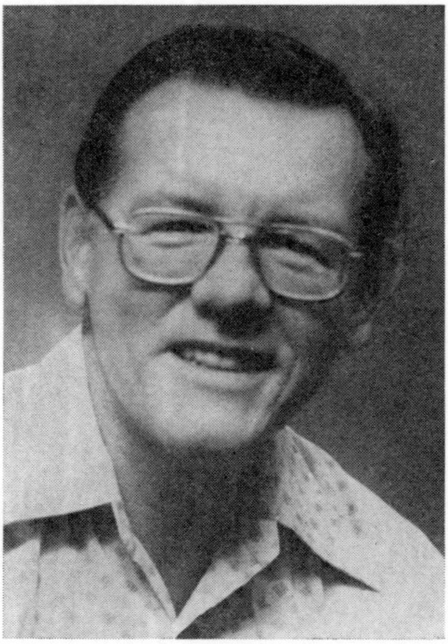

Ransom L. Baldwin, Jr. was born on September 21, 1935 in Meriden, Connecticut, U.S.A. He received a B.S. degree in 1957 from University of Connecticut and a Ph.D. degree in 1963 from Michigan State University. While at Michigan State University, he was a NSF Fellow in 1961–3.

Positions held include the following: Assistant Professor, Department of Animal Science, University of California, Davis, 1963–7 ; Associate Professor, 1967–70 ; Professor, 1970–present.

Some of the Societies of which he is a member include Sigma Xi, AIN, ADSA and he is an Associate Editor of the Journal of Nutrition.

Dr. Baldwin has received a number of awards including a Guggenheim Fellowship (1968) and an American Feed Manufactures Award (1970).

THE INITIATION AND MAINTENANCE OF LACTATION

R. L. BALDWIN, JR.

Department of Animal Science, University of California, Davis, California, USA

We became interested in studying mechanisms of hormone action associated with the initiation and maintenance of lactation in 1962. At that time, there were considerable data available regarding the hormonal requirements for mammary development and function (*20*). Also, many data were available indicating that extensive cell proliferation occurred in the mammary gland during pregnancy (*33*), that the rates and patterns of carbohydrate metabolism shifted markedly at lactogenesis, and that dramatic increases in the activities of enzymes in the pathways of lactose, protein, and fat biosynthesis occurred during pregnancy and lactation (*20*, *33*). However, only limited data were available concerning enzymatic and cellular changes during the critical periods immediately pre- and post-partum. Data concerning changes which occur during these critical periods were essential before possible relationships among increases in cellularity, enzyme changes, lactogenesis and lactation could be evaluated in terms of hormonal regulation. Thus, our first series of studies was directed at characterization of magnitudes and time sequences of changes in cellularity and enzyme activities during pregnancy and lactation in rats, guinea pigs, and dairy cows (*1*, *9*). Results of these studies, represented by the rat data depicted in Fig. 1, enabled us to define three events essential to lactogenesis and attainment of full lactation (*2*). The first essential event is the formation of functionally differentiated secretory cells. This event is characterized *in vivo* by extensive cell proliferation, lobuloalveolar development, and increases in DNA in late pregnancy and early lactation

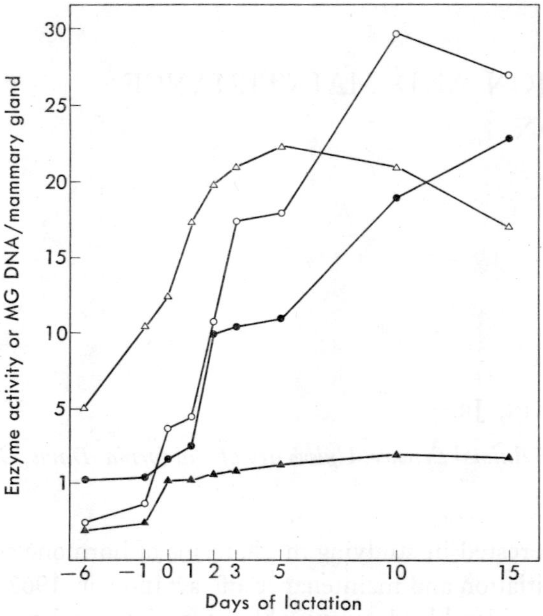

FIG. 1. Changes in rat mammary (MG) DNA and enzyme levels during pregnancy and lactation

Taken from Ref. *9*. UDPGPase, G6PD, and aldolase code UDPG pyrophosphorylase, glucose-6-P dehydrogenase, and fructose-1,6-diphosphate aldolase. ○ UDPGPase; ● G6PD; △ DNA; ▲ aldolase.

(Fig. 1). In *in vitro* (mammary explant) systems this event is characterized by lobuloalveolar development and an increase in DNA during the first 24 hr of culture (*40*). The second essential feature of mammary development is the formation of a characteristic complement of enzymes by the newly-formed secretory cells. In Fig. 1 this event is reflected by rapid increases in the activities of all mammary gland enzymes. These increases lag 18–24 hr behind increases in DNA. A similar pattern of development resulting in accumulation of milk components in explants has been observed *in vitro* (*40*). Much of the secretory cell development observed during this period appears to be inherent or constitutive in requiring only the formation of new cells since all enzymes studied appear to increase in a parallel fashion. The third essential event involves regulation of expression of capacity for milk synthesis resulting from the occurrence of the first two events. This process may involve the synthesis of a few key enzymes resulting in lactogenesis, as suggested by Bauman and coworkers

(*32*), hormonally induced increases in specific activities of biosynthetic enzymes, as represented by increases in glucose-6-P dehydrogenase and uridine diphosphate glucose (UDPG) pyrophosphorylase throughout lactation (Fig. 1) and as milk yield increases (*2*, *3*, *10*), and specific hormone actions upon secretory cell metabolic regulatory systems (*2–4*, *6*).

Most of our early studies were specifically directed at elucidation of hormone actions related to the three events described above. Results of several of these studies will be discussed in subsequent sections. More recent studies have been directed at understanding acute mechanisms of hormonal regulation of mammary metabolism, quantitative and dynamic analyses of mammary function, and effects of lactation upon functions of extramammary tissues. These will also be considered briefly.

Hormone Actions in Early Lactation

The hormonal requirements for mammary development and function *in vivo* were established prior to 1960 as a result of the classical studies of Lyons, Meites, Nandi, Cowie, Folley and others (*20*). Based on this knowledge and the temporal patterns of mammary cellular and enzymatic development established as a result of our first studies (*1*, *9*), we designed a series of *in vivo* experiments with hypophysectomized rats receiving various hormone replacement therapies. It was hoped that these would allow us to sort out specific actions of hormones of the lactogenic complex.

It should be noted prior to discussion of our data that numerous *in vitro* studies (*40*) of hormone actions upon mammary gland explants from mid-pregnant rodents were conducted and reported at about the same time as our *in vivo* experiments. Results from the *in vivo* and *in vitro* experiments were, largely, in agreement even though interpretations of the respective data changed as knowledge increased. However, some data were not completely consistent. Most of these differences are attributable to differences in the stages of mammary development studied. Most *in vitro* studies were conducted with mammary explants from mid-pregnant animals while our *in vivo* studies were conducted with rats hypophysectomized on the first or tenth day of lactation. *In vitro* techniques for the culture of mammary explants from lactating animals have not been developed; rapid losses of metabolic activity occur *in vitro*, presumably due to the accumulation of milk in the alveoli.

Several data from an experiment with animals hypophysectomized on the first day of lactation are presented in Table I. As expected, treatment

TABLE I. Effects of Several Hormone Replacement Therapies on the Characteristics of Mammary Glands from Rats Hypophysectomized during Early Lactation[a]

	Hormone treatment				
	O	CO	PO	CPO	S
Av. change in pup wt. (g)	−1.2	−1.0	−0.6	+0.6	+2.2
DNA (mg/g)	0.7	0.6	0.8	1.0	0.9
DNA (S.A.)[b]	0.5	0.4	1.0	1.1	1.5
RNA (mg/g)	1.3	1.3	2.1	2.4	3.0
Nuclear RNA (S.A.)[b]	6.3	16.4	20.6	25.2	25.6
RNA I (S.A.)[b]	1.3	1.4	2.3	3.4	2.1
RNA II (S.A.)[b]	1.4	2.1	4.5	5.6	5.9
G6PD (u/gl)[c]	0.14	0.16	0.32	1.3	1.6
Casein (cpm)[b]	1.8	3.5	3.8	11.5	12.0

[a] Data compiled from Ref. *8*. Rats were hypophysectomized on the 1st day of lactation and were administered 0.5 U oxytocin (O), 0.5 U oxytocin plus 0.25 mg cortisol (CO), 0.5 U oxytocin plus 10 U prolactin (PO), and 0.5 U oxytocin, 0.25 mg hydrocortisone plus 10 U prolactin (CPO) four times daily for 2.5 days before sampled. Sham (S) operated animals were administered saline.

[b] One hour prior to killing the experimental animals, $^{32}PO_4$ and leucine-^{14}C were injected intraperitoneally. DNA-^{32}P, nuclear RNA-^{32}P, casein-^{14}C, and two fractions of RNA (I and II)-^{32}P were isolated. Specific activities (S.A.) of the DNA and RNA are expressed as cpm$\times 10^{-3}$/mg nucleic acid. Casein synthesis is expressed as total cpm in casein.

[c] Activity of glucose-6-P dehydrogenase (G6PD) is expressed in units/gland.

with both cortisol and prolactin was required to achieve milk production sufficient to produce weight gains in nursing pups. Mammary gland DNA values and rates of DNA synthesis were higher in animals treated with prolactin, as might be expected based on the classical study of Lyons (*28*), which indicated that prolactin stimulated mammary growth and lobulo-alveolar development *in vivo*.

Prolactin seemed to be primarily responsible for the development and/or maintenance of normal RNA levels in mammary glands even though cortisol also stimulated nuclear RNA synthesis (Table I). The RNA fraction I, isolated from mammary homogenates, comprised the bulk of tissue RNA and judging from base composition appears to be, primarily, ribosomal RNA. RNA fraction II, comprised 4–7% of mammary cell RNA and had a base composition comparable with DNA. Methods for separating various species of cellular RNA available at the time these experiments were conducted were not as sophisticated nor as dependable as those currently available. Therefore, the designation of RNA

I as largely ribosomal RNA, and RNA II as largely messenger-type RNA was considered tentative. The data in Table I were interpreted as indicating that prolactin acts in a general fashion in stimulating RNA synthesis in mammary tissue, while cortisol acts in a specific fashion in stimulating the synthesis of messenger-type RNA. This conclusion is consistent with results of subsequent experiments; however, it should be reexamined using modern techniques.

Both glucose-6-P dehydrogenase activity and rates of casein synthesis were markedly depressed by hypophysectomy and were only restored to normal when both cortisol and prolactin were administered (Table I). Based on this observation, the RNA data discussed above and on concurrent studies with fully-lactating rats (*7*), we speculated that cortisol stimulated the synthesis of messenger RNA for a number of key enzymes, including glucose-6-P dehydrogenase, while prolactin promoted the synthesis of ribosomal RNA required to translate the messages. This speculation appears to hold true but also requires further evaluation.

Hormone Actions during Mid-lactation

An early series of experiments with hypophysectomized mid-lactation rats receiving various hormone replacement therapies yielded results, conclusions, and speculations similar to those described above for early-lactation rats (*7*). In a subsequent experiment, rats were hypophysectomized on the 5th day of lactation and maintained on appropriate hormone therapies for 5 days (*5*, *22*). Patterns of RNA synthesis in nuclei isolated from the mammary glands of the experimental animals were investigated. Conclusions similar to those discussed above were reached and, in effect, implied that glucocorticoids regulated mammary nuclear RNA synthesis in a specific fashion and that the RNA most affected by glucocorticoids was in fractions with high levels of messenger-RNA activity. Also in this experiment, it became evident that the activities of many enzymes per gram tissue were virtually unaffected by hypophysectomy and the hormone treatments while others were dramatically affected. Data for two representatives of each group are presented in Table II. Malate dehydrogenase and isocitrate dehydrogenase activities were relatively independent of hormonal status, while fatty acid synthetase and citrate cleavage enzyme activities were highly dependent upon cortisol and prolactin. Several enzyme activities, typified by citrate cleavage enzyme (Table II), were elevated relative to the O and PO treatments when animals were treated with

TABLE II. Activities of Several Enzymes in Mammary Glands of Hypophysectomized Rats[a]

Enzyme[b]	Treatment				
	O	CO	PO	CPO	S
MDH	71.0	95.2	95.5	100.9	129.1
ICD-NADP	0.30	0.14	0.10	0.16	0.29
FAS	nil	nil	nil	0.27	0.78
CCE	0.07	0.37	0.06	1.4	1.2

[a] Tabulated from Ref. *22*. Treatment codes as for Table I.
[b] Activities of malate dehydrogenase (MDH), isocitrate dehydrogenase (nicotinamide-adenine dinucleotide phosphate (NADP)-linked; ICD-NADP), fatty acid synthetase (FAS), and citrate cleavage enzyme (CCE) expressed in units/mg tissue.

TABLE III. Effects of Adrenalectomy and Hormone Replacement Therapy upon Mammary Gland Enzyme Activities[a]

Enzyme	Treatment			
	N-5	AX	N-15	AX-C
αGPD	4.5	4.6	5.0	4.1
PGM	0.9	1.2	1.2	1.4
HK	0.19	0.22	0.19	0.23
CCE	0.5	0.3	1.0	1.1
UDPG	23.9	21.0	39.0	56.5
G6PD	10.0	10.0	21.3	26.2

[a] Taken from Ref. *23*. N-5 codes, normal 5 day lactating rats; AX codes, rats adrenalectomized on day 5 of lactation and sampled on day 15 of lactation; N-15 codes, normal 15-day lactating rats; and AX-C codes, rats adrenalectomized on day 5 of lactation which received cortisol therapy from day 5 through to day 15 of lactation when they were sampled.
[b] Activities of α-glycerol-P dehydrogenase (αGPD), phosphoglucomutase (PGM), hexokinase (HK), citrate cleavage enzyme (CCE), UDP-glucose phosphorylase (UDPG), and glucose-6-P dehydrogenase (G6PD) expressed in units/mg DNA.

cortisol. This is consistent with the adrenalectomy data presented in Table III, indicating that glucocorticoids are intimately involved in regulation of the synthesis of a number of mammary gland biosynthetic enzymes (*5*, *22*, *23*). The first three enzymes listed in Table III were not affected by treatment and are included to emphasize the specificity of the glucocorticoid action. Attainment of normal activities of the last three enzymes listed was glucocorticoid dependent. All enzymes whose activities appear to be glucocorticoid dependent increase markedly in activity after day 5 of lactation, as depicted for glucose-6-P dehydrogenase and UDPG pyrophosphorylase in Fig. 1. Enzymes whose activities are not affected by glucocorticoids increase only slightly in activity after the 5th day of lactation and might be considered constitutive enzymes as discussed above (Fig. 1). To date, 15 enzymes have been identified whose activities are partially glucocorticoid-dependent (*23–25*, *35*). All of these function in pathways related to milk biosynthesis.

An interesting aspect of the enzyme data presented in Table III is that activities of citrate cleavage enzyme, UDP glucose pyrophosphorylase, and glucose-6-P dehydrogenase in N-5 and AX animals are similar while N-15 and AX-C values are elevated. Thus, it appears that after adrenalectomy on day 5 of lactation the activities of glucocorticoid-dependent enzymes fail to increase normally. Milk production in adrenalectomized rats, as indicated by pup growth rates, also fails to increase normally during this period. If rats are adrenalectomized on days 13–15 of lactation, the activities of glucocorticoid-dependent enzymes decrease rapidly to approximately day 5 values (*25*). We took advantage of this observation to obtain estimates of the turnover rates of several mammary enzymes (*25*). The results obtained indicated half-lives ranging between 1 and 2 days, which is consistent with previous estimates obtained using specific antibody precipitation techniques (*18*). These observations support the view that glucocorticoids act upon mammary tissue in a specific fashion to increase the rates of synthesis of several enzymes in key biosynthetic pathways.

An observation possibly related to the observations regarding the glucocorticoid actions discussed above was made in a limited study of the cyclic AMP (cAMP) system of lactating rat mammary tissue. In normal animals as compared to adrenalectomized animals, mammary cAMP levels were decreased from 0.87 to 0.29 nmol/g (*26*, *27*). The possible significance of this observation with respect to mammary development and function requires further study.

Milk production decreases and mammary metabolic patterns change after adrenalectomy (*23*). After it was found that adrenalectomy led to decreases in the activities of a number of key biosynthetic enzymes, it was tempting to speculate that reduced milk yields and altered metabolic patterns could be attributed to reduced enzyme levels (*24*). This possibility was investigated in a series of studies using radioisotope tracer techniques and metabolite assays (*24*, *44*). Most of the decreases in rat mammary enzyme activities after adrenalectomy were found to have no direct (causative) relationship to depressed lactational performance after adrenalectomy. The data implied that the decreased fatty acid synthesis from glucose observed after adrenalectomy results from decreased formation of triose-P *via* the phosphofructokinase reaction (*44*). Mammary phosphofructokinase activity is not reduced after adrenalectomy (*23*). The possibility that the above-named alteration in cAMP metabolism after adrenalectomy is related to this effect should be investigated.

Discontinuing insulin therapy in diabetic lactating rats results in a rapid cessation of milk synthesis and within 2 days, irreversible losses of secretory cells (*29*). This observation emphasizes the unique dependence of mammary secretory cells upon insulin, not only for biosynthetic function but also for survival. We have reported several studies directed at identification of specific actions of insulin upon mammary secretory cells. Although the exact mechanism(s) of insulin action have not been established, several observations are of interest. Acute insulin insufficiency induced by administration of anti-insulin serum causes an increase in mammary cAMP levels from 0.82 to 1.22 nmols cAMP/g tissue within 1 hr (*26*). The primary site of action of insulin does not appear to be upon glucose transport or phosphorylation since mammary gland glucose and glucose-6-P levels are elevated 3- to 6-fold during insulin insufficiency (*29*, *30*). Mammary amino acid levels are also elevated during insulin insufficiency (*29*, *30*). Insulin insufficiency decreases pyruvate/lactate and acetoacetate/β-hydroxybutyrate ratios in the mammary gland, indicating that both the cytosol and mitochondria are more reduced in this condition. This occurs in spite of the fact that energy charge in the secretory cells $((2\times ATP+ADP)/2(ATP+ADP+AMP))$ is reduced from 0.73 to 0.58 (*30*, *31*). These observations were interpreted as indicating an interaction among insulin, cellular energy and redox state, and biosynthetic function. To test this interpretation, a study of insulin effects upon fatty acid synthesis from pyruvate, lactate, and glucose in isolated rat mammary cells was undertaken. A clear-cut interaction between the redox state of substrate used and insulin action upon fatty acid synthesis was observed as illustrated by the data in Table IV. Insulin stimulated fatty acid synthesis 2.7-fold when the more oxidized substrate, pyruvate, was used and depressed fatty acid synthesis 40% when lactate was the substrate (Table IV). When pyruvate and lactate were supplied together, creating an intermediate redox state, insulin induced a positive, 2.4-fold increase in fatty acid synthesis. The data in Table V indicate that this response pattern is directly related to the redox state. When the nicotinamide-adenine dinucleotide (NAD)-reducing effect of lactate was reversed

TABLE IV. Pyruvate-2-^{14}C and Lactate-2-^{14}C Metabolism in Mammary Cells[a]

Substrate	Fatty acid synthesis[b]	
	−insulin	+insulin
Pyruvate-2-^{14}C, 5 mM	3.2	8.6
Lactate-2-^{14}C, 5 mM	1.04	0.66
Pyruvate-2-^{14}C plus lactate, 2.5 mM each	1.8	4.4
Lactate-2-^{14}C plus pyruvate, 2.5 mM each	1.4	3.4

[a] From Ref. *43.*
[b] Data expressed as μg atoms labeled carbon incorporated by 1 ml of isolated (packed) secretory cells in 1 hr.

TABLE V. Effects of TMPD on Lactate and Pyruvate Metabolism and Responses to Insulin in Mammary Cells[a]

Substrate (5 mM)	TMPD (100 μM)[b]	Fatty acid synthesis[c]	
		−insulin	+insulin
Pyruvate-2-^{14}C	−	2.5	8.4
	+	0.5	2.6
Lactate-2-^{14}C	−	1.5	0.6
	+	1.4	2.4

[a] From Ref. *43.*
[b] TMPD is N, N, N′, N′-tetramethyl-P-phenylenediamine and acts as a specific oxidant of NADH.
[c] Data expressed as in Table IV.

by oxidizing NADH with N, N, N′, N′-tetramethyl-P-phenylenediamine (TMPD), the negative insulin action upon fatty acid synthesis became positive. Based upon the above-mentioned observations, we can conclude with certainty that insulin acts acutely at important sites other than or in addition to glucose transport in regulating mammary secretory cell metabolism and, particularly, fatty acid synthesis. We can also conclude that insulin actions upon fatty acid synthesis in mammary secretory cells are highly dependent upon or interactive with the cellular redox state and, possibly, cellular energy charge. The mechanisms or sites at which these interactions become manifest have not been identified.

Quantitative and Dynamic Aspects of Mammary Metabolism

During the course of our studies of rat and ruminant mammary metabolism, we collected a great many data on mammary enzyme and metabolite levels, mammary input-output (nutrient uptake and milk production) relationships, and matabolic rates and patterns. Also, based on available literature and on our own studies, a number of concepts and hypotheses regarding the regulation of mammary function were formulated. Several years ago it became evident to us that although our concepts, hypotheses, and data may seem, in the qualitative sense, to approach adequacy as explanations of variations in mammary metabolic function, the only truly rigorous and satisfactory test of the adequacy of current knowledge would require quantitative and dynamic analyses. In order to achieve this end, a number of data required for quantitative analyses were tabulated and summarized by Baldwin and Yang (*13*). Also, dynamic, computer simulation models of rat and cow mammary metabolism have been constructed (*12*, *36*, *38*). Progress in developing the simulation models has been slow due to the necessity of running experiments to collect additional, required data regarding several aspects of mammary metabolism. As a result, the models used in our analyses of mammary metabolism have not yet been published in full. However, the use of biomathematical techniques in support of our research on mammary metabolism has proven extremely useful in helping organize available data in a meaningful format, in identifying and interpreting required experiments and in evaluations of concepts and hypotheses. The models and attendant analyses will be published soon.

Effects of Lactation on Overall Animal Metabolism

In most mammalian species, food intake during lactation is three to five times greater than observed in non-pregnant, non-lactating adults. As well lactating animals often mobilize considerable body substance to support the lactation process. The magnitude of changes in amounts of nutrients which must be digested, absorbed, and metabolized during lactation suggests that changes must occur in the physiological and metabolic characteristics of tissues other than the mammary gland. With this view in mind, we undertook a number of studies to examine changes in extramammary tissue metabolism(s) during lactation (*11*, *14*, *16*, *19*, *21*, *37*, *39*, *41*, *42*).

Adipose tissue is a primary site of fatty acid synthesis and triglyceride storage in rats and ruminants. In addition, adipose fulfills an important role in the synthesis and release of fatty acids for subsequent incorporation into milk fat (*17*). Imperfect performance of the latter role by adipose has been implicated in the depression in milk fat which accompanies the feeding of high concentrate/low roughage rations to lactating cows (*17*, *34*). For these reasons, we have emphasized adipose function during lactation in several studies. Early experiments with lactating dairy cattle indicated decreased adipose lipoprotein lipase rates and increased adipose lipogenic and lipolytic rates during lactation (*11*, *41*, *42*). Adipose lipolytic rates were reduced to one-third of normal for lactating cows when high-concentrate diets were fed (*42*). These observations suggest that cow adipose tissue adapts during lactation in a fashion supportive of lactation (*i.e.*, increased synthesis and release of fatty acids for subsequent incorporation into milk fat). In a recent study of cows at peak lactation and in later stages of lactation, we found that lipolysis is elevated throughout lactation, consistent with the above suggestion that release by adipose of fatty acids for incorporation into milk fat is elevated during lactation, possibly due to the actions of hormones of the lactogenic complex (*21*). However, adipose lipogenesis was depressed relative to non-lactating animals during early lactation and elevated relative to normal during late lactation. The depression in lipogenesis during early lactation is comparable in magnitude to that observed during starvation and thus, may be related to the negative energy balance experienced during peak lactation rather than specific actions of hormones of the lactation complex. It is difficult to distinguish between these two possibilities. In late lactation, elevated rates of lipogenesis might be a starvation-refeeding type of response, might simply be a response to energy intakes in excess of needs for maintenance and lactation, or could reflect changes in hormonal status.

Lipogenesis in rat adipose tissue and liver is affected by nutritional status. Diets high in carbohydrate and low in fat stimulate lipogenesis, whereas starvation and high-fat diets depress lipogenesis (*14*). Lipogenesis in rat liver and adipose tissue seems to be influenced by physiological state or lactation in a fashion comparable to the peak lactation cow (*i.e.*, lipogenesis is depressed and lipolysis elevated during lactation (*14*)). In an experiment in which interactions among age, lactation, and diet were investigated, we were surprised to learn that the hyperlipogenic response commonly observed when high-carbohydrate/low-fat diets are fed to rats was absent in lactating rat liver, adipose, and mammary tissues (*19*). This observation implies that liver and adipose tissue perform only a small lipogenic role in support of lactation.

Brody (*15*) noted many years ago that the apparent maintenance requirements of lactating animals are elevated relative to non-lactating animals. The physiological and/or metabolic basis for this increase in maintenance requirements have been the subject of considerable speculation but have not yet been elucidated. In a series of experiments, currently ongoing, we are attempting to explain and utilize this observation as a probe to enable greater understanding of the effects lactation has upon the functions of extramammary tissues. One relevant set of observations has been that the relative weights (% body weight) of several "vital organs" including liver, heart, and gastrointestinal tract increase significantly during lactation. These tissues have very high energy expenditures per unit mass as compared with the body average. Maintenance energy expenditures per unit mass of liver do not change significantly when liver size increases during lactation (unpublished). Thus, increases in the relative weights of "vital organs" result in an increase in the body average maintenance requirement per unit mass. This explains part of the increase in maintenance requirements observed in lactating animals (*39*). Also, increases in "vital organ" weights and maintenance requirements appear to be highly related to food intake rather than to the lactation process *per se* (*16*).

SUMMARY

In this brief summary of our research experiences in the lactation area, we have attempted to provide an overview of our program; to characterize the flow of our program from considerations of fairly detailed aspects of secretory cell function to recent emphases on organismal function during lactation; and, to identify some of the contributions which have arisen from our studies.

REFERENCES

1. Baldwin, R. L. (1966). Enzymatic activities in mammary glands of several species. *J. Dairy Sci.* **49**, 1533–1542.
2. Baldwin, R. L. (1968). Development of milk synthesis. *J. Dairy Sci.* **52**, 729–736.
3. Baldwin, R. L. (1969). Enzymic and metabolic changes in mammary tissue at lactogenesis. In *Lactogenesis: The Initiation of Milk Secretion at Parturition*, ed. Reynolds, M. and Folley, S. J., pp. 85–95. Philadelphia: Univ. Penn. Press.
4. Baldwin, R. L. and Cheng, W. (1968). Metabolite changes associated with

initiation and maintenance of lactation in rats and cows. *J. Dairy Sci.* **52**, 523–528.

5. Baldwin, R. L., Korsrud, G. O., Martin, R. J., Cheng, W., and Schober, N. A. (1969). Effects of endocrinectomy and hormone replacement therapies upon RNA synthesis in isolated lactating rat mammary gland nuclei. *Biol. Reprod.* **1**, 31–40.
6. Baldwin, R. L. and Louis, S. L. (1975). Hormonal actions upon mammary metabolism. *J. Dairy Sci.* **58**, 1033–1041.
7. Baldwin, R. L. and Martin, R. J. (1967). Effects of hypophysectomy and several hormone replacement therapies upon patterns of nucleic acid and protein synthesis and enzyme levels in lactating rat mammary glands. *J. Dairy Sci.* **51**, 748–753.
8. Baldwin, R. L. and Martin, R. J. (1968). Protein and nucleic acid synthesis in rat mammary glands during early lactation. *Endocrinology* **82**, 1209–1216.
9. Baldwin, R. L. and Milligan, L. P. (1966). Enzymatic changes associated with the initiation and maintenance of lactation in the rat. *J. Biol. Chem.* **241**, 2058–2066.
10. Baldwin, R. L. and Plucinski, T. (1977). Mammary gland development and lactation. In *Reproduction in Domestic Animals*, 3rd ed., ed. Cole, H. H. and Cupps, P. T., pp. 369–400. New York, London: Academic Press.
11. Baldwin, R. L., Reichl, J. R., Louis, S., Smith, N. E., Yang, Y. T., and Osborne, E. (1973). Effects of age, pregnancy, and lactation of rat, guinea pig, and cow adipose enzyme activities and cow adipose metabolism. *J. Dairy Sci.* **56**, 340–349.
12. Baldwin, R. L. and Smith, N. E. (1971). Application of simulation modeling technique in analyses of dynamic aspects of animal energetics. *Fed. Proc.* **30**, 1459–1465.
13. Baldwin, R. L. and Yang, Y. T. (1974). Enzymatic and metabolic changes in the development of lactation. In *Lactation: A Comprehensive Treatise*, vol. 1, ed. Larson, B. L., and Smith, V. R., pp. 349–407. New York, London: Academic Press.
14. Baldwin, R. L., Yang, Y. T., Crist, K., and Grichting, G. (1976). Ruminant adipose tissue metabolism in relation to the whole animal. *Fed. Proc.* **35**, 2314–2318.
15. Brody, S. (1945). *Bioenergetics and Growth*. New York: Reinhold.
16. Cañas, R., Romero, J. J., Baldwin, R. L., and Koong, L. J. (1976). Lactational efficiency complex of rats: Provisional model for interpretation of energy balance data. *J. Dairy Sci.* **59**, 57–67.
17. Davis, C. L. and Brown, R. E. (1970). Low milk fat syndrome. In *Physiology of Digestion and Metabolism in the Ruminant*, ed. Phillipson, A. T., pp. 545–565. Newcastle-Upon-Tyne, England: Oriel Press.

18. Emergy, R. S. and Baldwin, R. L. (1967). Turnover of several mammary enzymes during lactation. *Biochim. Biophys. Acta* **136**, 223–232.
19. Farid, M., Baldwin, R. L., Yang, Y. T., Osborne, E., and Grichting, G. (1977). Effects of age, diet and lactation on lipogenesis in rat adipose, liver and mammary tissues. *J. Nutr.*, submitted.
20. Folley, S. J. (1961). Recent advances in the physiology and biochemistry of lactation. *Dairy Sci. Abstr.* **23**, 511–528.
21. Grichting, G. (1977). Effects of nutritional and physiological state on ruminant adipose tissue metabolism. Ph.D. Thesis, Univ. California, Davis.
22. Korsrud, G. O. and Baldwin, R. L. (1969). Effects of endocrinectomy and hormone replacement therapies upon enzyme activities in lactating rat mammary glands. *Biol. Reprod.* **1**, 21–30.
23. Korsrud, G. O. and Baldwin, R. L. (1972). Effects of adrenalectomy, adrenalectomy-ovariectomy, and cortisol and estrogen therapies upon enzyme activities in lactating rat mammary glands. *Can. J. Biochem.* **50**, 366–376.
24. Korsrud, G. O. and Baldwin, R. L. (1972). Hormonal regulation of rat mammary gland enzyme activities and metabolite patterns. *Can. J. Biochem.* **50**, 377–385.
25. Korsrud, G. O. and Baldwin, R. L. (1972). Estimations of rates of synthesis and degradation of several rat mammary gland enzymes from changes in enzyme activities. *Can. J. Biochem.* **50**, 386–391.
26. Louis, S. L. and Baldwin, R. L. (1975). Effect of adrenalectomy and insulin insufficiency upon the adenosine cAMP system of the rat mammary glands. *J. Dairy Sci.* **58**, 502–506.
27. Louis, S. L. and Baldwin, R. L. (1975). Changes in the cyclic 3′, 5′-adenosine monophosphate system of rat mammary gland during lactation cycle. *J. Dairy Sci.* **58**, 861–869.
28. Lyons, W. R. (1942). The direct mammotrophic action of lactogenic hormone. *Proc. Soc. Exp. Biol. Med.* **51**, 308–311.
29. Martin, R. J. and Baldwin, R. L. (1971). Effects of alloxan diabetes on lactational performance and mammary tissue metabolism in the rat. *Endocrinology* **88**, 863–867.
30. Martin, R. J. and Baldwin, R. L. (1971). Effects of insulin and anti-insulin serum treatments on levels of metabolites in rat mammary glands. *Endocrinology* **88**, 868–871.
31. Martin, R. J. and Baldwin, R. L. (1971). Effects of insulin on isolated rat mammary cell metabolism: Glucose utilization and metabolite patterns. *Endocrinology* **89**, 1263–1269.
32. Mellenberger, R. W., Bauman, D. E., and Nelson, D. R. (1973). Metabolic adaptations during lactogenesis—Fatty acid and lactose synthesis in cow mammary tissue. *Biochem. J.* **136**, 741–748.

33. Munford, R. E. (1964). A review of anatomical and biochemical changes in the mammary gland with particular reference to quantitative methods of assessing mammary development. *Dairy Sci. Abstr.* **26**, 293–304.
34. Optsvedt, J. and Ronning, M. (1967). Effect upon lipid metabolism of feeding alfalfa hay or concentrate ad libitum as the sole feed for milking cows. *J. Dairy Sci.* **50**, 345–354.
35. Plucinski, T. and Baldwin, R. L. (1976). Effects of adrenalectomy and glucocorticoid therapy on enzyme activities in mammary and adipose tissues from lactating rats. *J. Dairy Sci.* **59**, 157–160.
36. Plucinski, T. M. (1977). Biochemical regulation of rat mammary metabolism: Effects of hormones and 3′: 5′ cyclic adenosine monophosphates. Ph.D. Thesis, Univ. California, Davis.
37. Romero, J. J., Cañas, R., and Baldwin, R. L. (1975). A technique for estimating milk production in rats. *J. Nutr.* **105**, 413–420.
38. Smith, N. E. (1967). Quantitative analyses of ruminant metabolic functions: Basal; lactation; milk fat depression. Ph.D. Thesis, Univ. California, Davis.
39. Smith, N. E. and Baldwin, R. L. (1974). Effects of breed, pregnancy, and lactation on weights of organs and tissues in dairy cattle. *J. Dairy Sci.* **57**, 1055–1060.
40. Topper, Y. J. and Oka, T. (1974). Some aspects of mammary gland development in the mature mouse. In *Lactation: A Comprehensive Treatise*, vol. 1, ed. Larson, B. L. and Smith V. R., pp. 327–348. New York, London: Academic Press.
41. Yang, Y. T. and Baldwin, R. L. (1973). Preparation and metabolism of isolated cells from bovine adipose tissue. *J. Dairy Sci.* **56**, 350–365.
42. Yang, Y. T. and Baldwin, R. L. (1973). Lipolysis in isolated cow adipose cells. *J. Dairy Sci.* **56**, 366–374.
43. Yang, Y. T. and Baldwin, R. L. (1975). Effects of insulin upon fatty acids synthesis from pyruvate, lactate, and glucose in rat mammary cells. *J. Dairy Sci.* **58**, 337–343.
44. Yang, Y. T. and Baldwin, R. L. (1976). Effect of adrenalectomy on rat mammary metabolism. *J. Dairy Sci.* **59**, 620–626.

I–2

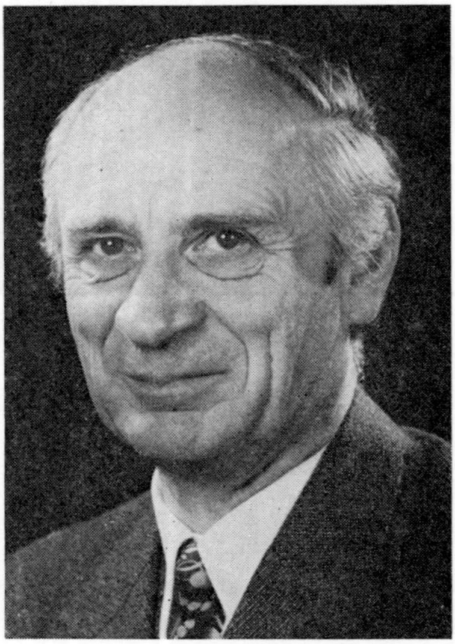

Georges Joseph Peeters was born in Overwinden, Belgium on November 25, 1919 and earned the degree of Bachelor of Science from the Catholic University of Louvain (1939). In 1940 he was in the Belgian army. In 1943 he was awarded the title of Doctor of Veterinary Sciences from the Veterinary College, State University of Ghent, Belgium. That same year he was appointed assistant to the Chair of Veterinary Obstetrics under the direction of Professor M. Vandeplassche. In 1946 he was appointed to the teaching staff of the Veterinary College in Ghent and was entrusted with the course of Physiology of the Domestic Animals. Two years later he was promoted to full-professorship. Since then, he has twice held the Presidency of the Board of the Veterinary College (1951, 1967). During the years of 1968 to 1970, he was elected Dean of the renamed Faculty of Veterinary Medicine, State University of Ghent.

In 1950 he worked at the Physiological Department of the National Institute for Research in Dairying at Shinfield, Reading, England (Director: Dr. S.J. Folley).

He has been doing research in the physiology of lactation in ruminants for almost 30 years. Immediately after the end of the war he began to develop an apparatus for the perfusion of isolated bovine udders. This technique led him to two major aspects of his research: the ejection of milk and studies of the precursors for synthesis of milk constituents. In his studies on milk ejection, he has been interested primarily in the hormones of the neurohypophysis, the plasmakinins, the innervation of the udder and the bloodflow through this gland. He studied the precursors for the synthesis of butterfat, lactose and casein by adding labelled substances to the perfusion blood of isolated cows and goats udders. Since growth hormone has an important function in the secretion of milk, he determined this hormone level in bovine blood plasma. He is a member of the Societies of Physiology, Biochemistry and Endocrinology in Belgium, of the Society of Endocrinology in London and of the Biochemical Society in London. He was laureate of several awards in Belgium (Gilbert Mullie Prize, 1954; J. Maisin Prize, 1975). He was also laureate of the Ludwig Schunk Prize (1961) awarded by the Faculty of Veterinary Sciences of the Justus Liebig University in Giessen, Germany.

MILK EJECTION AND SYNTHESIS OF MILK IN RUMINANTS

G. J. PEETERS

Physiological Department of the Veterinary Faculty, University of Ghent, Belgium

I was born in a very small Belgian village where agriculture and cattle-breeding were flourishing. It was not surprising, therefore, that I was attracted to veterinary medicine and hoped to start a practice in my home area. In September 1939, I started my studies at the Veterinary School of the State University in Ghent. Courses in physiology and biochemistry were taught there by Professor W. Libbrecht and his coworker Dr. L. Massart. They pointed out to me that besides careers in practice, veterinary science needs scientific research workers. In May 1940, I served in the Belgian army. Afterwards, at the age of 20, I started spending my free time during my veterinary studies working in a laboratory under the direction of Dr. L. Massart. At the end of my studies in 1943, Prof. Libbrecht was of the opinion that it was obvious that I should work a few years in a large animal clinic before starting a career in animal physiology. I worked under the skillful and dynamic direction of the young Prof. Marcel Vandeplassche, head of the Department of Obstetrics and Reproduction at the Ghent Veterinary School. In that Department, I obtained a good knowledge of several interesting aspects of the ruminant, *i.e.*, reproduction, lactation, and hormones. I liked that work and it became clear to me that fundamental research work oriented on a problem of great economic importance, would be most suitable for me. My choice fell on the study of the physiology of lactation in the ruminant. Since 1946 I have been teaching veterinary physiology in the Veterinary Faculty of Ghent.

In 1945, I started developing a technique for the perfusion of the isolated cows udder. Our first experiments were carried out in collaboration with Prof. L. Massart (*1*). Our technique was a modification of the one developed in American laboratories just before the war. In our method, the isolated udder was bisected into its symmetrical halves and each half was perfused independently. The blood circulation through the gland was considerably improved by adding a sympathicolytic drug (dibenamine) to the perfusate. Since 1962, we have concentrated upon the perfusion of the isolated sheep or goat udder, using the technique developed by Dr. J. Linzell in a modified form: the perfused gland produces considerable quantities of milk for a period of 10–15 hr.

During 1940's, the theory was advanced by Prof. W. Petersen in Minnesota that milk ejection was induced by reflex release of oxytocin. In the beginning, we used our perfusion technique for studies on milk ejection and we were able to confirm the results of Petersen. We perfused udder halves that were not milked out before slaughter and we used different perfusates for each symmetrical half. The teats were cannulated. We observed that during perfusion, certain substances are formed in the heparinized blood which cause ejection of milk and it is presently known that these activating products are plasmakinins (*2*). We also found that milk ejection activity was higher in the blood collected from a cow immediately after teat stimulation through milking than in the blood from a cow not stimulated (*3*). Thus it was postulated that during milking, there must be some substance in the blood which causes milk ejection. Through these experiments we became familiar with problems in connection with oxytocin, the neurohypophysis and the hypothalamus.

The circulation time in lactating cows was calculated through the intravenous injection of oxytocin (*4*). This causes a sudden swelling of the teats owing to the evacuation of milk from the alveolar region into the teat cisterns. The expansion of the teat volume was recorded by a plethysmographic technique. Nineteen seconds elapsed between the injection and the onset of the swelling.

In the years after the war, I often met Prof. C. Heymans, head of the Department of Pharmacology at the Ghent University. In 1939, Heymans received a Nobel Prize for his work on chemoreceptors and the carotid sinus. In these studies he often used the technique of cross-circulation on dogs. I often visited his institute and he always had time for long discussions, his advice being extremely useful to me. When we were talking about the oxytocin theory of Petersen, he suggested sheep experiments based on the cross-circulation technique: if two lactating sheep were connected by anastomoses of the blood vessels, milking of one animal should induce milk ejection in the other. However, preliminary experiments were unsuccessful.

In 1949, I met Prof. Verney, who lectured in Ghent. Prof. Verney having performed so much work in connection with antidiuretic hormone, suggested that I should study the effect of milking on water diuresis on the cow. Fifty liters of tepid water were infused by means of a pump into the rumen of a cow, a catheter was introduced permanently in the bladder and urine collected continuously in measuring cylinders (*5*). At the high point of diuresis, approximately 1 liter of urine was collected every 5 min. Handmilking induced a clear antidiuretic effect of the pituitary type: the urine secretion decreased while chloride content of the urine increased. Dr. B. Cross obtained similar results on hydrated rabbits in the same period at Cambridge.

From time immemorial, practices have existed in developing countries to induce milk ejection in indigenous cattle and buffalos by insufflation of air into the vagina. It seemed likely to me that this effect was due to reflexes described by Ferguson on the rabbit. At the end of 1950's, I decided to study this phenomenon further with my colleague Dr. M. Debackere. We established that distension of the vagina in lactating ruminants by means of an inflated balloon leads to a strong milk ejection response that begins after a latent period of 30 sec or more (*6*). This ejection was not blocked by denervation of the udder. In hydrated animals, distension of the vagina caused inhibition of diuresis. We then decided to carry out the cross-circulation experiments suggested many years before by Prof. Heymans. Two lactating ewes (A and B) were fixed on their back. Under local anaesthesia, the jugular veins of A and B were cross-connected by means of polyethylene tubing. Almost all the head blood of one animal flowed to the body of the other. When vaginal distension was performed on A, there was a spectacular milk ejection and rise of intramammary pressure in B after a latent period of 30 sec (*7*). This effect could be repeated a number of times during the same experiment. Oxytocin, when injected in doses of 20 to 150 mU into the polyethylene anastomosis that carried blood from A to B, caused identical effects 30 sec after injection. There remained no doubt whatsoever that vaginal distension induces the release of a hormone in the head having milk ejection activity. It was concluded that the Ferguson reflex was well developed in ruminants.

In a subsequent series of experiments, we combined a sexually mature ram in cross-circulation with a lactating ewe. This demonstrated that massage *via* the rectum of the seminal vesicles and ampullae of the ram induced milk ejection in the ewe after a 30 sec interval.

After severing the pelvic nerves, milk ejection was no longer induced by vaginal distension (*8*). In other cross-circulation experiments with ewe, ram, and wether, we have shown that the stimulation of several organs in the pelvic region such as vagina, deep pelvic cavity, retroperitoneal part of the rectum, anus, bladder, and seminal vesicles will also induce release of neurohormones (*9*). It is noteworthy that all these effective organs are innervated by the pelvic nerves. Apparently the pelvic nerves act as an afferent pathway in the transport of the stimulus to the spinal cord. Our knowledge about the physiological meaning and importance of these reflexes is still very incomplete. The release of oxytocin occurs in response to stimuli arising from distension of the vagina during parturition in cows. On the other hand, Sharma, Fitzpatrick, and Ward (1972) detected a release of oxytocin immediately after coitus in rams.

In the last few years, radioimmunoassay techniques were developed in the laboratory of Prof. Franchimont in Liège for estimating neurophysin I and neurophysin II separately in serum of cattle. In experiments carried out in collaboration with Dr. J.J. Legros of the Liège laboratory, we found that neurophysin I is released selectively in cows during milking and suckling (*10*). On the other hand, an important and specific release of neurophysin II was induced by hemorrhage in cows (*11*). Recently we estimated the levels of both neurophysins in serum of cows during and after parturition (*12*). Neurophysin I levels increased in all cases during the second stage of labour, reaching high peak values during the expulsive phase. Values returned to the normal level during the hours of the postpartum period. A similar pattern of release was observed previously for oxytocin at parturition in cows by other workers. Similar variations were observed in the neurophysin II levels: the effect was striking in several animals but slight or absent in others. Neurophysin II peaks were also detected sporadically at different stages of labour and these effects might be ascribed to pain and stress. Our results are in accord with the concept that in cattle, neurophysin I is associated with oxytocin and neurophysin II with vasopressin.

Our colleague, Dr. Rika Reynaert could not detect any increase of serum growth hormone levels in cows during milking or suckling. In many cows and heifers, an increase in this hormone was observed during parturition, the total duration of the phenomenon amounting to a few hours. The peak occurred within the period of expulsion or a few minutes later (*13*). A precipitous fall of the plasma-free fatty acid (FFA) levels, whatever the cause (insulin, nicotinic acid, glucose infusion, *etc.*), induces a release of serum growth hormone in cows (*14*). Such a decline of plasma FFA levels might act as a stimulus on a centre in the hypothalamus leading to growth hormone release. Growth hormone levels were highest in calves 8 to 14 days old and were higher in male than in female calves. The level decreased significantly during stress caused by transport (*15*).

We found that bradykinin is very active when it is injected directly into an artery of the mammary gland of sheep, giving rise to milk ejection and increase of blood flow through the udder artery (*16*). Kinins originate in tissues by the action of kallikrein enzymes and recently we have isolated very small quantities of kallikrein from mammary tissue of cows (*17*). Perhaps, this enzyme plays a physiological role in the mammary gland in the regulation of blood flow and in milk expulsion.

Our studies on the autonomic innervation of the udder were among the first experiments we carried out on the isolated perfused cow's udder. Stimulation of the external spermatic nerve in isolated and perfused udder preparations induced teat contractions and vasoconstriction but no milk ejection (*18*). These effects were blocked by sympathicolytic drugs. There was no indication as to the presence of ganglia in the udder, since neither nicotine nor tetraethylammonium had any effect. During the nerve stimulations, no trace of acetylcholine could be detected in the mammary venous blood. It was, therefore, concluded that the udder was innervated by sympathetic adrenergic nerves. Extirpation of the sympathetic chain in the right lumbar region in lactating sheep immediately led to a vasodilatation in the homolateral mammary gland producing a rise in local temperature, but had no adverse influence on milk secretion in this half (*19*).

The teats of the cows udder are abundantly provided with smooth muscle cells. We studied the behaviour of these muscles in the presence of catecholamines and blocking agents "*in vitro*" and concluded that they contain α- and β-adrenoceptors: stimulation of α-receptors induces contraction whereas stimulation of β-receptors elicits relaxation (*20*).

We also studied teat motility in the living lactating cow by means of a teat plethysmographic technique developed in our laboratory (*21*). When the teat is stretched (*e.g.*, by the presence of milk under pressure or by insufflation of air), rhythmic contractions of the organ occur and continue for hours. This motility is especially pronounced at the beginning of milking or after infusion of oxytocin, due to the passage of milk from the alveolar regions towards the teat cisterns which distends the musculature. Intravenous injections of adrenaline, isopropylnoradrenaline, and isoxsuprine temporarily inhibit teat motility (β-adrenoceptor stimulation) whereas noradrenaline and neosynephrine activate teat motility (α-adrenoceptor stimulation) (*22*).

During the last few years, we have made chronic recordings of the blood flow through the mammary artery in lactating goats and cows with an electromagnetic flowmeter and studied the effect of intravenous injection of many substances (*e.g.*, catecholamines, adrenoceptor blocking agents, kinins, *etc.*) (*23*, *24*). This research was carried out by Drs. A. Houvenaghel and G. Dhondt in our laboratory and is presently being continued by Dr. C. Burvenich. Mammary blood flow decreases during emotional stress and rises during massage of the udder and during handmilking (*25*, *26*). During milking, mammary blood flow frequently increases at the moment of milk ejection. Blood flow increases after intravenous injection of physiological doses of oxytocin. Oxytocin is a factor which contributes to the increase of flow during handmilking. Experimental acute mastitis induced by intramammary infusion of coli-endotoxins in cows and goats is accompanied by a strong increase of mammary blood flow (*27*). It is remarkable that this phenomenon is always characterized by two distinct peaks.

We found that in cows which are suckled by their calves, milk ejection is induced by the mere sight of their calves (*28*). This phenomenon was ascribed to a conditioned reflex. However, in unexperienced primiparous heifers which were not previously suckled, milk ejection is also often induced by the sight of their calves, a few hours after parturition (*29*). We ascribed this phenomenon to limbic system-hypothalamus interactions.

In order to better understand the mechanism of the release of neurohormones in the goat, our colleague Dr. Georgette Vandeputte began a series of studies on neurotransmission in the hypothalamus. Permanent cannulae were implanted stereotaxically in the 3rd ventricle of female goats and neurotransmitters and blocking agents were infused *via* this route in the conscious animal. Thus far, only the release of antidiuretic hormone (ADH) has been studied. It was found by this technique that muscarine receptors, α-adrenoceptors, nicotine receptors, and dopamine receptors have a stimulating activity upon the release of ADH (*30*, *31*). On the other hand, β-adrenoceptors inhibit ADH release.

In other experiments, Dr. G. Vandeputte implanted 1 mg perphenazine by the stereotaxic technique into the eminentia media of 6 one-year-old virgin female goats (*32*). Artificial lactation was induced, maximum productions of 1 liter milk per day being obtained. Sham implantations however were ineffective.

When I started working in Dr. S.J. Folley's department at Shinfield in 1950, a very important tracer experiment carried out by Dr. Folley, Dr. Popjak and their colleagues had just been completed. In that experiment, acetate-1-^{14}C was administered to a lactating goat and it was found that the short chain milk fatty acids were synthesized in the mammary gland from acetate. When I suggested that it might be interesting to perform a similar experiment on a perfused cow's udder, Drs. Folley and Popjak agreed and a perfusion experiment was planned. This perfusion which was carried out in Ghent in 1950 was one of the first ^{14}C experiments performed at our University. Two separated halves of a lactating cow's udder were independently perfused, one with blood containing acetate-1-^{14}C and the other with ^{14}C-labelled bicarbonate (*33*). Dr. Alfred Cowie, at the time one of the closest co-workers of Dr. Folley, came from England to help at the perfusion experiment. In order to avoid possible risks resulting from $^{14}CO_2$ production, the perfusion apparatus was mounted in the open air and gasmasks were used. Just as in the living goat experiment, fatty acid fractions, from the "acetate" half, isolated from the milk and udder glycerides after perfusion were highly labelled: a strong ^{14}C incorporation was observed in pure fatty acids from C_4 up to C_{16}. Lactose of milk from the "acetate" half was also appreciably radioactive. The results from the "bicarbonate" half indicated that the incorporation of $^{14}CO_2$ in butterfat and lactose was negligible.

The acetate-1-^{14}C experiment was the beginning of a long series of tracer studies carried out in perfused mammary glands from cows and later from sheep and goats. The isolations of amino acids and lipid fractions after perfusion were carried out by our colleagues Dr. Roger Verbeke and Dr. Monique Lauryssens. When they left the department, their task was taken over by Dr. Eddy Roets and Dr. Anne Marie Massart.

In other experiments, we added butyrate-1-^{14}C and -3-^{14}C, caproate-1-^{14}C, and isovalerate-1-^{14}C to the perfusion blood of the isolated cows udder (*34–36*). From a qualitative standpoint these precursors led to identical results as obtained with acetate-1-^{14}C, but from a quantitative standpoint, the incorporation was lower than that of acetate.

In 1956 we studied the metabolism of propionate-1-^{14}C in the perfused udder and we observed a moderate incorporation of ^{14}C into the fat. Dr. A.T. James in London had demonstrated the widespread occurrence of straight-chain odd-numbered acids in natural fats by means of gas-liquid chromatography. He suggested that propionate-1-^{14}C might have been incorporated in the odd-numbered fatty acids of the butterfat by the perfused udder. According to these expectations, he found the highest specific activities in the odd-numbered straight-chain fatty acids isolated from the udder after the propionate perfusion (*37*). Since acetate-1-^{14}C was also incorporated in these acids, it was suggested that odd-numbered straight-chain acids are synthesized by condensation of acetate with propionic acid.

Several organic acids were isolated from udder tissue perfused in the presence of butyrate-3-^{14}C, caproate-1-^{14}C, and propionate-1-^{14}C (*38*). The acids of the Krebs cycle (citrate, α-oxoglutarate, succinate, malate) had a very high specific activity, whereas pyruvate was less active. In all experiments the activity of succinate was localized in the carboxyl groups. On the other hand, distribution of ^{14}C in the carboxyl groups of casein-glutamic acid varied according to the precursor used. The results could be explained on the assumption that propionate enters the Krebs cycle *via* methylmalonate and succinate, whereas butyrate and caproate enter the cycle *via* acetyl CoA.

Stearic acid belongs to the FFA fraction which occurs in small quantities in bovine plasma. We added albumin-bound stearate-1-^{14}C to the perfusion blood of an isolated bovine udder (*39*, *40*). In the evening before the experiment, we did not succeed in dissolving the quantity of labelled stearate in plasma according to the plan despite hours-long efforts. Nevertheless, the perfusion experiment was carried out. Dr. Monique Lauryssens isolated significantly labelled stearate and oleate from the triglycerides of the udder tissue after the perfusion. This was an important experiment in that it was observed that oleic acid, which occurs in large concentrations in the triglycerides of the butterfat of cows, does not originate exclusively from the oleate fraction of the blood. The greatest part of oleate in milk fat actually originates from dehydrogenation of plasma stearate.

A series of perfusion experiments was carried out on isolated sheep and goat mammary glands in the presence of palmitate-1-^{14}C, oleate-1-^{14}C and myristate-1-^{14}C (*41*, *42*). All these FFA were very extensively incorporated into the triglycerides of milk fat. Palmitate and myristate were dehydrogenated to some extent to palmitoleate and myristoleate, respectively. The specific activity of the labelled FFA decreases during passage through the udder and this is in agreement with results obtained by other workers on living animals.

We confirmed the presence of the pentose cycle in the mammary gland by using methods other than those used by previous workers. In homogenates of mammary tissue of 8 different animal species, incubated at 38°C in the presence of glucose-6-phosphate, we detected the formation of a series of phosphate esters which are characteristic for the pentose cycle (sedoheptulose-7-phosphate, ribose-5-phosphate, *etc.*) (*43*). We also added glucose-1-^{14}C to the perfusion blood of one isolated bovine udder-half and glucose-6-^{14}C to the other symmetrical half, both halves being perfused separately (Verbeke and Peeters, unpublished). In the glucose-1-^{14}C half, the $^{14}CO_2$ production was much higher than in the glucose-6-^{14}C half. On the other hand, the ^{14}C incorporation into fatty acids, casein amino acids (alanine, cysteine, serine, glutamic acid, aspartic acid) and organic acids (citrate, succinate, malate, fumarate) of tissue and milk was much higher in the glucose-6-^{14}C half than in the glucose-1-^{14}C half. These results are typical for a high pentose cycle activity.

In the early 1950's, the mechanism of the synthesis of lactose in the mammary gland was still unknown but it was supposed that both hexose moieties of lactose were derived from the same precursor. If so, each moiety should have the same ^{14}C distribution in the 6C atoms. Wood and Schambye studied the ^{14}C distribution of both hexose moieties in a series of lactose samples derived from tracer experiments carried out in several laboratories using *Lactobacillus casei.* They found little difference between the total ^{14}C activities of glucose and galactose from the different lactose samples with the exception of the sample from the perfusion experiment carried out in Ghent in which acetate-1-^{14}C was added to the perfusate. The lactose from that experiment showed very little ^{14}C activity in the glucose moiety but high activity in the galactose. Other lactose samples which had little difference between the total ^{14}C activities of both hexose moieties, were derived from acetate ^{14}C experiments carried out on living animals. We then sent two other lactose samples to Dr. H.G. Wood (Cleveland, Ohio), one from a second acetate-1-^{14}C perfusion experiment and one from a propionate-1-^{14}C perfusion experiment. Wood and Schambye degraded the glucose and galactose moieties by fermentation using *Leuconostoc mesenteroides*. In every sample obtained from a perfusion experiment, more than 90% of the ^{14}C of lactose was localized in the galactose moiety (*44*). It was probable that the glucose and galactose moieties were not derived from the same precursor in the mammary gland. On the other hand, after intravenous injection of acetate-1-^{14}C to the living cow, due to incorporation of the precursor in glucose by the liver followed by passage of glucose to the udder, both hexose moieties of lactose had a similar total ^{14}C activity. On the basis of these results and other experiments in which he injected acetate-1-^{14}C directly into the artery of the udder in living cows, it was suggested by Wood in 1957 that lactose is synthesized in the mammary gland from UDP-galactose+free glucose. This prediction was borne out later when Watkins and Hassid in 1962 showed definitely by *in vitro* experiments that lactose is synthesized from glucose and uridine diphosphate (UDP)-galactose.

Other perfusion experiments carried out in collaboration with Dr. H.G. Wood, always led to the same conclusion where lactose synthesis was concerned. When the udder was perfused in the presence of glucose-2-^{14}C, the glucose moiety of lactose was exclusively labelled in C_2. Galactose was labelled in position 2, but also to an important degree in positions 1 and 3 (*45*). This is in complete agreement with the concept that free glucose of blood is incorporated directly into glucose of lactose, and that galactose is formed *via* phosphate esters, UDP-glucose and UDP-galactose. During its conversion through the esters, ^{14}C will randomize from position 2 to 1 and 3 under the influence of the pentose cycle. The stronger the activity of the pentose cycle, the greater the degree of this randomization. From the amount of randomization, it was calculated that 25 to 30% of the metabolized glucose molecules pass through the pentose cycle. The other metabolized glucose molecules pass into glycolysis or into the synthesis of lactose. Taking into account the radioactivity found in glycerol of milk fat in the glucose-2-^{14}C perfusion experiment and in glycerol in a glucose-6-^{14}C perfusion experiment (each of which was made on the symmetrical half of the same udder), it was calculated that less than 10% of the metabolized molecules of glucose pass through glycolysis. By difference, it was found that more than 60% of the metabolized glucose is converted into lactose.

When glucose-6-^{14}C+glucose-6-^{3}H or glucose-2-^{14}C+glucose-6-^{3}H were added to the perfusion blood, the ratio of ^{14}C to ^{3}H was identical in the administered glucose and in the glucose moiety of lactose. This was not the case in the galactose moiety that contained relatively much less ^{3}H.

During a perfusion experiment, glucose-2-^{14}C+glycerol-1,3-^{14}C were added to the blood (*46*). The glucose moiety of lactose was labelled in position 2 only, but galactose was labelled in positions 1, 2, 3, 4, and 6.

Glucose-6-phosphate, UDP-glucose, and UDP-galactose were isolated from the udder tissue after perfusion. Since the pattern of labelling of UDP-glucose and UDP-galactose was similar to that of the galactose of lactose, the UDP-hexoses do act as precursors for galactose. The activity of glucose-6-phosphate was 10 times lower than that of UDP-glucose and UDP-galactose indicating that there are two or more pools of glucose-6-phosphate in the udder.

In later experiments we became interested in the metabolism of fructose in the udder. We added fructose-U-^{14}C in physiological concentrations to the perfusion blood of isolated sheep and goat mammary glands. Fructose was only moderately incorporated into CO_2, citrate, alanine, and serine of casein (*47*). The specific activity of lactose was very low and identical to the activity of glucose of the plasma.

In studies on the precursors of milk proteins in ruminants, the technique of arterio-venous (AV) differences across the udder has been very valuable. We too have used this technique repeatedly. Moreover, in 1953, we estimated the concentration of 10 essential amino acids by a microbiological technique in blood samples which were taken at regular intervals from the perfused bovine udder (*48*). The concentrations of these amino acids decreased progressively during perfusion. Lysine, valine, leucine, and isoleucine particularly, which are found in important concentrations in milk protein, were taken up quickly. These results were in line with the results of tracer experiments carried out by other workers at that time who showed that milk proteins are synthesized from free amino acids of the plasma. We showed that many labelled amino acids are intensively incorporated by isolated udders into milk casein.

The first comprehensive study of amino acid AV differences across the udder *in vivo* was made by our laboratory (*49*). Blood samples were taken simultaneously from the bovine udder artery and the udder vein. Twenty two free amino acids were determined chromatographically in each sample. In a "dry" cow, almost no uptake of amino acids by the udder was found. On the other hand, most amino acids had a considerable decrease in concentration by passage across the lactating mammary gland. Estimates indicated that some amino acids were absorbed in sufficient quantities and others in inadequate amounts to account for their respective concentrations in milk proteins. The finding that large and significant quantities of ornithine were taken up from the blood by the udder, although this amino acid does not occur in milk protein, was unexpected. Citrulline, another noncasein amino acid, was often taken up by the udder to a small extent. These results were later confirmed and extended by Dr. Linzell and co-workers in goats and cows.

Several years ago we demonstrated in tracer experiments, carried out on perfused cow udders, that ^{14}C-labelled fatty acids such as acetate and propionate act as precursors for the synthesis of glutamate and aspartate of casein (*50*). The ^{14}C of labelled glucose was incorporated into alanine, serine, cysteine, glutamate, and aspartate. Strong indications were obtained that aspartate and glutamate act as precursors for the synthesis of asparagine and glutamine, respectively, by the perfused udder (*51*).

We also demonstrated that ornithine-2-^{14}C was converted into proline of casein by the isolated sheep udder. Chemical degradation of the synthesized proline indicated a metabolic scheme of ornithine conversion *via* glutamic-γ-semialdehyde to proline. Arginine-5-^{14}C is converted by the perfused sheep udder into ornithine and proline (*52–54*). Nearly one-quarter of the total amount of proline residues of the casein originates from these sources.

L-(Carbamoyl-^{14}C, 2-^{14}C) citrulline, added to the perfusion blood of isolated mammary glands of sheep and goats, acted as a precursor of arginine and proline of casein (*55*). In the plasma, we detected labelled arginine, proline, ornithine, urea, and unknown metabolites of the order of arginosuccinic acid. It appears that the udder metabolizes citrulline *via* arginine to urea, ornithine, and proline. An important part of the Krebs-Henseleit cycle, therefore, is present in udder tissue although the cycle is not complete.

Glycine-1-^{14}C was incorporated by the perfused sheep udder into casein of milk (*56*). The radioactivity was recovered primarily in glycine residues and little in serine.

L-Methionine-^{35}S was extensively incorporated by the isolated sheep udder into casein of milk (*57*). The highest radioactivity was recovered in the methionine residues but a small activity was also observed in cystine.

The perfused goat udder incorporated threonine-U-^{14}C and phenylalanine-U-^{14}C very efficiently into milk casein (*58*). All of the threonine residues and 1.5% of the glycine residues of casein were derived from free plasma threonine. Phenylalanine acted as precursor for the synthesis of tyrosine.

Our experiments demonstrate abundantly that the udder is able to synthesize the carbon portion of non-essential amino acids. Recently, we studied the origin of the nitrogen portion of the synthesized amino acids.

After administration of DL-ornithine [δ-^{15}N, 1-^{14}C] to the perfusion blood of isolated goat udders, incorporation of ^{15}N was detected in several amino acids of casein: glutamic acid, aspartic acid, alanine, serine, glycine, and the branched chain amino acids (*59*). The results indicated that the δ-amino group of ornithine is transaminated by the udder and may provide a large part of the α-amino N needed in the synthesis of non-essential amino acids.

Acknowledgments

I have given a presentation of experiments carried out in the Department of Physiology of Domestic Animals in the course of 30 years. I was very fortunate to have had very good assistants over the years with whom it was a pleasure to work in a friendly atmosphere. Experience has taught me that optimum results can be achieved by the collaboration between research workers from different laboratories. I have had the opportunity and the pleasure of co-operating with many eminent scientists from Belgium and from abroad and I greatly benefited from these collaborations. I must not forget to refer to the financial help our laboratory has received in the course of the last 25 years from different Foundations engaged in the support of scientific research: Institut pour l'Encouragement de la Recherche dans l'Industrie et l'Agriculture (Belgium); Fonds National de la Recherche Scientifique (Belgium); Actions de Recherches concertées (Belgium); National Institute of Health (USA). I wish to express my sincere gratitude to these Foundations.

REFERENCES

1. Peeters, G. and Massart, L. (1947). La perfusion de la glande mammaire isolée. *Arch. Int. Pharmacodyn.* **74**, 83–89.
2. Peeters, G., Sierens, G., and Silver, M. (1952). Expulsion of milk in the isolated perfused udder of the cow. *Arch. Int. Pharmacodyn.* **88**, 413–424.
3. Peeters, G., Massart, L., and Coussens, R. (1947). L'éjection du lait chez les bovidés. *Arch. Int. Pharmacodyn.* **75**, 85–89.
4. Vercruysse, R., Peeters, G., and Coussens, R. (1950). Circulation time of blood in the lactating cow. *Arch. Int. Pharmacodyn.* **82**, 93–98.
5. Peeters, G. and Coussens, R. (1950). The influence of the milking act on the diuresis of the lactating cow. *Arch. Int. Pharmacodyn.* **84**, 209–220.
6. Debackere, M. and Peeters, G. (1960). The influence of vaginal distension on milk ejection and diuresis in the lactating cow. *Arch. Int. Pharmacodyn.* **123**, 462–471.
7. Debackere, M., Peeters, G., and Tuyttens, N. (1961). Reflex release of an oxytocic hormone by stimulation of genital organs in male and female sheep studied by a cross-circulation technique. *J. Endocrinol.* **22**, 321–334.

8. Peeters, G., De Vos, N., and Houvenaghel, A. (1971). Elimination of the Ferguson reflex by section of the pelvic nerves in the lactating goat. *J. Endocrinol.* **49**, 125–130.
9. Peeters, G. and Houvenaghel, A. (1973). Reflex release of milk-ejection activity by stimulation of organs in the pelvic region in sheep as studied by cross-circulation experiments. *J. Endocrinol.* **58**, 53–66.
10. Legros, J. J., Reynaert, R., and Peeters, G. (1974). Specific release of bovine neurophysin I during milking and suckling in the cow. *J. Endocrinol.* **60**, 327–332.
11. Legros, J. J., Reynaert, R., and Peeters, G. (1975). Specific release of bovine neurophysin II during arterial or venous haemorrhage in the cow. *J. Endocrinol.* **67**, 297–302.
12. Legros, J. J., Peeters, G., Marcus, S., De Groot, W., and Reynaert, R. (1976). Independent release of neurophysin I and II during and following parturition in cows. *Arch. Int. Physiol. Biochim.* **84**, 887–888.
13. Reynaert, R., De Groot, W., Marcus, S., and Peeters, G. (1976). Serum growth hormone and free fatty acid levels in heifers and cows before, during and after parturition. *Ann. Endocrinol.* (Paris) **37**, 75–82.
14. Reynaert, R., De Paepe, M., Marcus, S., and Peeters, G. (1975). Influence of serum free fatty acid levels on growth hormone secretion in lactating cows. *J. Endocrinol.* **66**, 213–224.
15. Reynaert, R., Marcus, S., De Paepe, M., and Peeters, G. (1976). Influences of stress, age and sex on serum growth hormone and free fatty acid levels in cattle. *Horm. Metab. Res.* **8**, 109–114.
16. Peeters, G., Houvenaghel, A., Verbeke, R., and Van Sichem-Reynaert, R. (1972). Effects of bradykinin and kallikrein injected into the udder artery of sheep and goats. *Arch. Int. Pharmacodyn.* **198**, 397–414.
17. Peeters, G., Verbeke, R., Houvenaghel, A., and Reynaert, R. (1976). Isolation of kallikrein from mammary gland of cows. *Q. J. Exp. Physiol.* **61**, 1–14.
18. Peeters, G., Coussens, R., and Sierens, G. (1949). Physiology of the nerves in the bovine mammary gland. *Arch. Int. Pharmacodyn.* **79**, 75–82.
19. Peeters, G., Bouckaert, J., and Oyaert, W. (1952). The influence of unilateral lumbar sympathectomy on the udder of the sheep. *Arch. Int. Pharmacodyn.* **89**, 197–203.
20. Peeters, G., Petré, P., and Quintelier, W. (1977). Nature of adrenoceptor sites in bovine teat muscles. *Naunyn-Schmiedeberg's Arch. Pharmacol.* **296**, 111–115.
21. Peeters, G., Massart, L., Oyaert, W., and Coussens, R. (1948). Pletysmography applied to the teats of the bovine mammary gland. *Arch. Int. Pharmacodyn.* **75**, 243–255.

22. Peeters, G. and De Bruycker, R. (1975). Influence of sympathomimetic drugs on the motility of bovine teat muscles. *J. Dairy Res.* **42**, 11–19.
23. Houvenaghel, A. (1971). Electromagnetische bloedvloeimetingen aan de melkklierarterie bij niet geanesthesieerde lacterende kleine herkauwers. *Meded. Veeartsenijsch. Rijksuniv. Gent* **15**, 3–180.
24. Dhondt, G., Houvenaghel, A., Peeters, G., and Verschooten, F. (1973). Influence of vasoactive hormones on blood flow through the mammary artery in lactating cows. *Arch. Int. Pharmacodyn.* **204**, 89–104.
25. Houvenaghel, A. and Peeters, G. (1974). Influence d'hormones vasoactives et du stress sur le débit sanguin dans la glande mammaire de la chevre en lactation. *Ann. Biol. Anim. Biochim. Biophys.* **14**, 437–446.
26. Houvenaghel, A., Peeters, G., and Verschooten, F. (1973). Influences of manual udder stimulation and oxytocin on mammary artery blood flow in lactating cows. *Arch. Int. Pharmacodyn.* **205**, 124–133.
27. Dhondt, G. and Peeters, G. (1976). Influence of acute experimental mastitis on mammary blood flow in lactating ruminants. *Arch. Int. Physiol. Biochim.* **84**, 885–887.
28. Peeters, G., Stormorken, H., and Vanschoubroek, F. (1960). The effect of different stimuli on milk ejection and diuresis in the lactating cow. *J. Endocrinol.* **20**, 163–172.
29. Peeters, G., De Buysscher, E., and Vandevelde, M. (1973). Milk ejection in primiparous heifers in the presence of their calves. *Zbl. Vet. Med. A* **20**, 531–536.
30. Vandeputte-Van Messom, G. and Peeters, G. (1974). Effects of intraventricular administration of cholinergic drugs on water diuresis in goats. *Arch. Int. Pharmacodyn.* **211**, 80–98.
31. Vandeputte-Van Messom, G. and Peeters, G. (1975). Effect of intraventricular administration of noradrenaline on water diuresis in goats. *J. Endocrinol.* **66**, 375–383.
32. Vandeputte-Van Messom, G., Peeters, G., and Lauwers, H. (1976). Artificial induction of lactation by hypothalamic implantation of perphenazine in virgin goats. *J. Dairy Res.* **43**, 9–17.
33. Cowie, A. T., Duncombe, W. G., Folley, S. J., French, T. H., Glascock, R., Massart, L., Peeters, G., and Popjak, G. (1951). Synthesis of milk fat from acetic acid CH_3 $^{14}COOH$ by the perfused isolated bovine udder. *Biochem. J.* **49**, 610–615.
34. Lauryssens, M., Verbeke, R., Peeters, G., and Reinards, M. T. (1960). Incorporation of [1-^{14}C] and [3-^{14}C] butyrate into milk constituents by the perfused cow's udder. *J. Dairy Res.* **27**, 151–160.
35. Lauryssens, M., Verbeke, R., Peeters, G., and Donck, A. (1959). Incorporation of sodium [1-^{14}C] hexanoate and sodium hydrogen [^{14}C] carbonate into

milk constituents by the perfused cow's udder. *Biochem. J.* **73**, 71–75.
36. Verbeke, R., Lauryssens, M., Peeters, G., and James, A. T. (1959). Incorporation of DL [1-^{14}C] leucine and [1-^{14}C] iso-valeric acid into milk constituents by the perfused cow's udder. *Biochem. J.* **73**, 24–29.
37. James, A. T., Peeters, G., and Lauryssens, M. (1956). The metabolism of propionic acid. *Biochem. J.* **64**, 726–730.
38. Raafat, M. A., Verbeke, R., and Peeters, G. (1963). The metabolism of propionate in the isolated cow's udder. *Biochem. J.* **88**, 155–159.
39. Lauryssens, M., Verbeke, R., Peeters, G., Garton, G. A., Lough, A. K., and Duncan, W.R.H. (1960). Métabolisme du stéarate-1-^{14}C dans la glande mammaire bovine. *Arch. Int. Physiol. Biochim.* **68**, 511–512.
40. Lauryssens, M., Verbeke, R., and Peeters, G. (1961). Metabolism of stearate 1-^{14}C in the isolated cow's udder. *J. Lipid Res.* **2**, 383–388.
41. Massart-Leen, A. M., Florescu, S., Verbeke, R., and Peeters, G. (1970). Metabolism of [1-^{14}C] palmitate and [1-^{14}C] oleate by the isolated perfused mammary gland of the sheep or goat. *J. Dairy Res.* **37**, 373–387.
42. Massart-Leen, A. M., Roets, E., Verbeke, R., and Peeters, G. (1974). Incorporation de l'acide myristique-1-^{14}C dans les constituents du lait par la glande mammaire isolée. *Ann. Biol. Anim. Biochim. Biophys.* **14**, 459–469.
43. Peeters, G., Debackere, M., and Sierens, R. (1957). Etude du cycle oxydatif des hexose-mono-phosphates dans le tissu mammaire par la méthode de chromatographie sur papier. *Arch. Int. Physiol. Biochim.* **65**, 324–336.
44. Wood, H. G., Schambye, P., and Peeters, G. (1957). Lactose synthesis: The distribution of ^{14}C in lactose of milk from the perfused isolated cow's udder. *J. Biol. Chem.* **226**, 1023–1034.
45. Wood, H. G., Peeters, G., Verbeke, R., Lauryssens, M., and Jacobson, B. (1965). Estimation of the pentose cycle in the perfused cow's udder. *Biochem. J.* **96**, 607–615.
46. Hansen, R. G., Wood, H. G., Peeters, G., Jacobson, B., and Wilken, J. (1962). Lactose synthesis. VI. Labeling of lactose precursors by glycerol-1, 3-^{14}C and glucose-2-^{14}C. *J. Biol. Chem.* **237**, 1034–1039.
47. Verbeke, R., Massart-Leen, A. M., and Peeters, G. (1969). Metabolism of [U-^{14}C] D-fructose by the isolated perfused udder. *J. Dairy Res.* **36**, 233–239.
48. Bouckaert, J. H., Oyaert, W., Peeters, G., and Sierens, G. (1953). Uptake of plasma amino acids by the perfused isolated cow's udder. *Arch. Int. Pharmacodyn.* **93**, 443–449.
49. Verbeke, R. and Peeters, G. (1965). Uptake of free plasma amino acids by the lactating cow's udder and amino acid composition of udder lymph. *Biochem. J.* **94**, 183–189.

50. Verbeke, R., Aqvist, S., and Peeters, G. (1957). Acetate and propionate as precursors of amino acids in milk proteins of the perfused cow's udder. *Arch. Int. Physiol. Biochim.* **65**, 433–438.
51. Verbeke, R. and Peeters, G. (1960). The synthesis of amino acids by the perfused cow's udder. *Biochim. Biophys. Acta* **37**, 533–534.
52. Verbeke, R., Peeters, G., Cocquyt, G., and Lauryssens, M. (1965). Incorporation de l'ornithine-2-^{14}C dans les constituants du lait par la glande mammaire isolée de brebis. *Arch. Int. Physiol. Biochim.* **73**, 875–876.
53. Verbeke, R., Massart-Leen, A. M., and Peeters, G. (1966). Incorporation de l'arginine-5-^{14}C dans les constituants du lait par la glande mammaire isolée de la brebis. *Arch. Int. Physiol. Biochim.* **74**, 943–944.
54. Verbeke, R., Peeters, G., Massart-Leen, A. M., and Cocquyt, G. (1968). Incorporation of DL-[2-^{14}C] ornithine and DL-[5-^{14}C] arginine in milk constituents by the isolated lactating sheep udder. *Biochem. J.* **106**, 719–724.
55. Roets, E., Verbeke, R., Massart-Leen, A. M., and Peeters, G. (1974). Metabolism of ^{14}C citrulline in the perfused sheep and goat udder. *Biochem. J.* **144**, 435–446.
56. Verbeke, R., Feteanu, A., and Peeters, G. (1967). Incorporation de la glycine-1-^{14}C dans la caséine par la glande mammaire isolée de la brebis. *Arch. Int. Physiol. Biochim.* **75**, 675–684.
57. Verbeke, R., Simeonov, S., and Peeters, G. (1967). Incorporation de la L-méthionine-^{35}S dans la caséine par la glande mammaire isolée de la brebis. *Arch. Int. Physiol. Biochim.* **75**, 658–666.
58. Verbeke, R., Roets, E., Massart-Leen, A. M., and Peeters, G. (1972). Metabolism of [U-^{14}C]-L-threonine and [U-^{14}C]-L-phenylalanine by the isolated perfused udder. *J. Dairy Res.* **39**, 239–250.
59. Roets, E., Verbeke, R., Peeters, G., Axmann, H., and Proksch, G. (1976). Metabolism of DL-[δ-^{15}N; 1-^{14}C] ornithine in the perfused goat udder. In *Nuclear Techniques in Animal Production and Health*, pp. 327–334. Vienna: Int. Atomic Energy Agency.

I–3

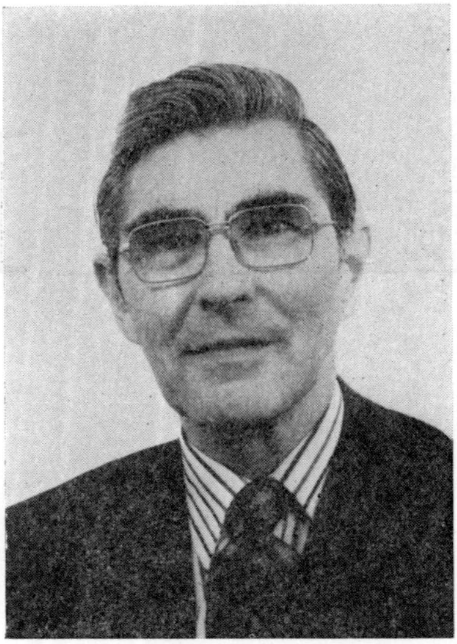

Alfred Tennant Cowie was born on August 16, 1916 in Aberdeenshire, Scotland. He received a B.Sc. degree of Veterinary Science from the University of Edinburgh and became a member of the Royal College of Veterinary Surgeons (M.R.C.V.S.) in 1938, a Ph.D. degree in 1947 and the degree of Doctor of Science in 1959 from University of Reading.

Dr. Cowie was a Centenary Postgraduate Fellow of the Royal (Dick) Veterinary College, Edinburgh in 1938–40. Positions held include the following: a Research Assistant of Animal Diseases Research Association, Moredun Institute, Edinburgh in 1940–41; on permanent staff, National Institute for Research in Dairying (NIRD) from 1947. Since 1970, he has been the Head of the Physiology Department of NIRD.

The awards and fellowships he has received include: Travel Grant from Rockfeller Foundation and Research Grant from Harvard University Medical School in 1952–3; Special Merit Promotion to Senior Principal Scientific Officer, Physiology Department, National Institute for Research in Dairying in 1962; Thomas Lawrance Pawlett Visiting Scholarship of University of Sydney, Royal Society and Nuffield Foundation Commonwealth Bursary in 1963. He held a Visiting Professorship in the Faculty of Agriculture, Nagoya University, Japan in 1975 and was elected a Fellow of the Institute of Biology in 1974 and a Fellow of the Royal College of Veterinary Surgeons in 1976.

Dr. Cowie was a Consultant, World Health Organization, Geneva, Scientific Group on the Physiology of Lactation in 1963; a member of the Editorial Board of the Journal of Endocrinology in 1966–72; a member of Committee of the Society for Endocrinology 1971–74; a member of the Veterinary Products Committee of the Ministry of Agriculture, Fisheries and Food, London (1970–77).

BACKWARD GLANCES

A. T. Cowie

National Institute for Research in Dairying, Shinfield, Reading, England

My entry into the field of physiology was entirely fortuitous. In 1938 I had qualified as a veterinary surgeon at the Royal (Dick) Veterinary College in Edinburgh and had taken concurrently a B. Sc. course in veterinary science at Edinburgh University; the latter had given me a taste for research. I was advised to get some preliminary experience in clinical practice but scarcely had I become an assistant in a veterinary practice in the south of Scotland when the Royal [Dick] Veterinary College offered me a research fellowship which for that year was allocated for studies in physiology. It was a condition of the fellowship that I spend several months gaining some insight into physiological research and it was my good fortune to be placed in the laboratory of Sir Joseph Barcroft in Cambridge where he and his colleague Professor D. H. Barron were in the midst of their studies on fetal physiology in sheep. Those were memorable months spent in the stimulating atmosphere of a very active research laboratory. I acquired some skill with the Van Slyke manometric blood-gas apparatus and began to feel I was making a slight contribution to the work. I received great kindness and encouragement from both Sir Joseph and Professor Barron and much daily help from a young biochemist who was also beginning his research career—now Professor Peter H. Forsham, Metabolic Research Unit, University of California (*1*). On my return to Edinburgh I began a study of the energy metabolism of pregnant sheep under the direction of Professor H. Dryerre but this had not progressed far when the respiration calorimeter was required for another purpose. With the outbreak of war alternative sources of cattle feed were under scrutiny and the Agricultural Research Council was anxious to get information on the energy value of sodium hydroxide treated straw—a new process said to increase the digestibility of straw. Under the supervision of Dr. James Stewart of the Moredun Institute I modified the calorimeter and set about determining in sheep the "starch equivalent" of the treated straw. The work was carried out and the findings, which I have long since forgotten, were reported to the Agricultural Research Council. I thought this method of treating straw had also passed into oblivion but only recently Sir Kenneth Blaxter, Rowett Research Institute, Aberdeen told me that, because of renewed interest in it, his staff were evaluating the energy value of hydroxide-treated straw by respiration calorimetry, and so, some 40 years after my fumbling attempts, a decisive conclusion on the metabolizable energy of this straw should soon be reached.

After my brief excursion into animal calorimetry there followed a short spell of clinical work in the veterinary college which gave me my first real interest in surgery.

In the autumn of 1941 I found myself at the National Institute for Research in Dairying working under the direction of Dr. S. J. Folley and Dr. G. W. Scott Blair on the development of a pregnancy test in cows based on the rheological properties of the secretions of the uterine cervix. Changes characteristic of pregnancy occurred in the flow properties of the secretion but unfortunately these were not sufficiently reliable in the first two months of gestation when an accurate test was required (*5*). During this period I decided that I was unlikely to become a rheologist; on the other hand I was greatly interested in the studies on lactation then in progress in Folley's department and I took every opportunity of participating in them. So by a somewhat circuitous route I entered the field of lactational physiology.

At that time the department was small, consisting of John Folley and Frank Malpress, together with the head laboratory assistant Stanley Watson and one or two junior assistants. Exciting developments were occurring in the field and the laboratory was a hive of activity (*11*, *12*). Folley, in collaboration with Prof. F. G. Young, had already demonstrated the galactopoietic effects of anterior pituitary extracts in cows in declining lactation; the synthetic oestrogens had recently become available and evidence was fast being obtained that these could be used to induce udder growth and lactation in non-pregnant ruminants; and milk yields in cows were being increased by administering iodinated proteins which had thyroxine-like activities. All these aspects were under study and in addition there were experiments in laboratory animals on the role of hormones in mammary growth and in milk secretion. My initial training was thus broadly based and included taking my turn to hand-milk the experimental heifers on Sundays when the animal attendant was off duty. My introduction to the importance of the milk-ejection reflex in cattle was far from theoretical!

Of the numerous aspects of lactational physiology in which I have been concerned I propose to consider only one or two problems of fairly general interest. The first is the induction of mammary growth and lactation in ruminants by suitable hormone therapy. Folley had initiated studies on induced lactation in the late 1930's, and when I became involved field trials (described in detail in *J. Endocrinol.*, **4** (1) (1944)) were being set up under the aegis of the Agricultural Research Council with Folley and Malpress conducting the work at Reading. With the co-operation of local farmers, infertile cows and heifers were treated with synthetic oestrogens, usually by tablet implantation, the owner being instructed to start milking the animal 10 days later. The daily milk yield was carefully watched, and when a peak had apparently been reached the implants were removed. Milk yields varied from negligible to 14 kg/day. I was soon to realize the value of such field trials in highlighting problems that had not become evident under laboratory conditions. Reports began to come in of treated animals that could only walk with difficulty or were lying down and could not get up. As I was a veterinarian this became my problem! It soon became apparent that the clinical signs were due to fractures of the pelvis; but what was the cause—could the oestrogen produce bone rarefaction? Autopsy followed by X-ray examination of the bones gave no support to this possibility; it was finally concluded that the fractures were occurring as the result of repeated trauma from the animals being mounted by others during the state of persistent oestrus induced by the oestrogen. The oestrogen also relaxed the pelvic ligaments and this probably increased the susceptibility to injury. Thereafter animals under experiment were kept singly during the period of treatment, as they had been under laboratory conditions, and no more fractures occurred.

There were unexpected incidents unrelated to the animals! Late one evening on the way home from a series of implantations Frank Malpress and I had to abandon the car after its entire electrical wiring suddenly fused. The wartime roads were completely deserted and we had to walk some 53 km to the Institute! On another occasion we arrived at a small farm to find the entrance bedecked with antivivisection posters. The owner was a charming old lady. With some misgivings we explained what we proposed to do. She agreed and held her two cows, watching with interest the operation of implanting the oestrogen tablets under the skin. On completion she thanked us and kindly entertained us to a meal. The cows responded well and we received details of the milk yields on notepaper decorated with antivivisection slogans and, moreover, containing a request to implant a cow belonging to her neighbour. I have yet to decide on the morality of our actions, but both the antivivisector and the experimenters were well satisfied with the responses!

The lactational responses in these trials were too uncertain to permit the widespread use of the procedure. While the results were disappointing from the view of practical application they nevertheless proved a most valuable stimulus to further studies of a more basic nature on the endocrine control of mammary growth in both this and other laboratories. The contemporary views and conclusions have been well set down by Folley and Malpress (*13*) and I shall not recapitulate them in any detail. Suffice it to say that the theory of two specific mammogenic factors secreted by the anterior pituitary—a duct growth factor and a lobulo-alveolar growth factor—put forward by Turner and his colleagues had aroused much controversy but usefully had focused attention to the role of the pituitary in mammary growth; in addition there was much discussion of the respective roles of oestrogen and progesterone. Folley had little brief for the specific mammogen theory and considered that the mammogenic effects of the pituitary could be explained on the basis of the known hormones. Studies on a broad front were planned to investigate the roles of oestrogen and progesterone in mammary growth in the goat and laboratory animals, the effects of different ratios of the ovarian hormones in mammary growth and, in due course, mammogenesis in the hypophysectomized goat. The studies were carried out over the years in collaboration with departmental colleagues, with staff in the Statistics department, and with a number of visitors from abroad including Don Flux, Sam Goldzveig, Motoo Naito, Akira Yokoyama (for references see Cowie and Tindal (*7*)).

The studies on cattle had indicated that poor lactational responses were associated with inadequate growth and development of the lobulo-alveolar tissue in the udder and a likely reason was that progesterone was also necessary for normal mammary growth. Progesterone was then a scarce and expensive hormone but thanks to the generosity of a drug company sufficient progesterone was obtained to start a study in goats. Later in the early 1950's when progesterone was synthesized from plant sterols it became available not in milligram but in kilogram quantities!

It was decided that the degree of lobulo-alveolar growth must be carefully assessed and in this we received the invaluable co-operation of Mr. K. C. Richardson, University College, London, who devised a method for measuring the surface area of the secretory epithelium. Our objective was to mimic the normal growth of the mammary gland and to this end we daily injected young goats, which had been ovariectomized to eliminate endogenous ovarian hormones, with oestrogen and progesterone over a period equivalent to normal gestation, 140–150 days. At intervals during the treatment the udders of the goats were photographed against a standard grid to record increases in size. It soon became apparent that the udders of the goats treated with oestrogen were enlarging much more rapidly than those on the combined treatment. After treatment ended, milking was started. At the peak of lactation an udder-half (*i.e.*, one mammary gland) was removed surgically for histometric study, and the contralateral half was removed and similarly examined at the end of lactation. The milk yields of the goats treated with oestrogen and progesterone were generally higher and less variable than those of goats receiving only oestrogen. It became apparent that the rapid increase in udder size in the goats receiving oestrogen by itself was due not to a more rapid growth of lobulo-alveolar tissue but to the early initiation of secretion which distended the alveoli. In the ruminant one must distinguish carefully between increases in udder size and true growth of the parenchyma. Histological examination, moreover, revealed that the structure of the alveoli was essentially normal in the goats on the combined treatment whereas alveoli tended to be cystic in those receiving only oestrogen. While the addition of progesterone resulted in somewhat higher and less variable milk yields these were still only two-thirds of the yield expected had the goats come normally into lactation. The effect of varying the duration of treatment (35, 70, and 140 days) was next investigated when one gland was removed at the end of the treatment period, *i.e.*, before milking was started, the other at the peak of lactation. In general the longer the period of treatment with the combined hormones the sooner after milking were the peak yields achieved; with oestrogen by itself the yields were usually lower and the duration of treatment did not affect the interval to peak yield. In short, higher milk yields can be induced in the goat when treatment with oestrogen and progesterone is given over 70–140 days, but if treatment over a long period is not feasible then oestrogen by itself for a short period (35 days) will give the better result. This study, however, revealed in a most striking fashion the fact, previously not fully appreciated, that much of the mammary growth was occurring after treatments had ended, *i.e.*, during lactation. As the goats had been ovariectomized we could only surmize that the mammary growth was a response to pituitary hormones released by the milking stimulus. This we later confirmed by showing that the regular application of the milking stimulus induced lactation in nulliparous ovariectomized goats and that this response was abolished if the pituitary stalk was surgically transected before regular "milking" was started. The milk yields so induced were considerably less than would have been expected had the animals been treated with oestrogen and progesterone and the lobulo-alveolar structure was somewhat abnormal. Clearly we had been at fault in not initially including a group of control animals that were not given hormonal treatment before milking. We have shown that the ovarian hormones do not cause mammary growth in the hypophysectomized goat and so it must be concluded that the anterior pituitary plays the key role in stimulating mammary growth when lactation is induced with ovarian hormones.

In the last few years there has been renewed interest in other laboratories in the induction of lactation in infertile cattle following upon the observation that lactation could be induced after ovarian-hormone treatment for only 7 days with high doses of oestradiol (for a 600 kg animal, 60 mg oestradiol and 150 mg progesterone/day) (*9*). The milk yields, however, do not appear to be superior to those obtained in earlier studies. It has been suggested that the low yields are associated with poor functional differentiation and synthetic activity of the alveolar cells but I am convinced that the basic cause is an overall deficiency of lobulo-alveolar tissue and can only concur with Howe *et al.* (*17*) that successful induced lactation requires the development of more alveolar cells. An interesting application of induced lactation in cattle has been investigated by Professor M. Naito and his colleagues (*24*) whereby the response is used for predicting the future dairy performance of the animal but they point out that associated reproductive problems indicate caution in such a use.

There remains much work to be done on the basic endocrine control of mammary growth. In ruminants at least it may not be possible to induce full mammary growth with the ovarian hormones because we may be calling on the anterior pituitary to perform a task which it does not normally perform. As Folley and Malpress (*13*) wrote some 30 years ago, "It seems quite possible that in most experiments showing the importance of pituitary mammogenic function this gland has been acting vicariously for the absent placentae of normal pregnancy." The presence of a placental lactogen in ruminants was first demonstrated a few years ago by my colleagues Hugh Buttle, Isabel Forsyth, and Geoffrey Knaggs (*4*). Unfortunately, facilities were not immediately available to exploit their observations and it was other laboratories who first obtained highly purified preparations of ruminant placental lactogens. However, I am very glad we can now devote more attention to placental lactogens which may have an important role in mammary growth and in metabolic functions in pregnant ruminants.

I now turn back to studies concerned with the hormonal control of the maintenance of lactation. There is confusion over the terminology concerning the onset of secretory activity in the mammary gland, the onset of copious lactation at or around parturition, the maintenance of lactation and the stimulation of an existing lactation (*7*) and I shall therefore avoid the term "lactogenesis" which has been used for one or more of these phases. Prolactin was the first of the pituitary hormones to be isolated in a highly purified state in the late 1930's (see review by Cowie and Tindal, *7*) and it immediately became designated as *the* lactogenic hormone. This concept was first challenged by Folley (*10–12*) who maintained that since prolactin would not induced milk secretion in hypophysectomized animals with suitably developed glands (with the possible exception of the rabbit) it was clear that other anterior pituitary factors were involved and he considered it was more correct to talk of a "pituitary lactogenic complex." When I joined John Folley's department considerable experimental evidence had been obtained by him in collaborative studies with Professor F. G. Young that anterior pituitary extracts would increase the milk yields of cows in declining lactation whereas purified prolactin preparations were ineffective. About this time Lyons (*22*) published his early studies on the use of hypophysectomized-ovariectomized rats to determine, by replacement therapy, the hormones involved in mammary growth. This work was greatly admired by John Folley who encouraged me to acquire the techniques of hypophysectomy so that we could carry out similar replacement studies in animals hypophysectomized during lactation. Thanks to the advice and help received from Dr. Max Reiss, Dr. Dora Jacobsohn, and Dr. K. Ferguson, satisfactory techniques for the rat, rabbit, and goat were acquired. I also had the good fortune to spend a year in the Laboratory for Surgical Research of the Harvard Medical School working with Dr. David M. Hume (who was tragically killed in an aeroplane accident in 1973) where I participated in studies on the effects of surgery on the pituitary-adrenal axis in the dog and learnt much about the craft of surgery and of the metabolic responses to surgery.

Replacement studies were first tackled in the rat. I knew that replacement of oxytocin to ensure milk ejection would be required in addition to anterior pituitary hormones but it was perhaps fortunate that I did not appreciate the complexities of milk ejection in the rat as were much later revealed by Lincoln and his colleagues (*21*) who demonstrated that there are long periods when milk ejection occurs regularly every 5–15 min, there being some 50–80 occurrences of milk ejection during 24 hr. Had I been aware of this I might well have been deterred from studying the rat. My colleague Keith Benson and I (*2*) had found, however, that we were able to remove the posterior lobe of the pituitary while leaving the anterior lobe *in situ*. This operation abolished normal milk ejection but the rats were able to raise their litter if injected with oxytocin three times a day although the growth rate of the young was subnormal. Nevertheless, this observation indicated that we should be able to demonstrate at least partial replacement responses in totally hypophysectomized rats receiving oxytocin three times a day when suitable anterior pituitary preparations were given. We also made the interesting observation that if these rats became pregnant again it was unnecessary to give oxytocin to induce milk ejection during the subsequent lactation. This was one of the early observations on the re-organisation that can occur in neurosecretory tissue—a subject later studied and reviewed by Daniel and Prichard (*8*). I observed that partial restoration of lactation was obtained with prolactin and adrenocorticotrophin, a finding that was confirmed when John Tindal and I carried out further replacement studies in rats from which on day 13 of pregnancy only the anterior lobe of the pituitary had been removed and in which the milk ejection reflex was functional when lactation started (*7*). Our observations in the rat were in good agreement with the independent studies by Lyons and his colleagues (*3*) who reported a 50% restoration of lactation after hypophysectomy when prolactin and adrenal corticoids were administered. Since complete restoration of lactation, so far as I am aware, still has not been achieved in the rat, and since ruminant hormones have been used, it would be unwise to arrive at firm conclusions on the hormonal complex required for maintenance of milk secretion in the rat but the evidence suggests that prolactin and adrenocorticotropic hormone (ACTH) may be of major importance.

The development of a satisfactory technique of hypophysectomy in the goat proved somewhat more difficult. In the goat the pituitary is partially enclosed by large venous sinuses within which lie the arterial carotid retia, the approach to the pituitary must therefore be precise and there is little margin for error. Because a complete view of the sella is seldom possible it is also essential that on autopsy the sellar region should be decalcified and serial sections examined for the presence of remnants. In studies in recent years Hugh Buttle and I have used radioimmunoassays to detect the presence of anterior pituitary hormones in the blood after the operation and any prolactin response to the administration of thyrotrophin-releasing hormone (TRH), procedures which are proving valuable checks on the completeness of hypophysectomy. In our experience the operation is considerably easier in the sheep as the base of the skull is less thick and a much better exposure of the pituitary is possible. There are, however, important differences in reproductive physiology between the two species and the sheep cannot be used as a model for the goat.

Initially oxytocin was administered to hypophysectomized goats before each milking but this proved to be unnecessary. Later studies by Alan McNeilly (*23*) confirmed that goats can be completely milked out in the absence of any detectable release of oxytocin. Having demonstrated that some restoration of lactation could be obtained after hypophysectomy with crude pituitary extracts we moved on to the use of purified hormones. Eventually complete restoration of milk yield was achieved by administering sheep prolactin, bovine growth hormone, triiodothyronine, insulin, and dexamethasone (*7*). The progress of these studies was slow as only a few goats could be handled at a time and the preparation and examination of serial sections of each sella was time consuming. The lactational responses in a few goats were such that we suspected incomplete removal of the pituitary and these we initially excluded from the study with the proviso that the sellae would be sectioned and examined at some later date. Thanks to the conscientious work of my colleague Alan Turvey these sellae were eventually processed and I was very surprised when at least one of these goats was found to be completely hypophysectomized. Responses in this goat revealed that insulin was not essential, that some restoration of milk yield could be obtained with the other three hormones in the absence of prolactin, that while prolactin was required for the rapid restoration of the yield, once full lactation was established the yields were maintained when prolactin injections were stopped provided growth hormone, triiodothyronine, and adrenal corticoid were continued. Although we had long recognized the important role of growth hormone in the maintenance of lactation in the ruminant its ability to maintain high yields in the complete absence of prolactin was surprising. Subsequent studies by Professor Karg and his colleagues (*19*) in Germany and by my colleague Ian Hart (*15*) on the lactational responses to the inhibition of prolactin release by bromocriptine have underlined the important role of prolactin in the onset of copious lactation in ruminants whereas its role is apparently less critical in the maintenance of lactation. It is of interest, moreover, that complete restoration of milk yield was achieved at the time when the normal yields were declining. Restoration to their pre-operative levels (*i.e.*, peak yield) clearly suggests that the normal decline in yield is at least in part associated with changes in endocrine activities and with growth hormone in particular.

In the early stages of these studies in goats there began a most fruitful collaboration with Professor Peter Daniel and Dr. Marjorie Prichard of the Nuffield Institute for Medical Research, Oxford, who were working on hypothalamic and pituitary studies (*8*) in a variety of species including small ruminants and who had developed a technique for surgical transection of the pituitary stalk in the sheep. Enthusiastic collaboration between such small groups each with their own expertise is, in my opinion, of great importance and has very real synergistic effects on achievements.

In referring to the concept of a lactogenic hormone complex I earlier indicated that prolactin alone might induce milk secretion in the hypophysectomized rabbit. This arose from an observation in 1939 by Fredrikson (*14*) which for long remained unconfirmed. In 1964, however, Kilpatrick *et al.* (*20*) while studying the maintenance of the corpus luteum after hypophysectomy in the rabbit noted that prolactin while failing to maintain luteal function induced milk secretion. The authors were apparently unaware of the significance of this observation in confirming Fredrikson's earlier study. I therefore embarked on a more detailed study of the maintenance of lactation in the hypophysectomized rabbit which included biochemical investigations by my colleagues Ted Jones and Peter Hartmann (*7, 18*). It was essential to give oxytocin to obtain milk ejection but as the rabbit normally nurses its litter once daily this presented no problem. Lactation could indeed be fully restored by administration of sheep prolactin in the absence of other anterior pituitary hormones, but the yield then began to decline despite the continued injections of prolactin, and this decline could only be reversed when injections of human growth hormone were substituted for those of sheep prolactin; moreover if initially human growth hormone was given full milk yields were restored but again could not be maintained unless the human growth hormone was replaced by sheep prolactin. These alternating responses were, I believe, due to the development of antibodies to the sheep prolactin and human growth hormone. I think, therefore, that some caution should be used in interpreting studies in which prolactin from one species is given to unrelated species. Clearly the components of the hormone complex involved in the secretory functions of the mammary gland differ in the few species that have so far been studied, ranging from the single hormone in the rabbit to some four hormones in sheep and goats, and generalizations about the hormonal control of lactation cannot therefore validly be made from results on one species —a fact that tends to be forgotten by some who work exclusively on one species! These species differences are puzzling since the alveolar cells, regardless of species, are ultrastructurally identical and the synthetic pathways similar, and it would be expected that the hormonal requirements would be common. One can speculate that the hormonal patterns may be common but that differences in receptor development and behaviour may require the hormones to be present at differing times or stages in the development of the gland. Work in progress on mammary receptors by my colleagues Isabel Forsyth and Tom Hayden is beginning to reveal the complexities of the development and maintenance of these specific binding proteins in the mammary alveoli and may soon shed light on the above problem.

Ruminant prolactins, as already noted, were among the first anterior pituitary hormones to be isolated and of their actions, both physiological and pharmacological, about one hundred are known in a variety of vertebrates. Ironically the functions of prolactin in ruminants are still ill-defined. While apparently essential for the onset of copious lactation, its role in the maintenance of lactation is uncertain and unknown in metabolic functions. It is essential to remember that environmental factors, the length of day and the ambient temperature, have a major effect on the concentration of prolactin in the blood of ruminants, and therefore studies in the spring will be carried out against a background of rising prolactin levels whereas studies in the autumn will encounter declining levels (*16*). If these seasonal changes are overlooked false correlations can readily emerge!

Ian Hart in my department, in collaboration with colleagues in the Feeding and Metabolism department, is carrying out fascinating studies on the hormonal patterns (prolactin, growth hormone, insulin, thyroxine) in the lactating cow and relating these to milk yields and to how the animals partition their energy intake between milk production and meat production (*6*). Striking differences occur in the patterns observed in high and low yielding cows but the physiological significance of these observations and their interpretation are matters for further research.

In returning to the studies of the 1950's and 1960's I cannot but wish that radioimmunoassays and radioreceptor assays for the anterior pituitary hormones had then been available; indeed it might well be informative to repeat some of the hormone replacement studies with regular monitoring of hormone levels in the blood.

These few backward glances concern a few aspects of the work of this laboratory on the endocrine control of mammary growth and function with which I have been much involved. Perhaps I should have misquoted James Joyce and entitled my contribution "Mamaries of Odder Times"! It has, moreover, been my good fortune and privilege to work alongside, and perhaps at times to assist in various ways, many colleagues who have made exciting advances in the physiology, endocrinology, and biochemistry of lactation and reproduction. The important studies on the central nervous system by John Tindal are reviewed by him later in this book (see Chapter II-7).

I have enjoyed my work and got satisfaction from it—perhaps I am easily satisfied! I believe it is important that research workers should enjoy their work if they are to possess the enthusiasms and determination to do good research—for it can be hard work. To the enjoyment of my research work I must add the great pleasure of the friendship of research workers in many parts of the world and from whom I have received great hospitality. I would also mention that over the last 14 years my colleagues and I have had meetings every 2 or 3 years with our French counterparts in the Laboratoire de Physiologie de la Lactation, Jouy-en-Josas, which have permitted the exchange of information and ideas to our mutual advantage although the benefits to foreign-language fluency have, I regret, been decidedly unilateral! No doubt such camarderie exists in all fields of research but I believe it flourishes unusually well in that of lactational physiology.

It is indeed an honour to be invited to contribute to this book and I can only apologize to the editorial members Professor Akira Yokoyama, Professor Hideo Mizuno, and Dr. Hiroshi Nagasawa for the inadequacies of my effort. I had the great pleasure of attending in Tokyo one of the meetings of their research group on the physiology of lactation and I take this opportunity of wishing their group and their book every success and of recording my thanks to them, to my great friend Professor Motoo Naito, and to the many other Japanese research workers for giving me so much of their time and so great hospitality when I visited their country and for making my visit most memorable and interesting. I confess that on my arrival the awareness of instant illiteracy was a little disconcerting—a second childhood indeed! The feeling, however, was later somewhat relieved by a flash of childish satisfaction when in Tokyo railway station the *katakana* caption on a sign slowly resolved into "a i su ku ri mu," and perhaps fitting that the word should denote a dairy product!

I must now end these backward glances and look to advancing attractions in the field!

REFERENCES

1. Barcroft, J., Barron, D. H., Cowie, A. T., and Forsham, P. H. (1940). The oxygen supply of the foetal brain of the sheep and the effect of asphyxia on foetal respiratory movement. *J. Physiol.* **97**, 338–346.
2. Benson, G. K. and Cowie, A. T. (1956). Lactation in the rat after hypophysial posterior lobectomy. *J. Endocrinol.* **14**, 54–64.
3. Bintarningsih, Lyons, W. R., Johnson, R. E., and Li, C. H. (1958). Hormonally-induced lactation in hypophysectomized rats. *Endocrinology* **63**, 540–548.
4. Buttle, H. L., Forsyth, I. A., and Knaggs, G. S. (1972). Plasma prolactin measured by radioimmunoassay and bioassay in pregnant and lactating goats and the occurrence of a placental lactogen. *J. Endocrinol.* **53**, 483–491.
5. Cowie, A. T. (1948). *Pregnancy Diagnosis Tests: A Review*, Commonwealth Agricultural Bureaux Joint Publication, No. 13. Great Britain.
6. Cowie, A. T. (1976). Hormones and the efficiency of lactation. *Arch. Int. Physiol. Biochim.* **84**, 879–885.
7. Cowie, A. T. and Tindal, J. S. (1971). *The Physiology of Lactation.* London: Arnold.
8. Daniel, P. M. and Prichard, M.M.L. (1975). Studies of the hypothalamus and pituitary gland. *Acta Endocrinol.* (*Copenh.*) Suppl. **201**, 1–203.
9. Erb, R. E. (1977). Hormonal control of mammogenesis and onset of lactation in cows—A review. *J. Dairy Sci.* **60**, 155–169.
10. Folley, S. J. (1938). The rôle of the anterior pituitary in lactation. *Lancet* **ii**, 389–390.
11. Folley, S. J. (1940). Lactation. *Biol. Rev.* **15**, 421–458.
12. Folley, S. J. (1945). The hormonal control of lactation. *J. Roy. Soc. Arts* **93**, 114–141.
13. Folley, S. J. and Malpress, F. H. (1948). Hormonal control of mammary growth. In *The Hormones*, vol. 1, ed. Pincus, G. and Thiman, K. V., pp 695–743. New York: Academic Press.
14. Fredrikson, H. (1939). Endocrine factors involved in the development and function of the mammary glands of female rabbits. *Acta Obstet. Gynecol. Scand.* **19** (Suppl. 1), 6–167.
15. Hart, I. C. (1973). Effect of 2-bromo-α-ergocryptine on milk yield and the level of prolactin and growth hormone in the blood of the goat at milking. *J. Endocrinol.* **57**, 178–180.
16. Hart, I. C. (1975). Seasonal factors affecting the release of prolactin in goats in response to milking. *J. Endocrinol.* **64**, 313–322.
17. Howe, J. E., Heald, C. W., and Bibb, T. L. (1975). Histology of induced bovine lactogenesis. *J. Dairy Sci.* **58**, 853–860.
18. Jones, E. A. and Cowie, A. T. (1972). The effect of hypophysectomy and

subsequent replacement therapy with sheep prolactin or bovine growth hormone on the lactose synthetase activity of rabbit mammary gland. *Biochem. J.* **130**, 997–1002.

19. Karg, H. and Schams, D. (1974). Prolactin release in cattle. *J. Reprod. Fert.* **39**, 463–472.
20. Kilpatrick, R., Armstrong, D. T., and Greep, R. O. (1964). Maintenance of the corpus luteum by gonadotrophins in the hypophysectomized rabbit. *Endocrinology* **74**, 453–461.
21. Lincoln, D. W., Hill, A., and Wakerley, J. B. (1973). The milk-ejection reflex in the rat: an intermittent function not abolished by surgical levels of anaesthesia. *J. Endocrinol.* **57**, 459–476.
22. Lyons, W. R. (1943). Lobulo-alveolar mammary growth induced in hypophysectomized rats by injections of ovarian and hypophysial hormones. In *Essays in Biology in Honor of Herbert M. Evans*, pp. 317–329. Berkeley: Univ. California Press.
23. McNeilly, A. S. (1972). The blood levels of oxytocin during suckling and hand-milking in the goat with some observations on the pattern of hormone release. *J. Endocrinol.* **52**, 177–188.
24. Naito, M., Kano, Y., Okubo, E., Nemoto, H., Miya, T., Kashiwagi, K., Sakurai, M., Katsuki, T., and Morita, K. (1968). The prediction of dairy performance of cows from the lactation induced by treatment with oestrogen. *J. Dairy Res.* **35**, 331–341.

I-4

Barry A. Cross was born in Surrey, England on 17th March 1925. He attended Reigate Grammar School from 1935–43 and graduated from The Royal Veterinary College, London in 1947. After brief spells in veterinary practice he went to St. John's College, Cambridge where he obtained the BA in Natural Sciences in 1949. He was successively Animal Health Trust Scholar and ICI Research Fellow in the Physiological Laboratory, Cambridge under G. W. Harris. He won the Gedge Prize for physiological research in 1952 and received the Ph.D. degree in 1951. Cambridge University appointed him in 1951 to a Demonstratorship in the Zoological Laboratory and he was promoted to a Lectureship in 1955 after he was later transferred to the Anatomy School. He held a Rockefeller Travelling Fellowship to UCLA in 1957–8 and was elected Fellow of Corpus Christi College, Cambridge in 1962. He was awarded the ScD degree in 1965 and four years later was appointed Professor and Head of the Department of Anatomy in Bristol University Medical School. He remained in Bristol until 1974 when he became Director of the ARC Institute of Animal Physiology, Babraham, Cambridge.

Dr. Cross has held office in various Scientific Societies including the Anatomical and Physiological Societies, the Society for the Study of Fertility, the Society of Endocrinology, the Association for the Study of Animal Behaviour and the Brain Research Association. He was elected Fellow of the Royal Society in 1975 and is currently President of the International Society for Neuroendocrinology.

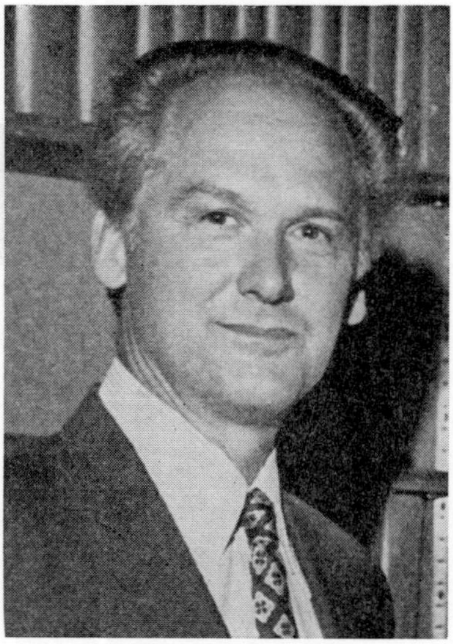

Barry A. Cross was born in Surrey, England on 17th March 1925. He attended Reigate Grammar School from 1933–43 and graduated from The Royal Veterinary College, London in 1947. After brief spells in veterinary practice he went to St. Johns College, Cambridge where he obtained the BA hons in Natural Sciences in 1949. He was successively Animal Health Trust Scholar and ICI Research Fellow in the Physiological Laboratory, Cambridge under G. W. Harris. He won the Gedge Prize for physiological research in 1952 and received the Ph. D. degree in 1953. Cambridge University appointed him in 1951 to a Demonstratorship in the Zoological Laboratory and he was promoted to a Lectureship in 1955 that was later transferred to the Anatomy School. He held a Rockefeller Travelling Fellowship to UCLA in 1957–8 and was elected Fellow of Corpus Christi College, Cambridge in 1962. He was awarded the ScD degree in 1963 and four years later was appointed Professor and Head of the Department of Anatomy in Bristol University Medical School. He remained in Bristol until 1974 when he became Director of the ARC Institute of Animal Physiology, Babraham, Cambridge.

Dr. Cross has held office in various Scientific Societies including the Anatomical and Physiological Societies, the Society for the Study of Fertility, the Society of Endocrinology, the Association for the Study of Animal Behaviour and the Brain Research Association. He was elected Fellow of the Royal Society in 1975 and is currently President of the International Society for Neuroendocrinology.

STUDIES IN SUCKLING

B. A. Cross

Institute of Animal Physiology, Agricultural Research Council, Babraham, Cambridge, England

Why choose lactational physiology as an area for research? I think the attraction for me was partly utilitarian and partly intellectual. Science was there to cure disease and to feed mankind, but also to understand the natural world. At the Royal Veterinary College I had been intrigued to learn about the wartime research on induction of lactation in virgin heifers by subcutaneous implantation of oestrogens, and the boosting of milk yields with thyroactive (iodinated) casein. But what most aroused my curiosity was the dramatic impact of the suckling (or milking) stimulus on the endocrinology and metabolism of the female. Apparently suckling could switch off oestrous and menstrual cycles, stimulate mammary growth and secretion and produce a gamut of changes in the pituitary and other vegetative functions. Even in the late forties the hypothalamus was implicated as a crucial site for the overall control of these various bodily adjustments and it was there that I determined to initiate my attack.

As I have suggested elsewhere (*8*), Cambridge was an excellent centre for commencing neuroendocrine research in 1949 and I was especially fortunate to be able to start work in the Physiological Laboratory with G. W. Harris while at the same time having the encouragement and active support of Sir John Hammond in the Department of Agriculture. Hammond (*15*) had hypothesised that "let-down" of milk in cows was a consequence of vascular engorgement of the udder produced by reflex vasodilation in a manner akin to erection of the penis. Another spinal-reflex hypothesis current in the thirties held that mammary smooth muscle was the effector tissue rather than blood vessels. Both views failed to explain the effects of spinal transections on the continuance of lactation (*19*) and Ely and Petersen (*13*) developed a neurohormonal theory according to which "let-down" resulted from an excess of oxytocin over adrenaline in the circulating blood. The data adduced in support of this theory were striking. Unilateral denervation of a cow's udder did not prevent "let-down" occurring synchronously on both innervated and denervated sides and injections of 40 IU Pitocin evoked a similar effect. On the other hand placing cats on the cow's back or bursting paper bags inhibited "let-down" and a comparable effect was observed when 5 mg adrenaline was injected intravenously (i.v.). In historical perspective, it is interesting that the evidence for a role for oxytocin had not significantly advanced from the time of Gaines (*14*), while the symptoms produced by the excessive doses of adrenaline were far more extreme than those occurring in emotional disturbance of "let-down." Nevertheless the impact of Petersen's work on dairy practice was wholly beneficial and more critical studies later proved his theory to be essentially correct.

My own attempts at enlightenment necessitated a laboratory animal that exhibited a "let-down" or milk-ejection reflex. With encouragement from Harris and Hammond I soon found that if separated from their litters overnight lactating rabbits would immediately nurse their young when allowed access to the nest. Suckling usually lasted only 3 or 4 min. No milk was obtained in the first 40–50 sec but thereafter rapid gulping occurred until the glands were virtually emptied and the litter had gained 100–200 g in weight. One such meal a day was sufficient to ensure normal weight gains and an average litter doubled its birth weight in 10 days. Clearly the rabbit was a good subject for analysing milk-ejection mechanisms.

Having learned about the physiology of anti-diuretic hormone from E. B. Verney I set an indirect test for the Petersen theory of milk ejection by seeing if the suckling stimulus in the rabbit elicited an antidiuresis of posterior pituitary origin. A small interruption of diuresis in water-loaded lactating rabbits was induced by suckling which had the qualitative features and approximate quantitative equivalence of the response to 0.5 mU of vasopressin given i.v. This evidence (*3*) supported the idea of stimulation of the neurohypophysis by suckling, but the loss of the anti-diuretic effect when escape of milk was prevented by painting the teats with collodion raised doubts as to whether the hormone were released before milk ejection (as required by the Petersen theory) or only after fluid loss from the body.

At about the same time, however, we developed the technique of cannulating the rabbit teat for intramammary pressure recording, and with this it soon became clear that the quantity of vasopressin released by suckling was well below the threshold dose for inducing milk ejection. Later experiments with the purified hormones (*12*) showed that the milk-ejecting potency of oxytocin was about six times that of vasopressin. Also with the cannulation procedure the way was open to explore the hypothalamic pathways for exciting the milk-ejection response. A rather primitive stereotaxic instrument was used to lower a glass-insulated platinum electrode through a drill hole in the skull at bregma into the brain. Stimuli were without effect on milk ejection until the electrode was lowered to about 1.9 cm from the skull surface when the infundibular stem was reached. At this point after a latent period of 25 to 40 sec stimulation elicited ejection of milk which with a 15 sec stimulus gave a response comparable to that following injection of about 50 mU oxytocin. Lowering the electrode tip further, into the adenohypophysis, eliminated the positive response to stimulation, which however could easily be recovered on raising the electrode into the infundibular region once more (*10*).

While these experiments were going on in Cambridge Bengt Andersson was performing elegant experiments with the Hess stimulation technique in unanaesthetised lactating goats, which showed that stimulation of both the supraoptic and paraventricular nuclei increased milk flow from cannulated teats (*1*). In the anaesthetised rabbit the smaller brain made it difficult to stimulate the paraventricular nucleus without at the same time exciting descending sympathetic pathways the effect of which was to block the mammary response to oxytocin (see below). However when steps were taken to eliminate the sympathetic effects stimulation of both magnocellular nuclei and their axonal projections to the posterior pituitary elicited clear milk-ejection responses.

With the use of the once daily suckling regime, stereotaxic stimulation and the teat cannulation technique we could then submit the Petersen theory to the crucial test by interrupting the final common path of the postulated reflex with electrolytic lesions in the supraoptico-hypophysial tract. This was done in rabbits that had for a week or more successfully ejected their milk to the sucklings in a daily nursing. After lesioning nursing behaviour was normal but the pups were unable to obtain the proper yield of milk and the glands remained full after the mother rabbit left the nest, but an i.v. injection of posterior pituitary extract (30–200 mU) given just before suckling restored milk withdrawal to normal (*10*). In these rabbits at a terminal experiment electrical stimulation of the neurohypophysis failed to induce milk ejection though oxytocin was still effective, and histological examination confirmed that the neurohypophysis had become atrophic. By contrast a group of lactating rabbits with similar electrolytic lesions placed in the dorsal hypothalamus showed no interference with maternal milk ejection reflex or with the electrically stimulated response.

I now felt reasonably certain that Petersen had been right about oxytocin mediating the natural milk-ejection reflex. To ascertain the amount of hormone discharged in the suckled rabbit I carried out replacement tests with varying doses of oxytocin given i.v. immediately before does aesthetised with sodium pentobarbitone to block milk ejection were suckled by their litters. From these experiments I estimated that 50 mU oxytocin was about the physiological dose. It was also clear that the ratio of the two neurohypophysial hormones released by suckling was of the order of 100: 1 in favour of oxytocin. Peeters and Coussens (*23*) reported a similar ratio for the cow which was very reassuring for at this time in contrast to the considerable knowledge about secretion of anti-diuretic hormone virtually nothing was published about the normal values for oxytocin secretion under physiological conditions.

What about the other part of the Petersen theory—the adrenaline block of "let-down" in cows engendered by crawling cats and bursting paper bags? It was not difficult to demonstrate in rabbits a comparable interference with milk removal as a consequence of emotional stimuli. Moreover i.v. injection of adrenaline during nursing crudely mimicked the blocking effect on milk ejection. Further experiments revealed that suitable stimulation of the sympathetic areas of the hypothalamus could release adrenaline from the adrenal medulla in sufficient quantity (1–5 μg) greatly to depress the mammary response to a physiological dose (50 mU) of oxytocin (*4*).

All the ingredients therefore were present for the Petersen mechanism to operate, but I was not satisfied that this was the real explanation of emotional inhibition of milk ejection, which was seldom accompanied by the profound arousal effects of exophthalmos, pupillo-dilation, and hyperpnoea that follow hypothalamic stimulation. Experiments in conscious rabbits soon showed that emotional inhibition of milk removal was usually not associated with any loss of responsiveness of the mammary glands to oxytocin. It could not therefore be the result of circulating adrenaline, but must be due to the failure of reflex release of oxytocin from the neurohypophysis (*5*).

Pickford (*24*) showed that intracarotid injection of adrenaline could block release of neurohypophysial hormones and some writers misinterpreted my conclusions in the rabbit as implying that adrenaline acts centrally rather than peripherally at the mammary gland. I had not shown this, indeed I felt it most improbable that if sufficient adrenomedullary adrenaline had been secreted to exert a central effect I would have failed to detect a peripheral action also. However another possibility in harmony with the known facts was that adrenergic nervous pathways were inhibitory to the hypothalamic neurosecretory neurones, and further evidence in favour of this idea has accumulated since.

My own work in the fifties and that of Linzell (*20*) placed the emphasis for the inhibitory effect of circulating adrenaline on its vasoconstrictor action on mammary blood vessels thus preventing access of the hormone to the contractile myoepithelium. Our interpretation of the findings was that the mammary blood flow, like that of the skin in general was exquisitely susceptible to sympathetico-adrenal discharge in various stressful situations such as emotion, cold, asphyxia or hypotension, as part of the circulatory homeostatic compensation mechanism. Ian Silver and I found for example that hypercapnia induced a sympathetic discharge and blocked the milk-ejection response to i.v. oxytocin. With gold cathode monitoring of mammary oxygen tension we further showed that the blockade was not due to mammary anoxia for comparable depression of pO_2 produced by breathing nitrogen did not affect the milk-ejection responses (*11*). The use of the gold cathode for tissue oxygen tension recording also showed us that the rise in intramammary pressure caused by myoepithelial contraction actually occluded mammary capillaries as evidenced by a fall in oxygen tension. If the pressure rise were prevented by allowing free escape of milk from a cut teat myoepithelial contraction produced no change in oxygen tension. That finding strengthened the view that the depressant effect of mammary engorgement on milk secretion was in part due to reduced blood flow, but recent evidence in rats has raised doubts on this score (*17*).

The existence of a powerful sympathetico-adrenal inhibitory effect on milk ejection raised problems for the tracing of afferent and efferent neural pathways for the milk-ejection reflex by electrical stimulation techniques. We needed a responsive mammary gland to monitor small endogenous releases of oxytocin and any sympathetic activation or hypotension would reduce mammary blood flow and diminish the chance of detecting oxytocin. However by acute adrenalectomy or thoracic spinal section the inhibitory effects could be sufficiently attenuated to reveal activation of oxytocin discharge from stimuli delivered to the midbrain tegmentum, subthalamus, fimbria of the fornix as well as the paraventricular and supraoptic nuclei

(*6*). John Tindal and his co-workers (see Chapter II-7) obtained evidence for a much more compact afferent pathway in the midbrain of the rabbit and guinea pig and there is still some disagreement about the degree of diffuseness of the pathway in the rabbit. However it seems clear that mixed excitatory and inhibitory connexions are present which may contribute to the varying effects observed on electrical stimulation with focal electrodes.

On reflection I am surprised to have spent so much time exploring sympathetico-adrenal phenomena in the mammary gland which have failed to command the interest of other workers. Perhaps it was the strong impression made upon me as a student by the work of W. B. Cannon of Harvard, followed by the hypotheses of W. E. Petersen referred to above. While working with Charles Sawyer in Los Angeles for example we discovered that intracarotid injections of hypertonic saline besides eliciting a release of oxytocin could also generate a sympathetic discharge and in consequence a diminished or absent milk-ejection response (*18*). As recently as 1975 (*26*) I returned to the topic in order to confirm that stimulation of sympathetic areas in the hypothalamus of the rat produced a comparable inhibitory effect on the mammary response to oxytocin to that in the rabbit.

Without question, however, a richer vein of exploration began in 1957 when with J. D. Green at the University of California at Los Angeles (UCLA) we made the first attempts to record with steel microelectrodes the action potential activity of supraoptic and paraventricular neurones (*9*). Hypothalamic neurones, including the presumptive neurosecretory cells of the magnocellular nuclei were unexpectedly easy to record from in this way and exhibited electrophysiological characteristics not too disimilar from spinal motor cells that had previously been studied most extensively. Mammary stimuli appeared to have no very specific effects on hypothalamic unit activity, though non-specific excitations like those elicited by ear pinches could be observed. Since our rabbits were anaesthetised with urethane it was not possible to induce a milk-ejection reflex with the suckling litter, and our labours were diverted to osmotic and other stimuli calculated to excite the vasopressin secretory neurones.

After a 10-year interval back in Cambridge with unit recording studies focussed first on hypoxic and hypercapnic stimuli with I. A. Silver, then on gonadal hormone feedback on the hypothalamus with C. A. Barraclough, D. W. Lincoln, and J. Kitay, I took a Professorship in the University of Bristol. Shortly after setting up our neuroendocrine laboratories in the Department of Anatomy there my interest in the magnocellular nuclei was reactivated by a collaborative visit from two Los Angeles scientists, J. W.

Sundsten and D. Novin. We developed a technique for antidromic identification of paraventricular nucleus neurones by electric shocks to the infundibular process delivered by an electrode inserted through a foramen in the basisphenoid bone. This enabled us to determine the conduction velocity of the neurosecretory cell axons as <1 m/sec and show that many axons from PV neurones did not extend into the neural lobe (*25*). We could not of course distinguish which cells were secreting oxytocin, though the hope was that we might succeed in monitoring unit activity in the conscious rabbit during suckling to observe which neurones were excited thereby. In the meantime with R. W. Moss a study was begun of the effect of various putative neurotransmitters delivered micro-iontophoretically into identified neurosecretory cells in the magnocellular nuclei. The results showed that acetylcholine was predominantly excitatory while noradrenaline was inhibitory to neurosecretory cell discharge (*22*). In the next door laboratory similar results were obtained in the rat (*21*). It seemed therefore reasonable to suppose that afferent synapses on the final common path neurones in the milk-ejection reflex were probably cholinergic, while those responsible for inhibition were noradrenergic, but final proof of this idea is still to come.

At about this time in our Bristol laboratories Wakerley and Lincoln (*27*) working with anaesthetised rats were able to seize the prize that had eluded the efforts with anaesthetised rabbits, *i.e.*, to record precisely the unit activity correlated with oxytocin release in the milk-ejection reflex. It took the highly dramatic form of a synchronous rapid volley of spikes from half the neurones in each magnocellular nucleus (oxytocin neurones) occurring some 18 sec before the resulting mammary pressure rise. Lincoln was able to calculate that approximately half a million action potentials were needed to release 1 mU oxytocin, *i.e.*, the physiological dose. A unique feature in the rat was the recurrence of this milk ejection every 5 or 10 min during prolonged periods when the litter attach themselves to the mother's teats. Since rats had been used intensively in lactation studies for several decades it is astonishing that this recurrent milk-ejection phenomenon had not been observed sooner, especially as it is accompanied by a pronounced stretch response in all the pups as they start to gulp milk from previously dry nipples.

A more urgent mystery, still unsolved, is how the intermittent discharge of oxytocin is mediated when there appears to be no correlated antecedent change in the suckling situation. It seems inescapable that some rhythmic fluctuation is occurring in the central nervous excitability that interacts with a relatively constant mammary afferent input. Nothing of the kind can be operative in the lactating rabbit which normally has only one milk ejection every 24 hr stimulated by the brief initial suckling activity of the litter and which is dependent upon afferent discharges in sensory nerves from the teats. It is possible, as I have argued in a recent article (*7*), that the milk-ejection mechanisms in the rat and rabbit represent distinct physiological solutions to the many varied problems posed for milk removal in different genera of mammals, where suckling habits can be as diverse as the northern fur seal which may nurse the calf only once a week, and the domestic pig which nurses once an hour.

Having spent the bulk of this essay on milk ejection it is perhaps time I reverted to the neuroendocrine mechanisms in milk secretion. Apart from some very early work on the role of the suckling stimulus on food intake in rats and the effect of pituitary stalk section on milk secretion I have not personally contributed much to this problem. At the Institute of Animal Physiology a recent discovery of much significance is the finding in rats that suckling greatly increases cardiac output and mammary blood flow as an indispensable part of its galactopoietic effect, and these responses are themselves almost certainly due to reflex secretion of prolactin and growth hormone (*16*). In our laboratory Wakerley and others have shown additionally that prolactin and thyrotrophin are both stimulated by suckling in rats but by neural mechanisms that are largely independent both from each other and from the milk-ejection reflex (*2*). We are now at last poised to attack the longstanding question of the reciprocal relationship between fertility and lactation at the hypothalamic level. R. G. Dyer has been developing increasingly powerful techniques for studying the activity of preoptic and anterior hypothalamic neurones that send axons to the mediobasal hypothalamus and with radioimmunoassay to monitor concomitant changes in prolactin and gonadotrophic hormone following suckling it may be possible to pinpoint some of the neuronal mechanisms that switch off gonadotrophins when galactopoietic hormones are stimulated.

Looking back over the last 30 years I am grateful for the personal encouragement I have received from many fine scientists who have illuminated our knowledge of lactation. They include Sir John Hammond, G. W. Harris, John Folley, L. Desclin, H. B. van Dyke, F. G. Young, A. S. Parkes, B. A. Houssay, A. T. Cowie, G. Peeters, C. H. Sawyer, B. Anderssonn, S. M. McCann, and J. Meites. With some of these I have had the additional pleasure of experimental collaboration. Scientific research is most enjoyable when both the ecstasies and the heartbreaks can be shared. I have happy recollections of laboratory lactational labours with Geoffrey Harris,

Mary Cotes, Harry van Dyke, John Green, Charles Sawyer, Bob Holland, Alan Findlay, C. E. Grosvenor, John Sundsten, Don Novin, Ivan Urban, Bob Moss, Richard Dyer, Richard Dyball, and Jon Wakerley. Perhaps my most vivid memories are the first time I saw milk rising up the cannula from a mammary gland after stimulating the infundibular stem of a lactating rabbit, the simple experiments that enabled me to study psychosomatic mechanisms interfering with milk removal, the discovery that neurosecretory cells show normal action potentials, and first experiencing the extraordinary volley of spikes from oxytocin cells, like a blast of machine gun fire, preceding milk ejection in the rat. If the future holds new pleasures to equal these I shall be more than content.

REFERENCES

1. Anderssen, B. (1951). The effect and localisation of electrical stimulation of certain parts of the brain stem in sheep and goats. *Acta Physiol. Scand.* **23**, 8–23.
2. Burnet, F. R. and Wakerley, J. B. (1976). Plasma concentrations of prolactin and thyrotrophin during suckling in urethane-anaesthetised rats. *J. Endocrinol.* **70**, 429–437.
3. Cross, B. A. (1951). Suckling antidiuresis in rabbits. *J. Physiol.* **114**, 447–453.
4. Cross, B. A. (1955). The hypothalamus and the mechanism of sympathetico-adrenal inhibition of milk ejection. *J. Endocrinol.* **12**, 15–28.
5. Cross, B. A. (1955). Neurohormonal mechanisms in emotional inhibition of milk ejection. *J. Endocrinol.* **12**, 29–37.
6. Cross, B. A. (1966). Neural control of oxytocin secretion. In *Neuroendocrinology*, vol. 1, ed. Martini, L. and Ganong, W. F., pp. 217–259. New York: Academic Press.
7. Cross, B. A. (1977). Comparative physiology of milk removal. *Symp. Zool. Soc. Lond.* No. 41, 193–210.
8. Cross, B. A. (1977). Brain, breast and gonads: A passage in neuroendocrinology. In *Pioneers in Neuroendocrinology*, vol. 2, ed. Meites, J., Donovan, B. T., and McCann, S. M. New York: Plenum (in press).
9. Cross, B. A. and Green, J. D. (1959). Activity of single neurones in the hypothalamus: Effect of osmotic and other stimuli. *J. Physiol.* **148**, 554–569.
10. Cross, B. A. and Harris, G. W. (1952). The role of the neurohypophysis in the milk-ejection reflex. *J. Endocrinol.* **8**, 148–161.
11. Cross, B. A. and Silver, I. A. (1962). Mammary oxygen tension and the milk-ejection mechanism. *J. Endocrinol.* **23**, 375–384.

12. Cross, B. A. and Van Dyke, H. B. (1953). The effects of highly purified posterior pituitary principles on the lactating mammary gland of the rabbit. *J. Endocrinol.* **9**, 232–235.
13. Ely, F. and Petersen, W. E. (1941). Factors involved in the ejection of milk. *J. Dairy Sci.* **24**, 211–223.
14. Gaines, W. L. (1915). A contribution to the physiology of lactation. *Am. J. Physiol.* **38**, 285–312.
15. Hammond, J. (1936). The physiology of milk and butterfat secretion. *Vet. Rec.* **16**, 519–535.
16. Hanwell, A. and Linzell, J. L. (1973). The time course of cardiovascular changes in lactation in the rat. *J. Physiol.* **233**, 93–109.
17. Hanwell, A. and Linzell, J. L. (1973). The effects of engorgement with milk and of suckling on mammary blood flow in the rat. *J. Physiol.* **233**, 111–125.
18. Holland, R. C., Cross, B. A., and Sawyer, C. H. (1959). Effects of intracarotid injection of hypertonic solutions on the neurohypophysial milk-ejection mechanism. *Am. J. Physiol.* **196**, 791–795.
19. Inglebrecht, P. (1935). Influence du systéme nerveux central sur la mamelle lactante chez le rat blanc. *C. R. Soc. Biol. Paris* **120**, 1369–1371.
20. Linzell, J. L. (1955). Some observations on the contractile tissue of the mammary glands. *J. Physiol.* **130**, 257–267.
21. Moss, R. L., Dyball, R.E.J., and Cross, B. A. (1971). Responses of antidromically identified supraoptic and paraventricular units to acetylcholine, noradrenaline and glutamate applied iontophoretically. *Brain Res.* **35**, 573–575.
22. Moss, R. L., Urban, I., and Cross, B. A. (1972). Microelectrophoresis of cholinergic and aminergic drugs on paraventricular neurons. *Am. J. Physiol.* **223**, 310–318.
23. Peeters, G. and Coussens, R. (1950). The influence of the milking act on the diuresis of the lactating cow. *Arch. Int. Pharmacodyn.* **84**, 209–219.
24. Pickford, M. (1960). Factors affecting milk release in the dog and the quantity of oxytocin liberated by suckling. *J. Physiol.* **152**, 515–526.
25. Sundsten, J. W., Novin, D., and Cross, B. A. (1970). Identification and distribution of paraventricular units excited by stimulation of the neural lobe of the hypophysis. *Exp. Neurol.* **26**, 316–329.
26. Wakerley, J. B. and Cross, B. A. (1975). Milk ejection in the rat: Reversible blockade of hypothalamo-neurohypophysial and sympathetico-adrenal pathways by radio-frequency currents. *J. Endocrinol.* **67**, 31P–32P.
27. Wakerley, J. B. and Lincoln, D. W. (1973). The milk-ejection reflex of the rat: A 20–40 fold acceleration in the firing of paraventricular neurones during oxytocin release. *J. Endocrinol.* **57**, 477–493.

I – 5

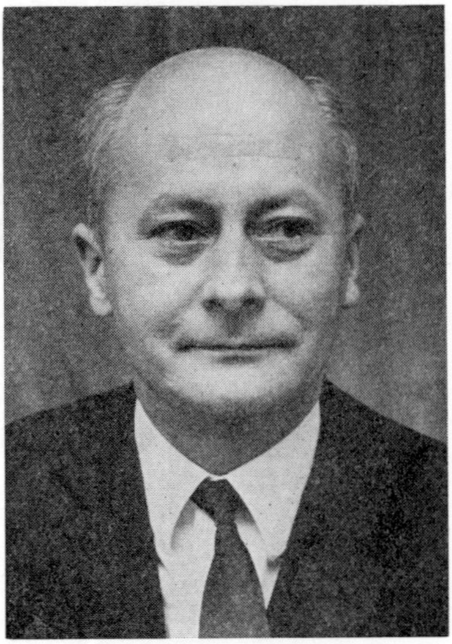

Edward Werner Flückiger was born on January 28, 1923 in Biel (Bern), Switzerland. He received Diploma of Natural Sciences (Biology) Federate Institute of Technology, Zürich in 1948 and Doctor of Natural Sciences (Zoology) = Dr. Sc. Nat., Federate Institute of Technology, Zürich in 1951.

Positions held include the following: Research Assistant in Pharmacology, University of Lund, Sweden in 1950–1; Research Assistant in Physiology, University of Basel in 1951–7; Privat-Dozent (= Lecturer) in Comparative Physiology, University of Basel in 1956; Research Pharmacologist, Department of Pharmacology, Sandoz Ltd., Basel in 1957–61; Senior Pharmacologist, Biological and Medical Research Division, Sandoz Ltd. since 1961; Lecturer in Physiology at the School of Pharmacy (University of Basel) in 1964–6. He has been Professor Extraordinary in Zoology and Comparative Physiology, University of Basel since 1964 and Assistant member of the board of management of Sandoz Ltd. since 1968.

Some of the Societies of which he is a member include; Schweizerische Zoologische Gesellschaft (Swiss Zoological Society), Schweizerische Gesellschaft für Endokrinologie (Swiss Endocrine Society), Schweizerischer Verein für Physiologie, Physiologische Chemie und Pharmakologie 1952–68 (Swiss Society for Physiology, Physiological Chemistry and Pharmacology), Schweizerischer Pharmakologenverein (Swiss Society of Pharmacologists), Schweizerische Naturforschende Gesellschaft, Schweizerische Gesellschaft für Physiologie (Swiss Society of Physiology), Deutsche Pharmakologische Gesellschaft 1970–(German Pharmacological Society), Deutsche Gesellschaft für Endokrinologie (German Society of Endocrinology).

LACTATION INHIBITION BY ERGOT DRUGS

E. W. FLÜCKIGER

Medical and Biological Research Division, Sandoz, Ltd., Basel

Progress in understanding in a particular field depends greatly on the tools and methods at the disposal of the investigators. Drugs used as tools have contributed widely to the understanding of many physiological processes. On the other hand, the understanding of the pharmacology of a particular drug depends on intimate knowledge of the physiology of the test function chosen to characterize the drug.

This interdependence of physiology and pharmacology is well illustrated by our early attempts to assess the prolactin secretion inhibitory activity of ergot alkaloids, particularly bromocriptine (CB 154), through their inhibitory action on lactation.

In the early 1960's, when we began to study the endocrine actions of ergot alkaloids and their derivatives, we entered a field which had been opened up by the work of M. C. Shelesnyak (*27–29*) several years before. He had shown that some ergot alkaloids can prevent uterine deciduoma formation in pseudopregnant rats, and inhibit ovum implantation with resumption of ovarian cyclicity in inseminated rats. Analyzing his early observations, Shelesnyak (*28*) had come to the conclusion that this effect could be due to inhibition of luteotropic hormone (prolactin) secretion. This hypothesis was later substantiated by the work of Zeilmaker and Carlsen (*35*) using ergocornine. In this paper it is further shown that ergocornine inhibits lactation and that this action could be antagonized by injection of prolactin. Thus, when carrying out structure-activity studies with various ergot compounds (*9*), we naturally chose ergocornine as the standard compound on which to improve if possible. Ovum implantation inhibition in the progestative rat (*10*) was the first test system applied and the compounds of interest were then tested for lactation inhibition in the same species.

Lactation inhibitory activity was assessed as follows: gravid rats of 180 to 200 g body weight were kept in single cages. Food and water were given *ad libitum*. The room temperature was kept at 22°C and the room artificially lighted for 14 hr a day. Postpartum, the number of young per litter was reduced to 8. Each litter was weighed daily between 8 and 9 a.m. to the nearest gram and the number of young with milk-spots, *i.e.*, with visible milk content in the stomach, was noted. Because of occasional deaths, the weights of the litters were divided by the number of young per litter, giving the average weight of each pup. At 5 p.m. on the 6th, 7th or 8th day postpartum the mothers were injected subcutaneously (s.c.) with either the test compound in different doses or with vehicle. Ten to 11 females were given each dosage and a total of about 30 females was used as controls. On the day after treatment the litters were weighed at 9 a.m. and at 5 p.m., and the milk-spots noted. On subsequent days, weighing and checking for milk-spots were performed only in the morning. The results from the experimental groups on the day after drug treatment were compared to those of the controls and expressed in two ways, *i.e.*, as percent of

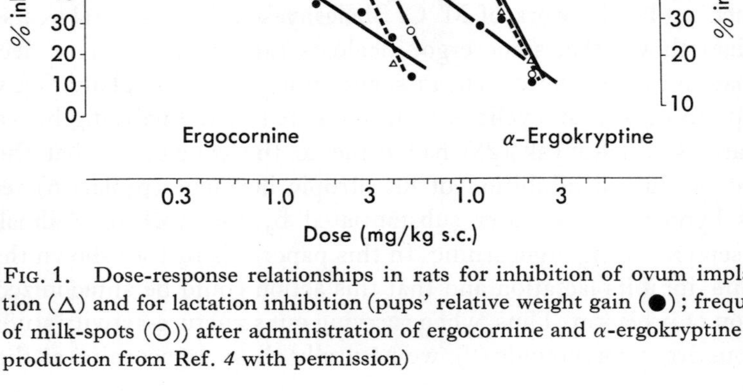

FIG. 1. Dose-response relationships in rats for inhibition of ovum implantation (△) and for lactation inhibition (pups' relative weight gain (●); frequency of milk-spots (○)) after administration of ergocornine and α-ergokryptine (Reproduction from Ref. *4* with permission)

reduction in weight gain in the pups and as percent of decrease in the numbers of milk-spots observed.

Ergocornine (*4*) and α-ergokryptine (*10*) produced good dose response curves with both criteria for lactation inhibition. As shown in Fig. 1, near maximal effects were reached at dosages which also produced a nearly maximal inhibition of ovum implantation in progestative rats. This convergence of the three dose response relationships on a common, maximally inhibitory dosage (*4*) seemed very logical. It suggested to us that both effects are due to one primary drug action, *i.e.*, inhibition of prolactin secretion. In agreement with the results of Zeilmaker and Carlsen (*35*), we were able to at least partially prevent the inhibitory effect of ergocornine on lactation by injecting prolactin. Although we were puzzled by the finding that prolactin was only partially effective in counteracting lactation inhibition by ergocornine, this did not lead us to analyze the observation further.

Several ergot derivatives which we studied did not result in a clear convergence of the dose response curves to one maximally effective dosage for implantation inhibition and lactation inhibition. 2-Br-α-ergokryptine (bromocriptine, CB 154) is one of these derivatives (*4*, *10*). As can be seen in Fig. 2, milk yield was only decreased by about 50% even at doses several

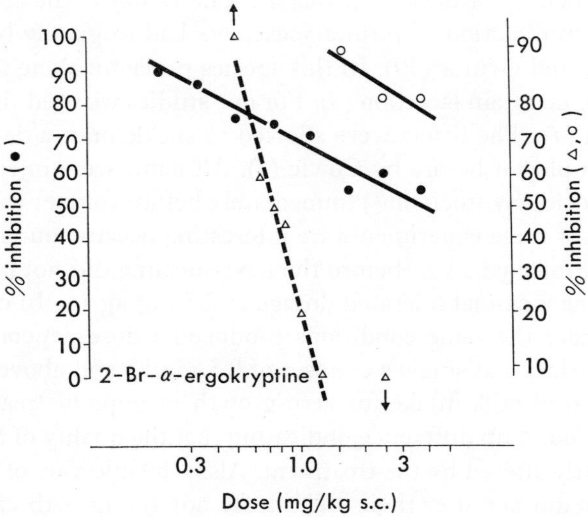

FIG. 2. Dose-dependent inhibitory action of 2-Br-α-ergokryptine in rats on ovum implantation (△) and on lactation (pups' relative weight gain (●); frequency of milk spots (○)) (Reproduced from Ref. *4* with permission)

times higher than needed for a complete inhibition of ovum implantation. In 1967 when we did these experiments, there was, of course, no possibility of measuring serum prolactin levels to resolve the puzzle. Also, we had accepted ergocornine as the standard compound for prolactin secretion inhibition and saw no reason to discard it. Therefore, we were led to consider an auxiliary hypothesis for the special case of bromocriptine: we concluded that the data obtained with bromocriptine were incompatible with the assumption of a single primary action responsible for inhibition of both lactation and implantation in the rat (*10*). We thought that bromocriptine inhibits prolactin response to the stimulatory inputs from copulation and from suckling at sites above the final common pathway, the inhibitory effect of the drug on the neuronal control of prolactin secretion being less effective against the repetitive sensory input from suckling young, than against the "hit and run" effect of copulation.

This situation momentarily raised grave doubts as to the potential of bromocriptine as a reliable inhibitor of prolactin secretion. On the other hand, we could not be certain of the validity of the rat lactation test as an indicator of prolactin secretion inhibition. Prolactin is not the only hormone required for maintenance of lactation in rats (*3*, *21*). Therefore, we extended our studies to further species.

In 1969 we took up studies with *rabbits*. The rabbit is the species in which the "prolactin" action of pituitary extracts had originally been detected by Stricker and Grüter (*30*). In this species prolactin alone is necessary to induce and maintain lactation (*3*). For our studies we used the "Yellow Fawn" strain (*4*). The litters were allowed to suckle once a day for 30 min, a method employed before by Cowie (*3*). All dams were injected s.c. with 0.5 IU oxytocin (Syntocinon®) immediately before contact with their litter. The results of these experiments are interesting because our standard drug ergocornine, injected 23 hr before the next suckling did not influence milk yield up to the maximal tolerated dosage of 2.5 mg/kg s.c. In contrast, bromocriptine under the same conditions produced a dose-dependent reduction in milk yield (*6*) at single s.c. doses of 0.5 mg/kg and above. When estimating the critical milk intake for zero growth in pups of treated and control dams, we found no difference, indicating that the quality of the milk was not significantly altered by the treatment. Also, the injection of bromocriptine into pups did not alter their milk intake nor the growth efficiency of the milk taken in. In view of this evidence we concluded that in rabbits bromocriptine-induced inhibition of lactation resulted from an inhibition of prolactin secretion.

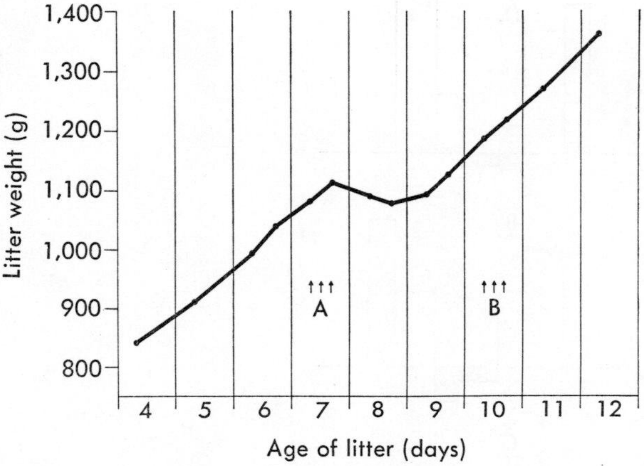

FIG. 3. Growth curve of a mini-pig litter of 5 between day 4 and 12 postpartum

At A, on day 7 postpartum, the sow was treated intramuscularly (i.m.) with 3×0.1 mg/kg bromocriptine (at 8 a.m., 0.30, and 5 p.m.) The suppression of growth of the piglets, who had no energy source other than the milk they suckled, is taken as indication of lactation inhibition. The effect was fully reversible. At B, on day 10 postpartum solvent for bromocriptine was injected without effect on the growth curve.

In 1969 we also performed studies on *pigs* and *mini-pigs*. Both responded to bromocriptine and showed dose-dependent lactation suppression (*4*) as illustrated for the mini-pig in Figs. 3 and 4. Later, the same was found in *dogs* (*22*).

Since we could not directly measure the milk volumes involved nor assess the quality in rats, pigs, or dogs we turned in 1970 to species which could easily be hand milked. We chose lactating *goats* of the Simmenthal breed for this purpose, and to our surprise we got no response to treatment. Ergocornine was poorly tolerated at 300 μg/kg s.c. and did not change milk yield. Bromocriptine, which was tolerated without visible side effects in dosages up to 900 μg/kg (14 mg total dose) s.c., also failed to alter milk yield or composition. We were of course greatly puzzled by this. In principle there were two possible explanations, either bromocriptine had not inhibited prolactin secretion, or lactation in goats was independent of prolactin. We favored the second possibility as an explanation to overcome our disappointment. Understandably we were greatly relieved when Hart (*17, 18*) later showed by the use of the RIA method that bromocriptine inhibits

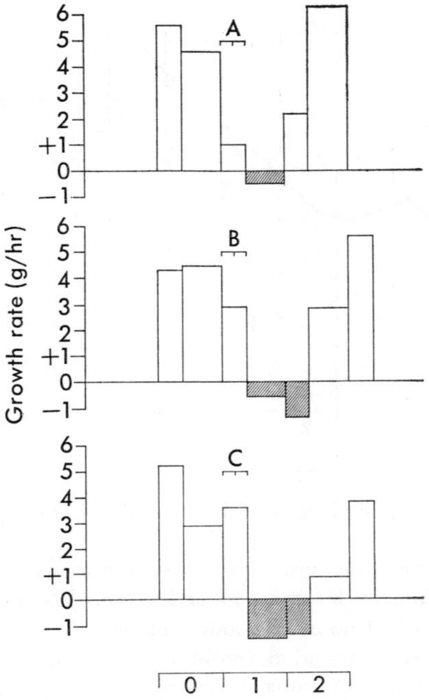

FIG. 4. Dose-dependent reduction of growth rate in the same litter of suckling piglets as in Fig. 3 by administration of bromocriptine

Growth rate (g/hr) was determined separately for daylight hours (8 a.m. to 5 p.m. = 9 hr) and night hours (5 p.m. to 8 a.m. = 15 hr) represented, respectively, by the narrow and the wide columns. Three experiments (A, B, C) performed respectively on the 7th, 14th, and 17th days postpartum are shown. Bromocriptine was applied i.m. in the following three dosages at 8 a.m., 0.30, and at 5 p.m.: A, 3×0.01 (mg/kg); B, 3×0.03; C, 3×0.1. Hatched columns represent periods with weight loss. (Reproduced from Ref. *4* with permission.)

prolactin secretion in goats but that established lactation is independent of this hormone. In the meantime similar observations in *dairy cows* had been published by Karg and his group: in cows of the Swiss Brown breed, suppression of prolactin secretion around parturition prevents lactogenesis, but once established, lactation was found to be quite insensitive to inhibition of prolactin secretion (*20*, *25*, *26*). These observations in goats and dairy cows raised the question (*6*) whether in species selected for high milk yield the selection process favored a genetic system ensuring independence of the mammary alveolar cells from the presence of prolactin after the induction phase. It is interesting to note that there exist great differences in the endocrinological and metabolic patterns between lactating dairy cows and lactating beef cows (*19*). Could it be that growth hormone in dairy breeds has taken over the mammotrope function of prolactin? These excursions into "comparative pharmacology of lactation" were very rewarding because they led to new insights into the physiology of lactation. Also, these experiences convinced us that the original rat lactation inhibition test is not optimal for indirect assessment of the potency of drugs as inhibitors of stimulated prolactin secretion.

Nicoll *et al.* (*24*) have pointed out that the difference in potency between α-ergokryptine and bromocriptine in inhibiting lactation in the rat may simply "indicate that bromination of the α-ergokryptine reduces its ability to depress oxytocin release . . .." Inhibition of the milk ejection reflex by ergotamine has been described by Grosvenor (*11*, *12*). Analysis of this action showed the reflex arc to have an important adrenergic link (*2*, *14*, *15*). Ergotamine, ergocornine and α-ergokryptine are quite potent α-adrenergic stimulants (*4*, *32*), while the 2-bromo derivative of the latter, bromocriptine, has only weak activity (*4*, *31*). The relative potencies of α-ergokryptine and bromocriptine as inhibitors of the milk ejection reflex have not yet been established (*36*).

In the meantime, methods to measure prolactin in rats had become available. Using polyacrylamide disc gel electrophoresis with subsequent photometric evaluation (*23*, *33*), Yanai and Nagasawa (*34*) had shown that both bromocriptine and ergocornine reduce the prolactin content of the pituitary in mice after prolonged administration. Using the same assay method in lactating rats, we found that bromocriptine also prevented the suckling-induced depletion of pituitary prolactin (*8*). This has been subsequently confirmed by radio-immunoassay and histological methods (*5*, *16*). Therefore, if prolactin is responsible for the maintenance of lactation in rats, bromocriptine would be expected to be an excellent inhibitor of lactation in this species. In 1973 Grosvenor and Mena published a paper with key information to our methodological problem (*13*). These authors, in analyzing the role of prolactin in maintaining lactation in rats, found a very significant time lag of 8 to 16 hr between the release of prolactin and the resulting rise in milk secretion. This means that our rat lactation inhibition test, which focused on weight gain by pups within the first 24 hr after injection of the drug into the mother must have been rather insensitive to effects of prolactin secretion suppression (*7*).

In order to escape the limitations of the original rat test system we then adopted the following procedure (*1*): The drug or its solvent were admin-

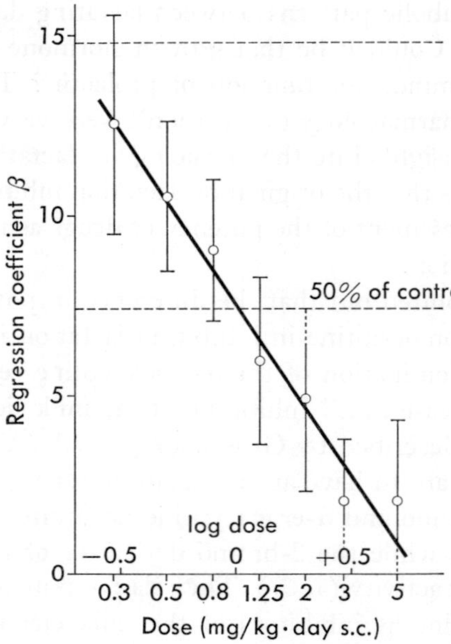

FIG. 5. Dose-response relationship for the inhibitory action of bromocriptine on weight gain of suckling rat pups

Bromocriptine was given 4 times subcutaneously (s.c.) to groups of lactating rats on days 5 to 8 postpartum. The regression coefficients β of daily weight gains of the pups are used as an indicator of milk intake (ordinate). Bromocriptine suppressed daily weight gain by 50% at 1 mg/kg·day s.c. $y=-9.60x+7.58$, $v=-0.853>-0.354(p<1\%)$.

istered to mothers 4 times, *i.e.*, on days 5, 6, 7, and 8 postpartum in the morning and the litters were weighed and checked for milk-spots daily in the morning from days 4 to 12. Regression coefficients for mean daily weight gain in the different treatment groups were then calculated for days 5 through 9. As shown in Fig. 5, a statistically highly significant log-linear relationship was found between these regression coefficients and the dosage of bromocriptine. In this test, bromocriptine inhibited the weight gain of the pups with an ID_{50} of 1 mg/kg·day s.c. (*7*). Also, the proportion of pups showing milk-spots diminished with increasing dosages (see Fig. 6). Up to the higest dosage used we observed reversibility of the lactation inhibition after cessation of bromocriptine treatment.

In contrast to the results which we reported in 1968 (*10*), the results in Table I reveal that the potency of bromocriptine in inhibiting weight gain

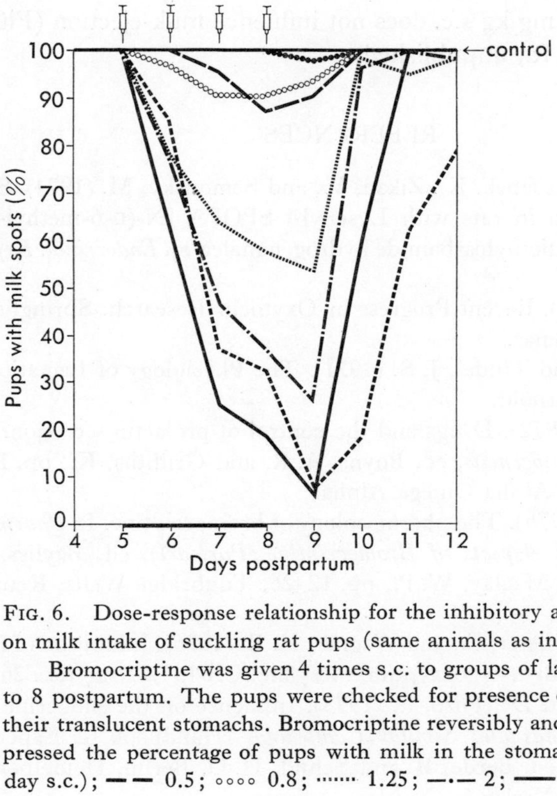

FIG. 6. Dose-response relationship for the inhibitory action of bromocriptine on milk intake of suckling rat pups (same animals as in Fig. 5)

Bromocriptine was given 4 times s.c. to groups of lactating rats on days 5 to 8 postpartum. The pups were checked for presence of milk (milk-spots) in their translucent stomachs. Bromocriptine reversibly and dose-dependently depressed the percentage of pups with milk in the stomach. •••• 0.3 (mg/kg·day s.c.); — — 0.5; ∘∘∘∘ 0.8; ······ 1.25; —·— 2; —— 3; ---- 5.

TABLE I. Comparison of 50% Effective Dosages of Bromocriptine in Different Tests Used to Estimate Its Prolactin Secretion Inhibitory Activity

Lactating rat; weight gain (4 days) of pups	ID_{50}=1.0 mg/kg·day s.c.
Female inseminated rat; ovum implantation (*9*)	ED_{50}=0.7 mg/kg s.c.
Adult male rat; serum prolactin level 24 hr post-drug (*9*)	ID_{50}=1.0 mg/kg s.c.

in rat pups correlates well with its potency as an inhibitor of prolactin secretion in other tests in this species.

Note Added in Proof

We have since observed that α-ergokryptine is a potent inhibitor of the milk-ejection reflex, as are ergotamine and ergocornine, while bromocriptine up to 3 mg/kg s.c. does not influence milk-ejection (Flückiger, E. and Wagner, H. R., unpublished).

REFERENCES

1. Aušková, M., Řežábek, K., Zikan, V., and Semonský, M. (1974). Suppression of lactation in rats with Lysenyl® SPOFA [N-(D-6-methyl-8-isoergolenyl) N′, N′-diethylcarbamide hydrogen maleate]. *Endocrinol. Exp.* **8**, 51–58.
2. Berde, B. (1959). Recent Progress in Oxytocin Research. Springfield, Ill.: Charles C. Thomas.
3. Cowie, A. T. and Tindal, J. S. (1971). The Physiology of Lactation. London: Edward Arnold.
4. Flückiger, E. (1972). Drugs and the control of prolactin secretion. In *Prolactin and Carcinogenesis*, ed. Boyns, A. R. and Griffiths, K., pp. 162–171. Cardiff, Wales: Alpha Omega Alpha.
5. Flückiger, E. (1976). The pharmacology of bromocriptine. In *Pharmacological and Clinical Aspects of Bromocriptine* (*Parlodel*), ed. Bayliss, R.I.S., Turner, P., and Maclay, W. P., pp. 12–26. Tunbridge Wells, Kent: MCS Consultants.
6. Flückiger, E., Billeter, E., and Wagner, H. R. (1976). Inhibition of lactation in rabbits by 2-Br-α-ergokryptine-mesylate (CB 154). *Drug Res.* **26**, 51–53.
7. Flückiger, E. and Del Pozo, E. (1978). Influence on the endocrine system. In *Ergot Alkaloids and Similar Compounds* (Handbook of Experimental Pharmacology), ed. Berde, B. and Schild, H. O. Berlin, Heidelberg, New York: Springer Verlag.
8. Flückiger, E. and Kovacs, E. (1974). Inhibition by 2-Br-α-ergokryptine-mesylate (CB 154) of suckling-induced pituitary prolactin depletion in lactating rats. *Experientia* **30**, 1173.
9. Flückiger, E., Marko, M., Doepfner, W., and Niederer, W. (1976). Effects of ergot alkaloids on the hypothalamic-pituitary axis. *Postgrad. Med. J.* **52** (Suppl. **1**), 57–61.
10. Flückiger, E. and Wagner, H. R. (1968). 2-Br-α-Ergokryptin: Beeinflussung von Fertilität und Laktation bei der Ratte. *Experientia* **24**, 1130.
11. Grosvenor, C. E. (1956). Effect of ergotamine on milk ejection in lactating rats. *Proc. Soc. Exp. Biol. Med.* **91**, 294–296.
12. Grosvenor, C. E. (1956). Some effects of ergotamine tartrate upon lactation in the rat. *Am. J. Physiol.* **186**, 211–215.
13. Grosvenor, C. E. and Mena, F. (1973). Evidence for a time delay between prolactin release and the resulting rise in milk secretion rate in the rat. *J. Endocrinol.* **58**, 31–39.

14. Grosvenor, C. E. and Turner, C. W. (1956). Ergotamine, oxytocin and milk let down in lactating rats. *Proc. Soc. Exp. Biol. Med.* **93**, 466–468.
15. Grosvenor, C. E. and Turner, C. W. (1957). Evidence for adrenergic and cholinergic components in milk let-down reflex in lactating rats. *Proc. Soc. Exp. Biol. Med.* **95**, 719–722.
16. Häusler, A. and Hodel, C. (1975). Morphological observations on pituitary mammotropes of lactating rats treated with 2-Bromo-α-ergokryptine (CB 154). *Acta Endocrinol.* Suppl. **193**, 66.
17. Hart, I. C. (1973). Effect of 2-Br-α-ergokryptine on milk yield and the level of prolactin and growth hormone in the blood of the goat at milking. *J. Endocrinol.* **57**, 179–180.
18. Hart, I. C. (1974). The relationship between lactation and the release of prolactin and growth hormone in the goat. *J. Reprod. Fert.* **39**, 485–499.
19. Hart, I. C., Bines, J. A., Balch, C. C., and Cowie, A. T. (1975). Hormone and metabolite differences between lactating beef and dairy cattle. *Life Sci.* **16**, 1285–1292.
20. Karg, H., Schams, D., and Reinhardt, V. (1972). Effects of 2-Br-α-ergokryptine on plasma prolactin level and milk yield in cows. *Experientia* **28**, 574–576.
21. Lyons, W. R., Li, C. H., and Johnson, R. E. (1958). The hormonal control of mammary growth. *Recent Progr. Horm. Res.* **14**, 219–248.
22. Mayer, P. and Schütze, E. (1973). Effect of 2-Br-α-ergokryptine (CB 154) on lactation in the bitch. *Experientia* **29**, 484.
23. Nicoll, C. S., Parsons, J. A., Fiorindo, R. P., and Nichols, C. W. (1969). Estimation of prolactin and growth hormone levels by polyacrylamide disc electrophoresis. *J. Endocrinol.* **45**, 183–196.
24. Nicoll, C. S., Yaron, Z., Nutt, N., and Daniels, E. (1970). Effects of ergotamine tartrate on prolactin and growth hormone secretion by rat adenohypophysis *in vitro*. *Biol. Reprod.* **5**, 59–66.
25. Schams, D. (1976). Hormonal control of lactation. In *Breast-feeding and the Mother* (Ciba Foundation Symposium), pp. 27–48. Amsterdam, Oxford, New York: Elsevier, Excerpta Medica, North Holland.
26. Schams, D., Reinhardt, V., and Karg, H. (1972). Effects of a synthetic ergot alkaloid on the peripheral blood level of prolactin in cows. *Acta. Endocrinol.* Suppl. **159**, 39.
27. Shelesnyak, M. C. (1954). The action of selected drugs on deciduoma formation. *Endocrinology* **55**, 85–89.
28. Shelesnyak, M. C. (1954) Ergotoxine inhibition of deciduoma formation and its reversal by progesterone. *Am. J. Physiol.* **179**, 301–304.
29. Shelesnyak, M. C. (1955). Disturbance of hormone balance in the female rat by a single injection of ergotoxine ethanesulphonate. *Am. J. Physiol.* **180**, 47–49.

30. Stricker, P. and Grüter, F. (1928). Action du lobe antérieur de l'hypophyse sur la montée laiteuse. *C. R. Soc. Biol.* (*Paris*) **99**, 1978–1980.
31. Stürmer, E. and Flückiger, E. (1974). *In vivo* smooth muscle stimulant activity of 2-bromo-α-ergokryptine mesylate (CB 154) as compared with that of ergotamine. *I.R.C.S.* **2**, 1591.
32. Weidmann, H., Müller-Schweinitzer, E., Salzmann, R., and Wagner, H. (1978). Basic pharmacological properties of ergot alkaloids and related compounds. In *Ergot Alkaloids and Similar Compounds* (Handbook of Experimental Pharmacology), ed. Berde, B. and Schild, H. O. Berlin, Heidelberg, New York: Springer Verlag.
33. Yanai, R. and Nagasawa, H. (1969). Quantitative analysis of prolactin by disc electrophoresis and its relation to biological activity. *Proc. Soc. Exp. Biol. Med.* **131**, 167–171.
34. Yanai, R. and Nagasawa, H. (1970). Effects of ergocornine and 2-Br-α-ergokryptine (CB 154) on the formation of mammary hyperplastic alveolar nodules and the pituitary prolactin levels in mice. *Experientia* **26**, 649–650.
35. Zeilmaker, G. H. and Carlsen, R. A. (1962). Experimental studies on the effect of ergocornine methane-sulfonate on the luteotrophic function of the rat pituitary gland. *Acta Endocrinol.* **41**, 321–335.

I-6

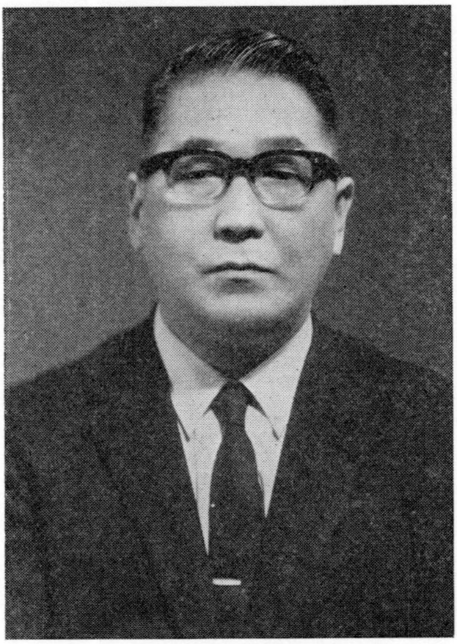

Masazumi Kawakami was born in Okayama Prefecture, Japan, in 1921. He graduated from Kiamsu Medical College as a top student in 1942. After joining to the military duty during 1943–45, he worked in Kobe University, Medical School, where in 1951 he was appointed Associate Professor in Physiology. In 1955, he obtained his Ph.D. from University of Tokyo and left for University of Minnesota for working with the late Prof. E. Gellhorn and next year moved to University of California at Los Angeles for working with Prof. C. H. Sawyer. In 1958 he came back from abroard and was appointed Professor of Physiology at Yokohama City University School of Medicine. He was elected Dean of the School of Medical in 1977.

At Kobe University, under supervision of the late Prof. R. Shoji, one of the founders of Japan Physiological Society, he was attracted profoundly by physiological mechanisms of adaptation of voluntary muscle to training. Later he originally uncovered the fact that sex steroid modified the muscular adaptation process to training.

In collaboration with Prof. Sawyer, he developed the electrophysiological principles of paradoxical sleep as the EEG After Reaction in the rabbit and discovered electrophysiologically the biphasic effects of progesterone on the hypothalamo-hypophysial-gonadal system. He eventually concentrated his interest to neuroendocrine encompassing reproductive biology. Since 1950, he has published more than 150 scientific publications. He edited the book "Biological Rhythms in Neuroendocine Activity."

Positions he has held in Japan include Executive Directors of Physiological Society, Japan Endocrine Society and Neuroendocrine Society. He has fullfilled editorial appointments in Endokrinologie (Leipzig) and Editor in Chief of Endocrinologia Japonica. He has been an active member of several Scientific Societies, *i.e.*, International Society of Neuroendocrinology, Endocrine Society (USA), Psychoneuroendocrinology Society, Neuroendocrine Section of IBRO, and, in 1977, he was elected the Honorable Membership of the Hungarian Society of Endocrinology and Metabolism.

HOW I BECAME A NEUROENDOCRINOLOGIST

Masazumi Kawakami

Department of Physiology, Yokohama City University School of Medicine, Kanagawa, Japan

My life as a physiologist began under the supervision of Prof. R. Shoji in 1944. He was a professor of the University of Kyoto, School of Medicine, and served concurrently as a professor of Kiamsu Medical College, where I was attracted by his lecture on pH theory and on the concept of adaptation mechanisms to cold. My intention of entering his laboratory after graduation from the school was interrupted by brief military service, but following the termination of World War II in 1945, I immediately went to his laboratory as a research assistant.

At that time, my interest was focused on the responsiveness of capillary vessels to alteration of skin temperature due to cold or heat stimuli. I also examined changes of pH and CO_2 reservation in the blood due to hyperventilation. In the course of those experiments, I became interested in how the organism can maintain constancy or aquire adaptation in a changing environment. I thought that the organism might have considerable reserves in its function which make the organism adjust or adapt to environment. I became fully convinced of this concept by the further observation that the abdominal muscle showed less action potential in the pregnant woman, suggesting a certain adjustment in the mechanism of stretch reflex of the abdominal muscle in order to adapt to an excess of extension. This experiment was dependent on my experience in an electrophysiological study investigating the relationship between changes in injury potential and electrolytes under Prof. K. Furusawa. He was the first investigator who noticed the deporalization phenomenon. I examined also discharge rates of action potential in the adbominal muscle at various stages during the menstrual cycle of women studying in the Kobe Pharmacological College. Through this study, I found that the discharge rate was decreased by administration of progesterone.

One problem which I had had in proving my theory was that Prof. Shoji believed that physiology in the medical field should be based on human research. However, when I presented those data to him, he allowed me to use animals in an experiment on the effect of hormones which I intended to investigate. I examined the effect of progesterone on the muscle spindle of the frog and on the action potential of the spinal cord in the cat, and confirmed a dependency of those parameters upon the hormonal environment. I think my future scientific direction was set in accordance with this finding on the action of sex hormones in the various organic functions. I had been an associate professor in Shoji's department since 1961.

Following T. Tokizane's advice, whom I happened to meet in a meeting on electromyogram (EMG), to extend my research to the brain function, I went to the University of Minnesota in 1955 as a Fulbright scholar to study under Prof. E. Gellhorn. I thought it was necessary to study autonomic nervous function for a better understanding of the brain control mechanism of hormones. This was right after I was awarded a Ph. D. by Tokyo University for a paper on a study of EMG entitled "Sex Hormone Control of Muscle Tension." Following one year's study in Minnesota, I moved to the University of California at Los Angeles (UCLA), where I studied with C. H. Sawyer.

I really think that this period was a "Golden Age," not only for me but also for the UCLA Brain Research Institute (BRI). My laboratory, *i.e.*, Sawyer's, was in a Quonset hut built on the grounds of Long Beach Veterans' Hospital. There were many other similar laboratories, *i.e.*, Quonset huts, for Profs. H. W. Magoun, D. F. Lindsley, J. D. French, and J. D. Green. Dr. E. Eldred was working actively and Drs. J. N. Hayward, E. Eidelberg, and J. S. Buchwald joined later. B. A. Cross's laboratory was next to mine. Several Japanese researchers, such as Drs. N. Yoshi, T. Kusama, K. Tasaki, B. Fujimori, and K. Otani were working there also. Sawyer drove over to Long Beach almost every day, even on Sunday, from Los Angeles, to check how the experiment was going. I remember that B. V. Critchlow and C. K. Haun came from Los Angeles sometimes. At lunch time, Prof. Magoun used to take us to a restaurant called the "Golden Lantern." It looked like all the members in this institute worked in unison at that time. During my next short stay in UCLA in 1961 I also got a chance to spend a pleasant time with Drs. B. Flerkó, J. S. Tindal, C. Bayer, S. Kanematsu, and N. Hagino.

In those days, we found that low-frequency stimulation of rhiencephalic-hypothalamic projections induced a phenomenon which we called an *electroencephalogram (EEG)-afterreaction*. It consisted of a period of slow wave sleep followed by what is now recognized as paradoxical sleep (PS)—a sequence occurring naturally only postcoitally in female rabbits under our recording conditions, hence the name EEG-afterreaction. Since it could be induced by electrical stimulation, it provided another response for threshold investigation. Testing the effects of progestins on these thresholds, we found that during the initial facilitation period both the EEG arousal and afterreaction threshold dropped and during the inhibitory stage they rose to heights far above normal-parallel biphasic effects.

Long acting derivatives of progesterone were found to extend both phases of the threshold curves, *i.e.*, the initial lowering and the secondary elevation. During the first phase the release of pituitary luteinizing hormone (LH) is readily induced but during the second the rabbit will not ovulate even if she mates. Interestingly, two of the longest acting progesterone esters, 17α-OH-progesterone caproate and dihydroxy progesterone acetophenide, have been used in women as long-acting antifertility agents—a single injection per month replacing daily ingestion of pills. A second series of antifertility steroids are comprised of nortestosterone derivatives, widely used in contraceptive pills. These steroids, like testosterone, elevated the EEG afterreaction threshold without lowering it and they did not change the EEG arousal threshold. Treated rabbits will mate but not ovulate. From these and other data it appeared that the EEG afterreaction threshold mirrors the threshold of pituitary activation and that antifertility steroids act on the brain to the extent that they elevate the threshold of rhiencephalic-hypothalamic activation. The EEG arousal threshold, on the other hand, does not seem closely concerned with pituitary secretion but rather with estrus—the appetitive phase of sexual behavior. The hormones, then, facilitate and inhibit pituitary activation and estrous behavior while lowering and raising brain thresholds (*16*, *33*, *34*).

The discovery that the postcoital EEG afterreaction in the female rabbit contained a phase of PS led to studies on hormones and sleep. We found that the whole afterreaction sequence of slow wave sleep and PS could be conditioned to occur in response to a tone if the rabbit was primed with estrogen. These findings were very exciting and directed my subsequent research interest to the feedback phenomenon of steroid

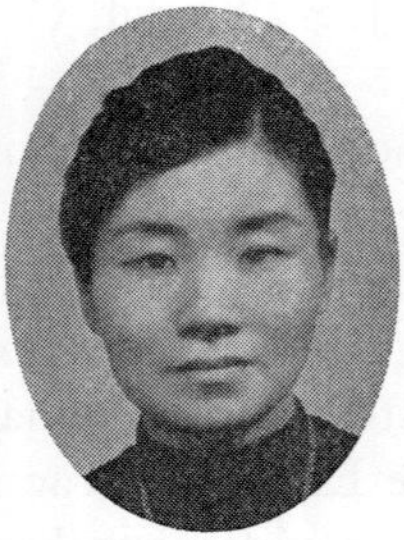

Dr. E. Terasawa

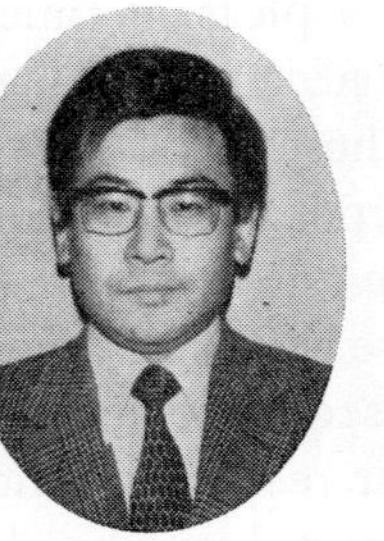

Dr. S. Ishida

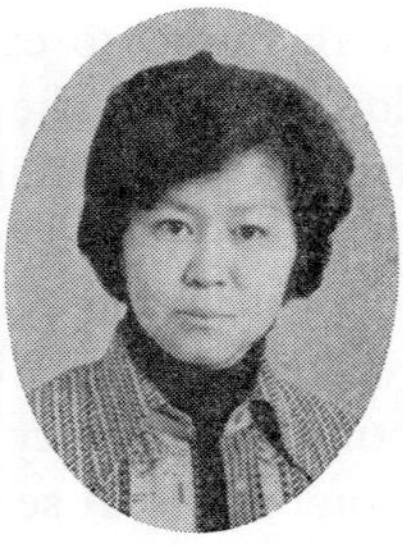

Dr. F. Kimura

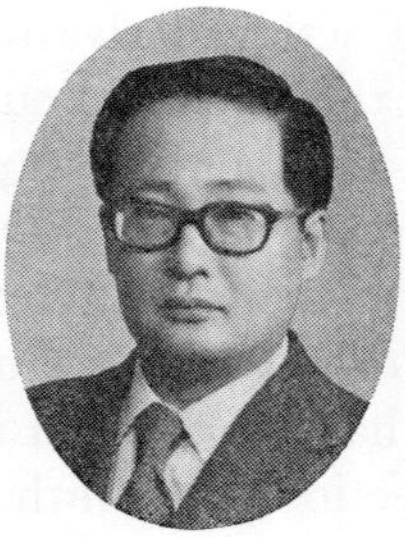

Dr. K. Yoshida

hormones upon brain activity analyzed either by electrophysiological study or by determination of pituitary hormones, directly or indirectly. I think this period in the United States was very valuable and the most fruitful and pleasant in my life.

It has been 16 years since I moved to Yokohama (December 1960) where I began to establish a new department. I was given a section in a new building which was almost empty with not a single teaching staff member available. I had only a stereotaxic instrument for the rabbit and cat, and some desks. With the beginning of my lectures that year, however, I got several third-year medical students who helped me with preparing for the experiment, and among them I had the chance to meet S. Yamaoka and F. Kimura. Next year, E. Terasawa, who is now at the University of Wisconsin, joined me as an instructor. She worked intensively with me for almost 13 years until she got married in the States in 1975. In the course of experiments which I arranged for the Medical Festival in my school according to a request by a small group of medical students, I also had a chance to meet H. Negoro, H. Saito, and S. Ishida.

Very luckily, in 1962, we got a grant from the National Institutes of Health, U.S.A., which continued for 5 years. At the same time, the Ministry of Education, Japan, granted us in 1964, which has continued until now. I would like to express my sincere thanks to both systems. I really think that the basis for research in my laboratory was established through the financial support offered by them. Getting an electroencephalograph with a frequency analyzer and electrical stimulator, I started an experiment on oxytocin-sensitive components in the cat reticular activating system with Terasawa, and got the result that the component has a close relationship with hippocampal activity (*24*). Successively, Terasawa analyzed the EEGs recorded from the female rabbit brain before and after copulation and found that with the progress of estrus, the integrated band values of the 2–8-Hz frequency components, including the high-amplitude spindle bursts as well as 20–30-Hz components in the amygdaloid complex, showed an increase. This was followed by a decrease of the components within 1 hr after copulation. In contrast, the 8–13-Hz regular rhythmic sinusoidal waves from the hippocampus decreased during the maximum stage of estrus and these components increased after copulation. It was shown that electrical activities in the hippocampus and amygdala changed in accordance with the progress of the reproductive process, and the changes of both areas were opposite (*26*).

During a period from 1963 to 1964, my department was enlivened by members who were studying the effects of estrogen and progesterone on the episodes of PS during the sleep phase in the rabbit. This group included S. Tsuchihashi, T. Uemura (graduate research fellows), K. Yoshida (first medical student), M. Yanase, and K. Ibuka (premedical students). Ishida supervised the students. They recorded EEGs day and night, and day by day, staying by the electroencephalograph to check the behavior of the rabbits and the recording paper. They slept alternately in the "Student Union," a room I arranged for them to rest in in my department. This exhaustive experiment extended the concept of the intimate relationship between sleep and hormones which I challenged with Sawyer following discovery of postcoital EEG-afterreaction. The ratio of the total amount of hours occupied by the episodes of sleep with spindle bursts to that of PS decreased paralleling the progress of estrus, and this ratio showed the lowest value during the period of the first several hours following injection of progesterone in the ovariectomized estrogen primed rabbit (*2*). In addition, Yamaoka, S.

Kyuma, and K. Kubo (medical students) were trying to set up a recording technique for single unit activity in the rabbit and rat hypothalamus, which was later completed by postgraduate student H. Saito.

With the increase of postgraduate students and medical students who wanted to study with me, by 1965 I was able to carry out several projects: recording of evoked potential and single unit activities for analyzing sex hormone feedback mechanisms (with Terasawa, Saito, and Kimura who joined us that year as a postgraduate student), recording EEGs under exposure to immobilization stress (with Negoro, who became an instructor in 1963, Yanase who was a postgraduate student, and M. Mohri who was a medical student), recording of EEGs under cold and heat stress (with Negoro, Yamaoka, and Mohri), investigating the sleep-inducing substances (with Yoshida), and so on. Throughout these experiments, our interest was in the attitude of the limbic system in response to steroid hormones and long-acting stress. We recognized that the hippocampus and the amygdala, as well as the reticular activating system, are profoundly concerned with the feedback and adaptation mechanism. Negoro (*29*), Saito (*32*), Yamaoka (*36*, *37*), Yanase (*38*, *39*), and Mohri (*28*) were awarded their Ph. D.'s from those works.

In close cooperation with K. Seto, who has been an associate professor since 1966, we started several series of studies measuring the incorporative rate of ^{14}C from ^{14}C-1-acetate into ovarian and adrenocortical steroids in the *in vitro* system, as an indicator for steroid biosynthetic activity. Yoshida worked very hard on these studies and got many interesing findings indicating the importance of the limbic system in the control of gonadotropins (*18*) and adrenocorticotropic hormone (ACTH) release. Most striking among them was the finding suggesting that the hippocampus is highly sensitive to corticosterone; implantation of corticosterone increased the biosynthesis of adrenal cortical steroids (*19*). This was later supported by autoradiographic studies showing that the hippocampus is the major site for corticosterone uptake. In this series of experiments, he also found that the hippocampus may change its ACTH release stimulating activity in normal conditions into an inhibitory one under stressful conditions. Developing these studies later, Kimura, Ishida, and Yanase exposed rabbits to 7 days' repeated immobilization stress and found that, after such stress, either the hippocampal or the amygdaloid stimulation decreased ACTH release, as indicated by a decrease of the ^{14}C incorporative rate into corticosterone. Considering that the ACTH release response to immobilization stress was reduced markedly after 7 days' stress, we deduced that the central nervous system (CNS) adaptation to this kind of stress is obtained by the alteration of the hippocampal and amygdaloid functions (*17*).

In 1968, Kimura began to use rats for a study on reproduction in an experiment checking the vaginal estrous cycle after hippocampal stimulation. She found that stimulation may delay ovulation. I began a study with Terasawa recording multiunit activity (MUA) in the rat. She had returned from UCLA, where she had worked under Sawyer's instruction. From chronic recordings of MUA in the cyclic rat, we noticed characteristic bursts in the arcuate nucleus, the medial preoptic area and the medial amygdala during the ovulatory quota of gonadotropin release (*22*). Since electrical stimulation of the medial preoptic area was effective in inducing ovulation, associated with an increase of MUA in the arcuate nucleus, we thought that those bursts might be related to neural excitation responsible for activating gonadotropin release (*23*). Later, M. Manaka, who joined us in 1969, made an effort to analyze a large amount of MUA data he had carefully recorded. Many brain areas showed a diurnal variation in their MUA, which was higher in the afternoon than morning. There were two types of cyclical variations superimposed on this diurnal variation. In the arcuate nucleus, medial preoptic area, and bed nucleus of stria terminalis, the level increased in accordance with the progress of estrus to reach its peak in the afternoon of proestrus. The MUA in the medial amygdala started to increase in the afternoon of diestrus 1 or early morning of diestrus 2 and attained its peak in the morning of proestrus, preceding maximum elevation in the former two areas. In the hippocampus, fornix and lateral amygdala, levels demonstrated a nadir on the day of proestrus (Fig. 1) (*27*).

Through these experiments, we felt keenly the necessity to determine gonadotropin levels in serum and the pituitary gland. Getting kind help from Dr. K. Wakabayashi at the National Institute of Radiological Sciences, and with the efforts made by Terasawa and Kimura, we introduced the radioimmunoassay technique into my laboratory in 1971. Terasawa confirmed that stimulation of the medial preoptic area on each day of the cycle was effective in inducing LH release (*25*), and Kimura found that stimulation of the hippocampus inhibited the ovulatory release of LH, follicle stimulating hormone (FSH), and prolactin (*9*). Later she also found that stimulation of the lateral amygdala or the central gray matter inhibited it (*7*). That the stimulation of those areas decreases MUA in the arcuate nucleus and the medial preoptic area was confirmed by N. Konda, who was a postgraduate student (*8*).

In the meantime, Terasawa, who was much interested in the limbic

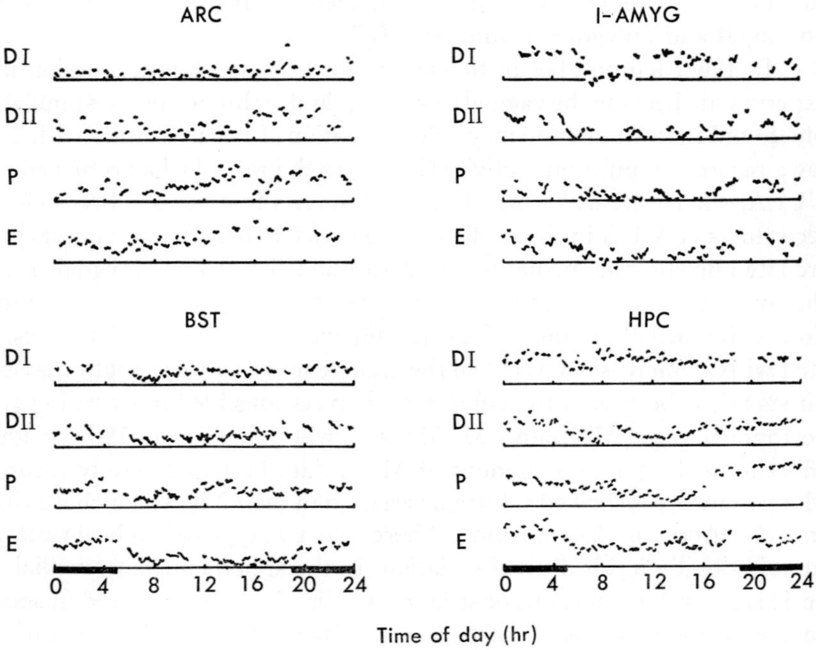

FIG. 1. Integrated multiple unit activity in the arcuate nucleus (ARC), bed nucleus of stria terminalis (BST), lateral part of amygdala (l-AMYG), and hippocampus (HPC)

system, made an acute horizontal cut just above the medial preoptic area, which sectioned or destroyed the medial amygdaloid efferents and the bed nucleus of stria terminalis, on the day of diestrus 1, and found that the cut prevented the progress of gonadal activity and ovulation (*21*). This observation was followed by an experiment which showed that electrical stimulation of the medial amygdala or the bed nucleus of stria terminalis on the day of diestrus 2 induced FSH release. Those findings suggested to us the crucial role of the estrogen neuron system, such as the medial amygdala and the bed nucleus of stria terminalis, in the mechanisms responsible for stimulating the release of gonadotropins.

Subsequently, our attention was focused on the positive feedback sites of estrogen and progesterone in the release of gonadotropins. The double canula implantation method, which we have utilized since 1974 for implanting solid hormones or chemical substances into localized brain areas without any surgical procedure or anesthesia, was so useful that we could localize several brain areas as the sites. Estradiol benzoate implanted in the medial amygdala or in the bed nucleus of stria terminalis induced ovulation in the progesterone-blocked 4-day cyclic rat (*35*) and advanced ovulation in the 5-day cyclic rat (*6*). In the 5-day cyclic rat, implantation in the arcuate nucleus was also effective, whereas that in the medial preoptic area was not. MUA in the arcuate nucleus showed an afternoon elevation on the day of implantation (diestrus day 2) into the medial amygdala or the bed nucleus of stria terminalis as well as on the day following, while it did not induce such change on the day of implantation when implanted into the medial preoptic area.

We speculated that the induction of ovulation by estradiol implantation into the medial amygdala or the bed nucleus of stria terminalis depends on the stimulation of folliculotropin release, as indicated in a brain transection experiment. Subcutaneous injection of estradiol at 12.00 hr on the day of diestrus 2 in the 5-day cyclic rat, which might be effective in advancing ovulation, induced an acute release of FSH and prolactin concomitantly with an inhibition of LH release in the afternoon of the same day. It was found, as expected, that this estradiol effect was achieved by implantation into the above two areas, although an effect on LH release was not observed. As a result, the implantation advanced cyclic changes in vaginal smears, indicating an acute estrogen release, and only those rats which showed an advancement of vaginal cycle ovulated early. More interestingly, when implantation in the bed nucleus of the stria terminalis was done for shorter periods of time on the day of diestrus 2 (from 12.00 to 20.00 hr), an advancement of those parameters was similarly observed.

It was considered that the medial amygdala and the bed nucleus of stria terminalis in mid-diestrus in the 5-day cycle, responding to estradiol, stimulated FSH and prolactin release without affecting LH, which triggers a chain of reproductive events, including the release of ovarian steroid, responsible for early ovulatory gonadotropin release (*5*). The electrical activity of the medial amygdala and the bed nucleus of stria terminalis elevates in accordance with the estradiol rise in the blood, which is single spread during the estrous cycle and thus stimulates the preoptic-hypothalamic system with 4- or 5-day periodicity.

Our next problem was the role of the medial preoptic area in the neural apparatus for ovulatory LH surge. We thought that this area might integrate the neural stimuli from the medial amygdala and the bed nucleus of stria terminalis, and might give them the feature of 24-hr rhythmicity. Therefore, the limbic neural impulses would reach the hypothalamus only

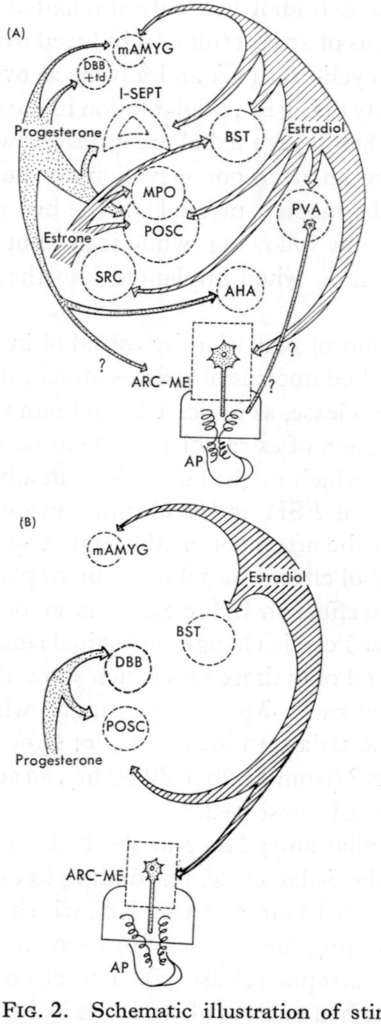

FIG. 2. Schematic illustration of stimulatory feedback sites of estrogen and progesterone which regulate LH release (A) and FSH release (B) with special reference to the location

mAMYG, medial amygdala; DBB+td, diagonal bund of Broca; l-SEPT, lateral septum; PVA, anterior basal area of the third ventricle including organum vasculosum laminae terminalis; POSC, periventricular suprachiasmatic area and adjacent area; MPO, medial preoptic area; SRC, retro-suprachiasmatic area; AHA, anterior part of hypothalamus; ARC−ME, arcuate nucleus and median eminence of hypothalamus; AP, anterior pituitary gland.

during a period of its circadian excitation. Our idea was that a certain kind of ovarian steroid, other than estradiol, should exert an influence on the manifestation of the medial preoptic circadian rhythm. Kimura first tested the effect of estrone. The result was as speculated. Implantation of estrone into the medial preoptic area in ovariectomized estradiol-primed rats was effective in inducing LH release during the afternoon of implantation. This correlated with an increase in MUA in the arcuate nucleus. However, we found from this experiment that implantation in the cycling rat was not so effective in advancing ovulation. Only 2 out of 6 animals ovulated in advance. This indicated to us that excitation by implantation of estrone is not enough to induce early LH surge, and excitatory impulses from the limbic system may be needed.

In this regard, the arcuate nucleus seemed to behave like the medial preoptic area. An increase of LH by implantation of estradiol in the ovariectomized estradiol-primed rat occurred in the afternoon of the same day, whereas in the case of implantation into the medial amygdala or the bed nucleus of stria terminalis the release occurred on the following day. Estrone implantation in the arcuate nucleus induced LH release in the afternoon of the same day. Additionally, anterior deafferentation simultaneous with estradiol implantation in the area prevented estradiol's effect in induction of early ovulation. Thus, it appeared that the arcuate nucleus requires facilitatory inputs from the medial preoptic area, either of circadian or of 4- or 5-day nature, for stimulating the LH surge in response to estrogen. However, the medial preoptic-arcuate nucleus system itself seems to manifest a circadian nature rather than a 4- or 5-day cyclic one. The rat with a cut just above the medial preoptic area revealed more significant circadian fluctuations of MUA in the preoptic-hypothalamic areas than those left intact. It was considered that preovulatory gonadotropin release undergoes two complex rhythms, one based on 4- or 5-day periodical excitation of the limbic system and the other on circadian excitation of the preoptic-hypothalamic system.

We think we partly resolved the problem resulting from the fact that in the chronically sectioned rat at the level of anterior commisure cyclic gonadotropin release is maintained, which was demonstrated first by Halász (*1*). It was found that medial preoptic implantation of estradiol was effective in inducing LH release after the chronic section of the limbic afferents, which shows that the medial preoptic-arcuate nucleus system might compensate for the function of the limbic-forebrain system by aquiring responsiveness to estradiol (*3*). Our tentative concept on the mechanism of

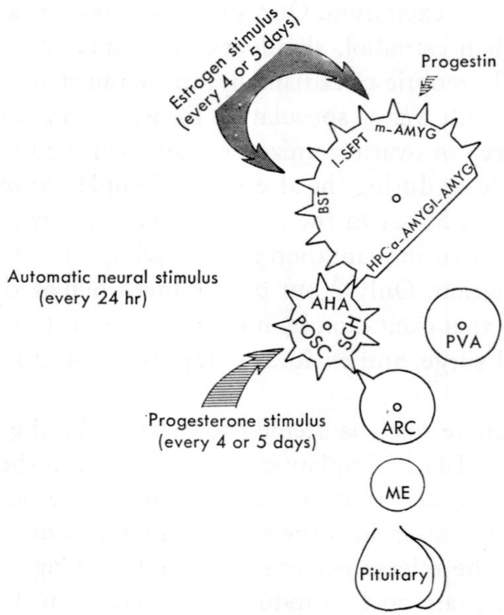

FIG. 3. Schematic illustration of estrogen and progesterone feedback mechanisms with special reference to the functional relationship between the locations for stimulating 4-day and 24-hr rhythmic LH release

The neural substrates which underline the LH release mechanism are mainly comprised of the extrahypothalamic and the hypothalamic centers. Among the extrahypothalamic elements, the limbic septal system plays an important role. Included in the system are both stimulatory and inhibitory loci and mechanisms regulating LH release. m-AMYG, BST, and l-SEPT comprise the stimulatory system. l-AMYG, a-AMYG (anterior part of amygdala), and HPC comprise the inhibitory system. Those two systems work antagonistically and in a reciprocal fashion. When the stimulatory influence is high the inhibitory influence is low. The summated activity gradually increases and reaches an appropriate level to cause the hypothalamic center to release LH within a cycle of 4 or 5 days. The hypothalamic center includes MPO, POSC, and SRC. This center is driven daily by automatic 24-hr rhythmic stimuli initiated within themselves and from somewhere else in the brain. Every 24 hr, the center is ready to transmit the neuronal message for LH release to the common LH-RH pool in ARC. PVA is possibly another LH-RH pool. The ARC and possibly PVA transmit the humoral message LH-RH through the ME to activate the anterior pituitary for LH release. The gonadal steroids estrogen and progestin, from the target organ (ovary) of LH feedback to the two centers. Estrogen primarily activates while progestin questionably activates the limbic systems in terms of their positive feedback actions. Progestin highly activates the hypothalamic center for LH release. (The description for the positive feedback actions of estrogen and progesterone on the anterior pituitary gland were omitted in Figs. 2 and 3.)

cyclical gonadotropin release is, therefore, that the estrogen neuron system in the limbic forebrain structure composes a facilitatory mechanism with the preoptic-hypothalamic axis, and the activation of this mechanism depends on the ovarian steroid hormones on one hand, and, on the other hand, on the activity of an inhibitory mechanism composed of limbic structures sparse in estrogen neurons. This was strengthened by the finding of Kimura that the acute sectioning of fornical fibers resulted in advancement of ovulatory LH release (Fig. 3) (*4*).

Our next subject was to localize the site of positive feedback of progesterone. A trial to determine if ovulation would be advanced by the implantation of progesterone into the brain failed. No implantation into the medial amygdala, the bed nucleus of stria terminalis, the medial preoptic area or the hippocampus induced ovulation in advance when they were implanted on diestrus day 3 in the 5-day cyclic rat. However, in the ovariectomized estradiol-primed rat, the implantation into the medial basal preoptic suprachiasmatic area was highly effective in inducing LH release in the afternoon. Implantation into the other areas described above was ineffective (unpublished). These results indicate that the action of progesterone responsible for fine determination of timing of the critical period is mediated largely by a region in the hypothalamus (Fig. 3).

We believed that the medial basal prechiasmatic area, including the area surrounding the preoptic recess of the third ventricle and thus the organum vasculosum laminae terminalis, might be intimately involved in the control of gonadotropin release, when we found in 1972 that this area showed a dramatic change of MUA around the critical period on the day of proestrus. Later, it was found that electrical stimulation of this area increases LH and prolactin release (*10*), and neurons with a neurosecretory nature terminate in the arcuate nucleus-median eminence without a synapse in between (*12*). That this area contains a considerable amount of LH-releasing hormone (RH) was also confirmed. However, since this area did not show any positive response to implanted estradiol or progesterone, unlike the arcuate nucleus, we now think the function of this area is rather constant and independent of other brain areas.

Another approach to clarify the brain mechanism for cyclic gonadotropin release in the female rat uses acyclic rats, such as neonatally androgenized or estrogenized rats, and male rats. It was apparent that, in those rats, the limbic structures such as the medial amygdala and the hippocampus, instead of the medial preoptic area, have functions different from those of the female (*20*). We suppose that the lack of cyclical gonadotropin release is largely dependent on the feature of limbic structures. Furthermore, in our opinion, the male brain is already male at the time of birth, and is not determined by androgen at that time. Kimura found that in the neonatally castrated male rat, the positive feedback effect of estrogen was not observed, while it was observed in rats castrated as adults.

Saito, Kubo, and Y. Sakuma who were postgraduate students, were much interested in a study utilizing single unit recordings and have obtained interesting results. It was Saito who found rhythmic discharge in the ventromedial neurons in the hypothalamus and he was awarded his Ph. D. with this paper (*13*). Studying the effect of vaginal stimulation and brain electrical stimulation on unit activity in the brain, Kubo found that: (1) unit discharges in the arcuate nucleus and the medial preoptic area were facilitated but those in the ventromedial nucleus and anterior hypothalamic area were inhibited; (2) discharges in the midbrain reticular formation, dorsal hippocampus and medial complex of the amygdala were facilitated by vaginal stimulation; (3) electrical stimulation of the anterior hypothalamic area or the medial preoptic area increased the unit discharges in the arcuate nucleus, whereas it decreased those in the ventromedial nucleus; and (4) stimulation of the dorsal hippocampus increased the unit discharges in the anterior hypothalamic area and decreased those in the medial preoptic area, whereas that of the medial amygdala exerted converse effects. Similarly, the stimulation of the hippocampus increased, and that of the medial amygdala decreased, discharges in the arcuate nucleus, while they exerted a reverse influence on ventromedial unit activity. From those findings, he proposed that the dorsal hippocampus mainly activates the anterior hypothalamic area-arcuate nucleus circuit and the medial amygdala activates the medial preoptic-arcuate nucleus cricuit, while both the hippocampus and amygdala may participate in different functional reorganizations activated by responses to vaginal stimulation (*11*).

Sakuma noticed that medial preoptic stimulation facilitated 31% of the arcuate nucleus units, which had been identified antidromically by electrical shocks to the medial eminence, and that hippocampal stimulation inhibited 24% of the units. Stimulation of the medial amygdala facilitated 22% of the arcuate neurons. Furthermore, 88% of the units which had been facilitated by medial preoptic stimulation was accelerated by noradrenaline applied iontophoretically and 83% of the units which had been inhibited by the hippocampal stimulation reduced their activities in response to acetylcholine. It was suggested that the facilitatory neural afferents which locate along the medial preoptic area are mediated by noradrenergic synapses in the medial basal hypothalamus and the inhibitory effect of the hypothalamus is mediated by the cholinergic system (*14*). At the same time, Sakuma indicated some doperminergic neural mechanism projecting from the medial basal hypothalamus to the median eminence which might exert a depolarizing effect on axons of a particular type of neuron characterized by fractionating spikes (*15*).

Negoro has been engaged in a study on the periventriculoneurohypophyseal system since he worked in the Mahidol University in Thailand with Prof. R. C. Holland. He found the existence of recurrent collaterals in the periventricular neurons, which may act in the auto-regulation of oxytocin release, and also a significant variation of spontaneous unit activity in accordance with the estrous cycle as well as with the progress of pregnancy (*30, 31*). Negoro has also acted as a go-between Thai and Japanese scientists: Prof. M. Kantaputra came to our laboratory in 1972 to work for 4 months on EMG, and S. Visessuvan, who came in 1975, is now a postgraduate student in my school.

The experiment on body temperature, which was first started in a study concerning adaptation to cold or heat stress, has also been continued. This has been developed to study the interaction between hormones and the thermo-regulatory center. Mohri found that dehydroepiandrosterone administration to castrated rats is effective in maintaining body temperature during exposure to cold stress. An ovariectomy lowered the basal temperature without affecting the pattern of diurnal rhythm, which has a nadir at 15.00 hr, and administration of estradiol restored it on the following day. Implantation of estradiol into the filiforma nucleus and its vicinity, which have been considered to be a heat loss center, on diestrus day 2 in the 5-day cyclic rat advanced the appearance of minimal temperature otherwise observed on the day of proestrus. Implantation of progesterone raised the temperature within 2 hr.

The voluminous research of my staffs, colleagues, postgraduate students, research fellows, and visiting investigators, both in the past and at present, can't be summarized here. These workers include Kawamura, Kawachi, Yamaguchi, Nakagawa, Fukuzawa, Ono, Takahashi, Koshino, Tsukiyama, Otsuka, Manabe, Ibuki, Shinohara, Matsuyama, Hiyama, Arita, Akema, and Sakanishi. I would like to say that R. A. Gorski is a most unique visitor to my laboratory. He came to Yokohama in 1969 as a visiting professor and worked with us for 6 months. Although his stay here was very short, his presence in our laboratory was highly stimulatory and influential because of his excellence in the field of reproduction, and also because of the friendship he showed to us. He has offered the members in my laboratory a chance to study in his laboratory at UCLA.

REFERENCES

1. Szentágothai, J., Flerkó, B., Mess, B., and Halász, B. (1968). *Hypothalamic Control of the Anterior Pituitary*. Budapest: Akadémiai Kiadó.
2. Kawakami, M., Ishida, S., Yoshida, K., Ibuka, K., Terasawa, E., and Negoro, H. (1964). The effect of brain lesions upon the spontaneous EEG-afterreaction in rabbits treated with sex hormones. *Gunma Symp. Endocrinol.* **1**, 221–241.
3. Kawakami, M. and Kimura, F. (1975). Possible roles of CNS estrogen- neuron system in the control of gonadotropin release. In *Anatomical Neuroendocrinology*, ed. Stumpf, W. E. and Grant, L. D., pp. 216–231. Basel: Karger.
4. Kawakami, M. and Kimura, F. (1975). Acute and chronic effects of the fonix section on cyclic gonadotropin secretion and ovulation in the rat. *Endocrinol. Japon.* **22**, 43–48.
5. Kawakami, M., Kimura, F., and Higuchi, T. (1973). Effect of electrical stimulation of the brain on gonadotropin secretion in male rats. *Endocrinol. Japon.* **20**, 447–454.
6. Kawakami, M., Kimura, F., and Higuchi, T. (1975). Localization and mechanism of stimulatory feedback action of estrogen: Effect of limbic forebrain implantation of estradiol benzoate on advancement of ovulation. *Endocrinol. Japon.* **22**, 327–338.
7. Kawakami, M., Kimura, F., and Kawagoe, S. (1976). Cholinergic and serotonergic links and the inhibitory effects of hippocampus, lateral amygdala and central gray matter on gonadotropin release. *Endocrinol. Japon.* **23**, 11–21.
8. Kawakami, M., Kimura, F., and Konda, N. (1976). Role of forebrain structures in the regulation of gonadotropin secretion. In *Neuroendocrine Regulation of Fertility*, ed. Anand Kumar, T. C., pp. 101–113. Basel: Karger.
9. Kawakami, M., Kimura, F., and Wakabayashi, K. (1972). Electrical stimulation of the hippocampus under the chronic preparations and changes of LH, FSH and prolactin levels in serum and pituitary. *Endocrinol. Japon.* **19**, 85–96.
10. Kawakami, M., Kimura, F., and Yanase, M. (1973). Involvement of the circumventricular organ in the regulation of gonadotropin and prolactin. In *Biological Rhythms in Neuroendocrine Activity*, ed. Kawakami, M., pp. 167–186. Tokyo: Igaku Shoin.
11. Kawakami, M. and Kubo, K. (1971). Neuro-correlate of limbic-hypothalamopituitary-gonadal axis in the rat: Changes in limbic-hypothalamic

unit activity induced by vaginal and electrical stimulation. *Neuroendocrinology* **7**, 65–89.
12. Kawakami, M., Negoro, H., Kimura, F., Higuchi, T., and Asai, T. (1975). Neural control of LH release in anterior periventriculo-median eminence-pituitary system. *Neuroendocrinology* **19**, 137–149.
13. Kawakami, M. and Saito, H. (1967). Unit activity in the hypothalamus of the cat: Effect of genital stimuli, luteinizing hormone and oxytocin. *Japan. J. Physiol.* **17**, 466–486.
14. Kawakami, M. and Sakuma, Y. (1977). (unpublished observation).
15. Kawakami, M., Sakuma, Y. and Akema, T. (1978). Effects of estrogen and aminergic drugs on the thresholds of medial basal hypothalamic axons in the median eminence of the rat. *Brain Res.* **156** (in press).
16. Kawakami, M. and Sawyer, C. H. (1967). Effects of sex hormones and antifertility steroids on brain thresholds in the rabbit. *Endocrinology* **80**, 857–871.
17. Kawakami, M., Seto, K., Kimura, F., and Yanase, M. (1971). Brain mechanisms involved in adaptation to the immobilization stress. *Gunma Symp. Endocrinol.* **8**, 171–197.
18. Kawakami, M., Seto, K., and Yoshida, K. (1966). Influence of the limbic system on ovulation and on progesterone and estrogen formation in rabbits. *Japan. J. Physiol.* **16**, 254–273.
19. Kawakami, M., Seto, K., and Yoshida, K. (1968). Influence of corticosterone implantation in limbic structure upon biosynthesis of adrenocortical steroid. *Neuroendocrinology* **3**, 349–354.
20. Kawakami, M. and Terasawa, E. (1972). A possible role of the hippocampus and the amygdala in the androgenized rat: Effect of electrical or electrochemical stimulation of the brain on gonadotropin secretion. *Endocrinol. Japon.* **19**, 349–358.
21. Kawakami, M. and Terasawa, E. (1972). Acute effect of neural deafferentation on timing of gonadotropin secretion before proestrus in the female rat. *Endocrinol. Japon.* **19**, 449–459.
22. Kawakami, M., Terasawa, E., and Ibuki, T. (1970). Changes in multiple unit activity of the brain during the estrous cycle. *Neuroendocrinology* **6**, 30–48.
23. Kawakami, M., Terasawa, E., Ibuki, T., and Manaka, M. (1971). Effect of sex hormones and ovulation-blocking steroids and drugs on electrical activity of the rat brain. In *Steroid Hormones and Brain Function*, ed. Sawyer, C. H. and Gorski, R. A., pp. 79–93. Berkeley: Univ. California Press.
24. Kawakami, M., Terasawa, E., and Kawachi, J. (1964). Studies on the oxytocin sensitive component in the reticular activating system. *Japan. J. Physiol.* **14**, 104–121.

25. Kawakami, M., Terasawa, E., Seto, K., and Wakabayashi, K. (1971). Effect of electrical stimulation of the medial preoptic area on hypothalamic multiple unit activity in relation to LH release. *Endocrinol. Japon.* **18**, 13–21.
26. Kawakami, M., Terasawa, E., Tsuchihashi, S., and Yamanaka, K. (1966). Differential control by sex hormones of brain activity in the rabbit and its physiological significance. In *Steroid Dynamics*, ed. Pincus, G., Nakao, T., and Tait, J. F., pp. 237–302. New York: Academic Press.
27. Manaka, M. (1976). The role of limbic forebrain structures on electrical activity rhythm of the brain with special reference to their dual modes of actions on gonadotropin release. *J. Steril. Fertil.* **21**, 9–22.
28. Mohri, M. (1974). Study on the neurohumoral mechanism of the thermoregulation: Role of the hypothalamus on the thermoregulatory mechanisms under extreme cold. *Yokohama Igaku* **24**, 161–175 (in Japanese).
29. Negoro, H. (1968). Electro-physiological changes in the limbic-hypothalamic system in response to cold in the rabbit. *Yokohama Igaku* **19**, 299–316 (in Japanese).
30. Negoro, H. and Holland, R. C. (1972). Inhibition of unit activity in the hypothalamic paraventricular nucleus following antidromic activation. *Brain Res.* **42**, 385–402.
31. Negoro, H., Visessuwan, S., and Holland, R. C. (1973). Unit activity in the paraventricular nucleus of female rats at different stages of the reproductive cycle and after ovariectomy with or without oestrogen or progesterone treatment. *J. Endocrinol.* **59**, 545–558.
32. Saito, H. (1968). Effects of luteinizing hormone and oxytocin upon hypothalamic unit activity in female cat. *J. Physiol. Soc. Japan* **30**, 1–12 (in Japanese).
33. Sawyer, C. H. and Kawakami, M. (1961). Interaction between the central nervous system and hormones influencing ovulation. In *Control of Ovulation*, ed. Villee, C. A., pp. 79–100. New York: Pergamon Press.
34. Sawyer, C. H., Kawakami, M., and Kanematsu, S. (1966). Neuroendocrine aspects of reproduction. *Endocr. Cent. Nerv. Syst.* **43**, 59–85.
35. Terasawa, E. and Kawakami, M. (1974). Positive feedback sites of estrogen in the brain on ovulation: Possible role of the bed nucleus of stria terminalis and the amygdala. *Endocrinol. Japon.* **21**, 51–60.
36. Yamaoka, S. (1969). Relationship between brown adipose tissue and the brain activity. I. EEG activity. *J. Physiol. Soc. Japan* **31**, 127–154 (in Japanese).
37. Yamaoka, S. (1969). Relationship between brown adipose tissue and brain activity. II. Effect of electrical stimulation of the brain on brown adipose tissue. *J. Physiol. Soc. Japan* **31**, 199–208 (in Japanese).
38. Yanase, M. (1973). A study on the role of brain for the establishment of adaptation to the repeated immobilization stress. I. Changes in brain activity

and several functions of the body under the repeated immobilization stress. *J. Physiol. Soc. Japan* **35**, 109–124 (in Japanese).

39. Yanase, M. (1973). A study on the role of brain for the establishment of adaptation to the repeated immobilization stress. II. A role of the limbic-midbrain system in the repeated immobilization stress. *J. Physiol. Soc. Japan* **35**, 171–178 (in Japanese).

I – 7

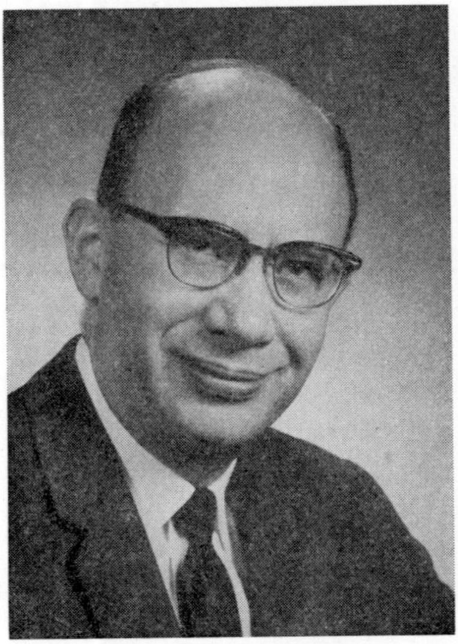

Joseph MEITES was born on December 22, 1913 in Kishinev, Russia and came to USA in 1920 (St. Joseph, Missouri). He received a B.S. degree in 1938 and a Ph.D. degree in 1947 from University of Missouri.

Positions held are Assistant Professor in 1947–50, Associate Professor in 1950–3 and Professor since 1953 at Department of Physiology, Michigan State University (MSU).

Dr. Meites has received a number of awards, fellowships and honors including Junior Award, MSU, Chapter of Sigma Xi (1953); Senior Award, MSU, Chapter of Sigma Xi (1967); Weizmann Fellowship (postdoctoral) (1955–6); Vice President and President, Michigan Section, Society for Experimental Biology and Medicine (1959–60); Distinguished Faculty Award, MSU (1970).

Dr. Meites was or is a member of Editorial Board of Neuroendocrinology (1967–76), Cancer Research (1972–present), Psychoneuroendocrinology (1975–present), Endocrinology (1953–6 and 1966–74) and Comparative and General Endocrinology (1968–71), Endokrinologie (1975–present). Furthermore, he was or is a member of Endocrinology Study Section, NIH (1966–70), Subcommitee on Use of Hormones in Domestic Animals, National Academy of Sciences—National Research Council (1960–70), National Pituitary Agency, NIH (1969–76) and Committee on Anti-Fertility Drugs, NICHD (1971–2); Chairman, IUPS Commission on Neuroendocrinology (1971–present) and President, International Society of Neuroendocrinology (1972–6).

The Scientific Societies in which he is a member include; The Endocrine Society, American Physiological Society, Society for Experimental Biology and Medicine, International Society for Neuroendocrinology, International Society for Psychoneuroendocrinology, International Brain Organization, American Association for Cancer Research, European Society of Comparative Endocrinology, Society for the Study of Reproduction, Gerontological Society, Sigma Xi and International Union of Physiological Sciences, Commission on Neuroendocrinology.

EARLY STUDIES ON CONTROL OF INITIATION OF LACTATION AND PROLACTIN SECRETION

Joseph Meites

Department of Physiology, Neuroendocrine Research Laboratory, Michigan State University, East Lansing, Michigan, USA

My initiation into the endocrinology of lactation and prolactin began while I was an undergraduate student at the University of Missouri. I was fortunate enough in 1937 to become a part-time technician in Professor C. W. Turner's laboratory in the Department of Dairy Science, and remained to become a graduate student. Dr. Turner had achieved an international reputation for his pioneer investigations on the endocrinology of the mammary gland. His laboratory attracted many graduate students and postdoctoral fellows, and it was a lively and stimulating place to work. Dr. Turner permitted his students maximum freedom in the choice of problems, and he was ever ready to provide ideas, advice, and encouragement. Everyone felt free to express their views, and Dr. Turner never took offense when his students occasionally disagreed with him. He retained his scholarly interests to the end of his life in 1975, and probably more than anyone else, helped lay the foundations for our present knowledge of lactational physiology.

Control of Lactation

The research I did for my Ph. D. thesis was concerned with the mechanisms controlling the onset of lactation at the end of pregnancy. I had read theories developed by earlier investigators on the control of lactation, and found much that was controversial or unproven. Some believed that the developing fetus during gestation inhibited lactation, others that it was the placenta or the corpus luteum, but the most widely-held view was that advanced by the late Warren Nelson, namely that the large amounts of estrogen secreted during gestation inhibited secretion of prolactin. Nelson showed that large amounts of estrogen could indeed inhibit lactation, and this could largely be overcome by injecting prolactin preparations. This appeared to be contradicted by the work of Ralph Reece who, as a graduate student under Turner in 1936, showed that estrogen actually could increase pituitary prolactin content and initiate lactation in rats, suggesting that estrogen stimulated prolactin release. Later we and others reported that administration of moderate doses of estrogens could induce lactation in rabbits, guinea pigs, goats, and cows. Even when I injected estrogen in relatively huge doses to rats, guinea pigs or rabbits, only increases and never decreases in pituitary prolactin content were found, although high doses were less effective than low doses. Later, David Chen, who was then a graduate student in my laboratory, showed that a wide range of estrogen doses only elevated and never depressed serum prolactin levels as measured by radioimmunoassay in ovariectomized rats, although again low doses were more effective than high doses (*1*). We therefore concluded that estrogens were only stimulatory to the secretion of prolactin. Similar observations have been reported in recent years in other species, including primates.

Based in part on work on the effects of different combinations of estrogen and progesterone on pituitary prolactin content and on the resultant mammary secretion, we theorized that the ratio of estrogen to progesterone which prevailed during gestation inhibited prolactin secretion and prevented the onset of lactation during pregnancy, but at the end of gestation estrogen became predominant and stimulated the pituitary to increase prolactin secretion and initiate lactation (*7*). The necessity for adrenal cortical steroids in addition to prolactin for initiating lactation was not ignored, but the action of prolactin was considered to be primary whereas that of adrenal steroids was believed to be mainly supportive in lactation.

Additional work in rabbits on this problem after I came to Michigan State University in 1947 indicated that estrogen and progesterone together, or even high doses of estrogen alone, could inhibit the peripheral lactational action of prolactin on the mammary gland, and that relatively large doses of prolactin could overcome this inhibition. Warren Nelson actually had suggested such a possibility, but apparently considered it secondary to the inhibition of prolactin secretion by estrogen. I modified our theory to state that lactation is not initiated during pregnancy because high levels of estrogen and progesterone secretion interfered with the peripheral lactational action of prolactin and adrenal steroids on the mammary gland and also inhibited pituitary prolactin secretion. Near the time of parturition these restraints were removed, permitting prolactin secretion to increase and to initiate lactation (*4*). This hypothesis apparently does not apply in its entirely to all species. In pregnant rats, for example, Yoshinaga reported that estrogen secretion remains very low until a few days before parturition, when it increases significantly. This appears to parallel the serum levels of pituitary prolactin although placental prolactin rises in the pregnant rat, as shown by Friesen and his colleagues. In other species both estrogen and progesterone increase during gestation. In pregnant women, unlike other species, pituitary as well as placental prolactin increase in the blood, but copious lactation usually does not begin because of the restraining influence of the high estrogen and progesterone levels on the peripheral action of prolactin. The mechanisms responsible for preventing lactation during gestation and its onset at about the time of parturition still are not completely understood, and the role of the hypothalamus in this process remains to be studied.

Control of Prolactin Secretion

My first serious effort in neuroendocrinology began with studies on the effects of central acting drugs on prolactin secretion. In addition to the work of Markee, Sawyer, and Everett on induction of ovulation with drugs, I read with great interest the reports by French workers and by Professor Felix Sulman and his colleagues of the Hebrew University of Jerusalem on the action of tranquilizing drugs on the endocrine system. In 1956, I attended a meeting where I was fortunate to see Bob Gaunt, whom I had known of for some years because of his significant contributions on the relation of the adrenal cortex to lactation. Bob was then a Research Director of Ciba, and had studied the endocrine effects of reserpine, and he offered to make reserpine available to me to see whether it could initiate lactation in rabbits as it had been reported to do occasionally in women. Since I knew that virgin female rabbits had only rudimentary mammary glands, I first injected them with estrogen for 2–3 weeks or made them pseudopregnant to develop their mammary secretory (alveolar) tissue, and then gave them a single intravenous injection of reserpine. This produced lactation in most of the rabbits, which I attributed to the release of prolactin (*3*). Charles (Tom) Sawyer in the same year independently observed the same phenomenon with reserpine in rabbits. Estrogen-treated female rats also responded with onset of lactation when injected with reserpine or chlorpromazine, and we subsequently used initiation of lactation in estrogen-pretreated female rats as a semi-quantitative assay for prolactin release.

Interestingly, when pigeons were injected with reserpine or chlorpromazine, crop milk secretion was not elicited, as might have been expected if prolactin was released. This was another indication to us that hypothalamic control of prolactin secretion in birds was probably different from that in mammals. An earlier observation of a difference in the control of prolactin secretion in pigeons was that injections of testosterone, estrogen, and progesterone did not increase pituitary prolactin levels in the pigeon as they did in rats and other laboratory mammals (*8*). We subsequently reported in a series of papers that hypothalamic extracts from pigeons, chickens, Japanese quail, and turkeys promoted prolactin release when incubated *in vitro* with pituitary tissue from these species (*6*). There is as yet no full understanding of the mechanisms involved in control of prolactin release in birds.

C. H. Nicoll, P. K. Talwalker, A. Ratner, and I found that many drugs could initiate lactation in estrogen-primed rats or rabbits, whereas others had no apparent effect. Thus serotonin, acetylcholine, pilocarpine, eserine, atropine, meprobamate, morphine sulfate, amphetamine, insulin, amphetamine and several carcinogens (3-methylcholanthrene, 3, 4-benzpyrene, and 9, 10-dimethyl-1, 2-benzanthracene), and a corticotropic hormone releasing factor (CRF) preparation obtained from Roger Guillemin, were effective in producing lactation, whereas lysergic acid diethylamide (LSD) had no effect (*5*). Later we showed that LSD inhibited prolactin release. Two of the most active drugs for evoking lactation were morphine sulfate and serotonin, both subsequently shown to elevate serum prolactin levels as measured by radioimmunoassay. In 1964, Mizuno, Talwalker, and I (*11*) reported that iproniazid, a monoamine oxidase (MAO) inhibitor, suppressed postpartum lactation, and later Nagasawa and I (*12*) found that it produced regression of carcinogen-induced mammary cancers in rats. However, we did not fully understand the central mechanism involved at that time.

One of the most fascinating group of drugs we worked with was the ergot derivatives. In 1955–1956, while on a sabbatical leave at the Weizmann Institute of Science in Israel, I did some collaborative research with M. C. Shelesnyak (see his chapter in "Pioneers in Neuroendocrinology," 1975), who was studying the effects of ergot drugs on implantation of fertilized eggs and deciduoma formation in pseudopregnant rats. Since the ergot drugs inhibited implantation and deciduoma formation, "Shelly" correctly deduced that they probably inhibited prolactin secretion and thereby depressed progesterone secretion by the ovaries. We proceeded to test this by injecting rats with various ergot drugs, and then removed the pituitaries and assayed them for prolactin by the pigeon crop sac assay. To our disappointment, we found no significant change in pituitary prolactin content. The pigeon assay was not sufficiently sensitive to assay prolactin in the blood.

Years later, Sandoz A. G. in Basel, Switzerland, offered to make some ergot drugs available to me, and together with Dr. H. Nagasawa, a mammary cancer researcher from Tokyo who was on a fellowship in my laboratory, we tested the effects of ergocornine on growth of carcinogen-induced mammary cancers and on serum prolactin concentration by the newly developed radioimmunoassay for rat prolactin (*14*). We found that ergocornine induced marked regression of mammary cancers in the rats and profoundly depressed serum prolactin levels (*12*). We also reported that ergot drugs induced regression of prolactin-secreting transplantable pituitary tumors and reduced extraordinarily high serum prolactin to normal levels (*15*).

Subsequently, ergot drugs generally were reported to have limited or no effect on the growth of breast cancer in human patients, but to induce remission in patients with prolactin-secreting pituitary tumors. Ergot drugs also have been shown to be useful in inhibiting postpartum and inappropriate lactation in women.

Wolfgang Wuttke and John Lu, who were in my laboratory during the early work with the ergot drugs, showed that ergot drugs had no effect on the estrous cycle of rats when given in moderate doses, but could inhibit luteinizing hormone (LH) release when given in high doses. By the use of ergocornine, Wolfgang Wuttke and I were able to determine the purpose served by the prolactin rise during the afternoon of proestrus in the rat, and later in the mouse (*10*). Apparently the proestrous surge of prolactin produced luteolysis of the old corpora lutea from the previous cycle every 4–5 days. When ergocornine was given daily during successive estrous cycles in the rat and mouse, the ovaries became loaded with corpora lutea which did not disappear. We reported that ergot drugs acted directly on the pituitary as well as on the hypothalamus to inhibit prolactin release.

For several years, Karl Nicoll, P. K. Talwalker, and I were engaged in a friendly debate with John Folley, Keith Benson, and Alfred Cowie of the National Institute for Research in Dairying, Reading, England, as to whether oxytocin could stimulate prolactin release from the anterior pituitary (AP). In 1956, Benson and Folley first suggested that oxytocin stimulated prolactin release, based on their observation that administration of oxytocin into postpartum lactating rats after litter removal retarded involution of the mammary glands. Since prolactin injections previously had been shown to inhibit mammary involution in similarly treated postpartum rats, they concluded that oxytocin acted by promoting prolactin release. This appeared to be an attractive idea since the work of Bargmann (see his chapter "Pioneers in Neuroendocrinology," 1975) suggested that nerve tracts from the supraoptic and paraventricular nuclei might deposit some oxytocin and vasopressin into the portal vessels on their way down to the posterior pituitary. Soon there were many reports claiming that oxytocin induced pseudopregnancy and vaginal mucification, presumably indicative of prolactin release and luteal stimulation. Martini and others also had reported that vasopressin could induce release of several other AP hormones, and Geoffrey Harris agreed that oxytocin might act similarly on prolactin release. As a graduate student in Turner's laboratory, I had injected a posterior pituitary preparation (Pituitrin) and Pitocin (both Parke-Davis products) into guinea pigs and rabbits, and could neither initiate lactation nor alter pituitary prolactin content (*7*). Apparently this had been overlooked.

Although we confirmed the result by Folley and his colleagues that oxytocin could inhibit mammary involution in postpartum rats after litter removal, we presented evidence that this was due to a direct action of oxytocin on the mammary alveolar apparatus causing evacuation of milk into the ducts and not to increased prolactin release. We showed that oxytocin had no effect on mammary involution in the absence of milk in the glands. In hypophysectomized postpartum rats, we reported that oxytocin alone did not retard mammary involution, but when given together with prolactin and adrenocorticotropic hormone (ACTH), it acted synergistically to prevent mammary involution. Karl Nicoll and I also reported that culture of rat pituitary with oxytocin or vasopressin did not result in enhanced prolactin release, an observation confirmed by Pasteels. Subsequently it was shown by radioimmunoassays of prolactin that oxytocin did not increase serum prolactin concentrations in several species including the rat and cow. At the conclusion of the "Symposium on Neuroendocrinology" in Miami in December 1961, where both John Folley and I gave talks, Roy Greep in his summary of the meeting stated his belief that the controversy had been resolved in our favor (*13*).

The work with central acting drugs has continued to fascinate me, as it appeared then and even more now as a promising approach for controlling release of pituitary hormones in animals and man. The evidence is overwhelming that some of the neurotransmitters in the brain (catecholamines, serotonin, acetylcholine, and others) are involved in regulating release of pituitary hormones, and many laboratories are engaged in trying to unravel their actions. Many drugs are available to either inhibit or enhance the activity of these brain neurotransmitters. What is particularly needed are drugs that can alter secretion of single rather than several pituitary hormones at one time. Several drugs already have been shown to be useful in controlling various clinical endocrine disorders.

Until about 1960, the few reports that the hypothalamus contained hypophysiotropic releasing factors dealt almost exclusively with CRF and release of ACTH. We were interested in testing the effects of extracts of hypothalamus on prolactin release, and soon published our first work on this subject (*9*). Using the estrogen-primed female rat as our prolactin test model, we observed that hypothalamic extracts could initiate mammary secretion, whereas large doses of cerebral cortex (the control brain tissue used at that time) induced lactation in only a few rats. We concluded in this report that the hypothalamus contains prolactin-releasing factor. Although this was the first claim for a prolactin releasing factor (PRF) in the hypothalamus, we did not follow this up except in birds. Later Mishkinsky *et al.* (*2*) used a similar estrogen-primed rat preparation to show that hypothalamic extracts could initiate lactation and therefore contained a PRF.

More recently, the laboratories of Nicoll and Reichlin have presented further evidence for the presence of a PRF in mammalian hypothalamic extracts, but its structure is unknown. Thyroid stimulating hormone releasing hormone (TRH) can release prolactin, but work in our and other laboratories makes it appear doubtful that it is the principal PRF of the hypothalamus. Prolactin and thyroid stimulating hormone (TSH) release usually do not occur together under most endocrine states.

We presented our first *in vitro* evidence for the presence of prolactin release-inhibiting activity in hypothalamic homogenate and extract at the Symposium on Neuroendocrinology in Miami in December 1961, and at the annual meeting of the Endocrine Society in 1962. A full report was published a year later (*17*). Independently, Pasteels also reported *in vitro* evidence for prolactin release-inhibiting activity in rat hypothalamus. We named the presumed prolactin release inhibitor "prolactin inhibiting factor (PIF)," but its chemical identity remains unknown to the present day. The presence of PIF activity in hypothalamic extracts was confirmed by other workers, notably Sulman and colleagues, Schally, and by Grosvenor and McCann. The latter used an *in vivo* method to demonstrate its existence.

An interesting question was raised by John Everett and Tom Sawyer soon after the reports of the presence of PIF and luteinizing hormone releasing factor (LRF) in hypothalamic extracts, namely whether the two were not identical, since LH and prolactin release usually did not go together but in opposite directions. In a collaborative study (*16*), we reported that partially purified LRF of bovine and ovine origin did not contain PIF activity. More recently, Schally's laboratory reported that the pure decapeptide, luteinizing hormone releasing hormone (LRH), also did not inhibit prolactin release. The role of the biogenic amines and of other neurotransmitters in the hypothalamus on prolactin release was unknown in the early 1960's, but in subsequent years we presented evidence that catecholamines could increase PIF release from the hypothalamus and presumably thereby inhibit prolactin release. The ability of serotonin to increase serum prolactin levels may be mediated by decreasing PIF or increasing release of PRF.

The relation of dopamine to PIF has been of particular interest since there is some evidence that the two may be the same. Probably the most cogent evidence for this view was provided by two of my former students, Carl Shaar and Jim Clemens. They reported that when the catecholamines were removed from rat hypothalamic extracts by aluminum oxide or by incubation with monoamine oxidase, all of the PIF activity disappeared from their extracts. However, it is possible that a peptide PIF was also removed from the extracts by these procedures. One reason for believing that this may be the case is that their procedures also removed all prolactin-releasing activity from their hypothalamic extracts. Their extracts were completely inactive after treatment. In addition, the laboratories of Andrew Schally and Karl Folkers both have reported some evidence for a separate PIF in hypothalamic extracts which is not a catecholamine. However, it must be admitted that practically all of our studies on the effects of different stimuli on the release of prolactin could be explained as easily on the basis of a change in hypothalamic dopamine as in PIF activity. Since dopamine can act directly on the pituitary to inhibit prolactin release, it will be necessary to show that dopamine actually is discharged into the portal vessels when prolactin release is inhibited. Thus, although I'm still biased in the view that a separate peptide PIF is present in the hypothalamus, I'm maintaining an open mind on this problem.

REFERENCES

1. Chen, C. L. and Meites, J. (1970). Effects of estrogen and progesterone on serum and pituitary prolactin levels in ovariectomized rats. *Endocrinology* **86**, 503–505.
2. Mishkinsky, J., Khazen, K., and Sulman, F. G. (1968). Prolactin-releasing activity of the hypothalamus in post-partum rats. *Endocrinology* **82**, 611–613.
3. Meites, J. (1957). Induction of lactation in rabbits with reserpine. *Proc. Soc. Exp. Biol. Med.* **96**, 728–730.
4. Meites, J. (1966). Control of mammary growth and lactation. In *Neuroendocrinology*, vol. 1, ed. Martini, L. and Ganong, W. F., Chap. 16, pp. 669–707. New York: Academic Press.
5. Meites, J. (1963). Pharmacological control of prolactin secretion and lactation. In *Proceedings of the First International Pharmacological Meeting*, vol. 1, ed. Guillemin, R., pp. 151–181. New York: Pergamon Press.
6. Meites, J. and Nicoll, C. S. (1966). Adenohypophysis: Prolactin. *Ann. Rev. Physiol.* **28**, 57–88.
7. Meites, J. and Turner, C. W. (1942). Studies concerning the mechanism controlling the initiation of lactation at parturition I, II, III. *Endocrinology* **30**, 711–733.
8. Meites, J. and Turner, C. W. (1947). Effect of sex hormones on pituitary lactogen and crop glands of common pigeons. *Proc. Soc. Exp. Biol. Med.* **64**, 465–468.
9. Meites, J., Talwalker, P. K., and Nicoll, C. S. (1960). Initiation of lactation in rats with hypothalamic or cerebral tissue. *Proc. Soc. Exp. Biol. Med.* **103**, 298–300.
10. Meites, J., Lu, K. H., Wuttke, W., Welsch, C. W., Nagasawa, H., and Quadri, S. K. (1972). Recent studies on functions and control of prolactin secretion in rats. *Recent Prog. Horm. Res.* **28**, 471–516.
11. Mizuno, H., Talwalker, P. K., and Meites, J. (1964). Inhibition of mammary secretion in rats by iproniazid. *Proc. Soc. Exp. Biol. Med.* **115**, 604–607.
12. Nagasawa, H. and Meites, J. (1970). Suppression by ergocornine and iproniazid of carcinogen-induced mammary tumors in rats; effects on serum and pituitary prolactin levels. *Proc. Soc. Exp. Biol. Med.* **135**, 469–472.
13. Nalbandov, A. V. (1963). *Advances in Neuroendocrinology*, pp. 515. Urbana: Univ. Illinois Press.
14. Niswender, G. D., Chen, C. L., Midgley, A. R., Jr., Meites, J., and Ellis, S. (1969). Radioimmunoassay for rat prolactin. *Proc. Soc. Exp. Biol. Med.* **130**, 793–797.
15. Quadri, S. K., Lu, K. H., and Meites, J. (1972). Ergot-induced inhibition of pituitary tumor growth in rats. *Science* **176**, 417–418.
16. Schally, A. V., Meites, J., Bowers, C. Y., and Ratner, A. (1964). Identity of

prolactin inhibiting factor (PIF) and luteinizing hormone releasing factor (LRF). *Proc. Soc. Exp. Biol. Med.* **117**, 252–254.

17. Talwalker, P. K., Ratner, A., and Meites, J. (1963). *In vitro* inhibition of pituitary prolactin synthesis and release by hypothalamic extract. *Am. J. Physiol.* **205**, 213–218.

II. RECENT ADVANCE IN THE PHYSIOLOGY OF MAMMARY GLANDS

II – 1

I - II

NORMAL AND ABNORMAL GROWTH OF THE MAMMARY GLAND

Hiroshi NAGASAWA and Reiko YANAI

Pharmacology Division, National Cancer Center Research Institute, Tokyo, Japan

This chapter will not attempt a comprehensive survey of the literature and a review of all studies completed to date. An attempt will be made, rather, to elaborate on specific studies largely done in our laboratory, both published and unpublished. The reader can get more detailed information and references from the reviews and original articles cited in each section. Moreover, a book extensively surveying the research on "prolactin" has been issued every year since 1973 (*42–45*) and includes chapters on receptors, mammary growth, lactation, cancer, and on clinical medicine.

1. Methods for Evaluating Mammary Growth

There are several methods for evaluating mammary growth on which a number of modifications have been performed to estimate growth more accurately. The most well-known methods are:

a) Wholemount preparations, which can be employed for glands developing in two dimensions, such as the glands of mice, rats, and hamsters;

b) Light and electron microscopic observations;

c) Deoxyribonucleic acid (DNA) content assessments;

d) DNA synthesis or labelling index estimated by [^{3}H] thymidine incorporation into mammary DNA.

These methods are not always adequate if employed alone, because each of them has its disadvantages and advantages and estimates only one aspect of mammary growth. For instance, using mammary DNA content to estimate total mammary parenchymal values would provide no information on the structure of the glands. By contrast, morphological structure can be observed by the wholemount or histologic preparation of the glands, but this would indicate nothing about the amount of parenchyma. If a specific method highly correlates with another method, it would be considered to be more reliable for estimating growth than methods lacking correlation.

From this point of view, we have studied the relationship between several procedures for determining indices of normal or neoplastic mammary growth. The correlation between mammary gland area (MGA), the area bounded by a line joining the periphery of the ducts in the wholemount preparation, and DNA content was highly significant in any age group of C57BL/6 strain female mice whose mammary growth is restricted to duct systems unless they are pregnant. However, the relationship between these methods was not significant in the C3H/He strain from 90–150 days of age when the development of the mammary end-bud system is conspicuous. Ovariectomy (ovx) or ovx plus steroid hormone injections also resulted in no significant correlations between these methods. It was concluded that MGA would be a fairly good index of the quantitative growth of mammary glands only during the sharp growing phase of the mammary duct system (*101*, *106*).

Some methods for determining normal mammary growth can also be employed for evaluation of development and growth of mammary tumors. Furthermore, wet and dry weights of excised tumors or the sizes of tumors (area or volume) calculated from the mathematical or geometrical mean of the largest one to three diameters are simple and widely employed methods for evaluation of tumor growth. The correlation coefficients between the indices of mammary tumor growth, *i.e.*, arithmetical or geometrical mean of the major two diameters, wet or dry weight, total DNA content and DNA content/mg dry weight, were calculated using spontaneous mammary tumors in 4 inbred strains of mice (*82*). The methods examined were highly correlated with each other in every strain, except for DNA/mg dry weight. The growth characteristics of spontaneous mammary tumors in mice generally vary greatly, unlike those of transplanted tumors. Moreover, necrosis of the central part is often seen in spontaneous tumors when the tumors are more than 1 cm in diameter. A precise estimate of size, therefore, is difficult in these tumors. Nevertheless, these results strongly suggest the validity of applying these measures even to this type of tumor.

The relationship between morphology in the wholemount preparations or DNA content and DNA synthesis was studied in normal mammary glands of mice (*85*, *86*) and rats (*83*). Generally, there was little correlation between these measures. Structure and DNA content represent the static state of the gland, while DNA synthesis is a good indicator of the dynamic aspects of the gland. In essence, the results of these studies indicate that these methods should be regarded as complementary, but not as alternative.

2. *Normal Mammary Growth*

There are several reviews on normal mammary growth and its hormonal control in animals (*2*, *14*, *18*, *41*, *122*, *137*) and in humans (*117*, *120*, *125*, *139*). Experimental analysis of hormonal control of prenatal growth of mammary glands has also been discussed (*53*, *121*).

Normal mammary growth is a preceding condition for mammary tumorigenesis, *i.e.*, mammary tumorigenesis is dependent upon full development of the normal mammary gland. Therefore, analysis of the pattern of growth of normal mammary glands in relation to mammary tumorigenesis is of particular interest. Several characteristics of mammary growth were, therefore, compared between high and low mammary tumor strains of mice at several ages and under different conditions.

1) *Normal mammary growth in a high and a low mammary tumor strains of mice*

Mice used were C3H/He and SHN for high mammary tumor strains and C57BL/6 and SLN for low mammary tumor strains, respectively. SHN and SLN strains have recently been established in our laboratory from the same basal stock of Swiss albino. These mice are not related to the established high and low mammary tumor strains of mice at all (*112*).

a) *During virginal period*

The most distinct difference in normal mammary growth between the high and the low mammary tumor strains has been observed during the virginal period.

C3H/He females, when compared with C57BL/6 females, always had greater mammary DNA content from 1 to 7 months of age, while there were only slight differences between these strains in MGA and the branching of ducts. The formation of end-buds or lobulo-alveoli became marked at 2–3 months of age in the glands of C3H/He mice, but the glands of C57BL/6 mice consisted only of a duct system even at advanced ages (Fig. 1 a, b)

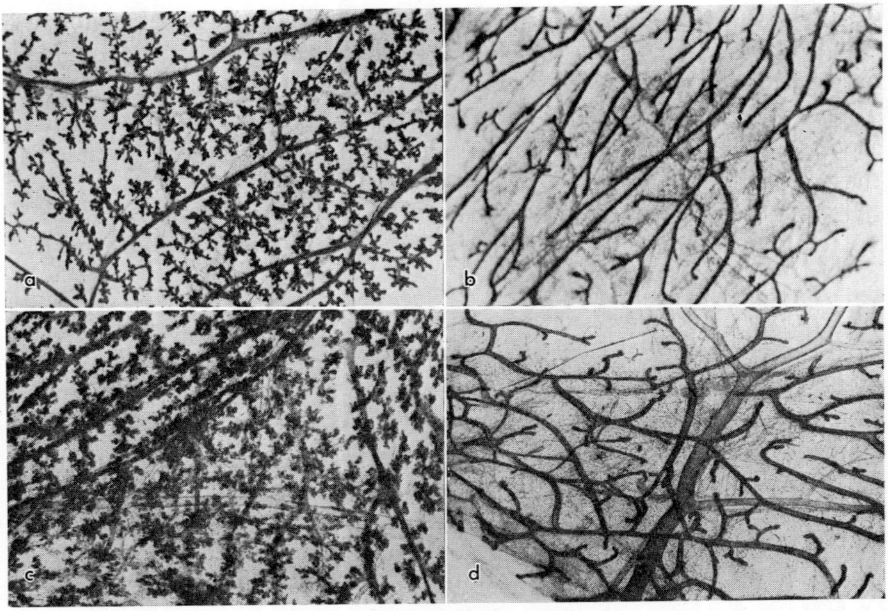

FIG. 1. Representative wholemount preparations of the third thoracic mammary glands of high and low mammary tumor strains of female mice

(a) C3H/He, 4-month-old; well-developed duct system with many endbuds. (b) C57BL/6, 4-month-old; glands are composed only of ducts. (c) SHN, 3-month-old; similar to a. (d) SLN, 3-month-old; similar to b. Stained with hematoxylin (×5).

(*105*). The mammary growth patterns of SHN and SLN mice were quite similar to those of C3H/He and C57BL/6 mice, respectively (Fig. 1 c, d) (*112*). Furthermore, there was a distinct difference between the pattern of relative growth of the mammary glands to body growth in the C3H/He and C57BL/6 strains (*105*).

b) *During pregnancy*

While there was no difference in the number of placentae, mammary gland ratings for lobulo-alveolar formation and mammary DNA content were significantly higher in C3H/He than in C57BL/6 on days 7, 14, and 19 of pregnancy (*150*). On the other hand, SLN was little different from SHN in mammary growth or in the number and weight of placentae at the end of pregnancy (*112*).

c) *During lactation*

C3H/He was significantly higher than C57BL/6 in mammary DNA

content on day 12 of lactation, not only in primipara but also in dipara (*92*). This was also the case when the litters were exchanged between these two strains (*110*).

C3H/He was also much better than C57BL/6 in reproductivity (*90*) and lactational performance (*92*, *110*). Similar differences were observed between SHN and SLN (*112*).

2) Causes of the strain-difference in normal mammary growth in mice

a) Secretion of prolactin and placental mammotropins

Pituitary prolactin levels were determined by disc electrophoresis on polyacrylamide gel (*147*, *163*) during virginal and pregnant stages and on day 12 of lactation in C3H/He and C57BL/6 strains of female mice (*151*). Both pituitary content and concentration were significantly higher in C3H/He than in C57BL/6 during the virginal and pregnant periods, while these levels declined gradually with the advance of pregnancy in both strains. On the other hand, no strain-differences existed in the level of this hormone either before or after 1 hr of suckling preceded by 8 hr litter removal on day 12 of lactation. The difference in the level between before and after suckling was significant only in C3H/He mice.

No distinct tendency was observed in plasma prolactin levels determined by radioimmunoassay between SHN and SLN; the level was significantly higher in SHN than in SLN during the virginal periods, but the opposite was the case on day 19 of pregnancy (*112*). Furthermore, there was no strain-difference in the level of this hormone after 30 min suckling following 1 hr litter removal on day 12 of lactation (Nagasawa, H. and Yanai, R. (1978). *Acta Endocrinol.* **87**, 94–98).

Sinha *et al.* (*128*) also found no consistent pattern in plasma prolactin levels in relation to the incidence of mammary tumors between C3H/St mice and C57BL/St mice under different environmental conditions. They have inferred that the essential difference between the two strains is their ability to metabolize prolactin.

Placental lactogen (*25*) is another important mammotropin, although it is effective only during pregnancy. In an experiment in which number of placentae was adjusted to 1–12 on day 8 of pregnancy in mice, the number and weight of placentae had positive correlations with total DNA content and the rating for lobulo-alveolar development of mammary glands on day 19 of pregnancy (*76*). This indicates that placental mammotropins, including placental lactogen, contribute quantitatively to mammary growth during pregnancy in mice. However, there was little difference between C3H/

He and C57BL/6 mice in the mammogenic activity of extracts of placentae either on day 14 or day 19 of pregnancy (*150*).

b) Mammary response to pituitary mammotropin

Mammary growth in response to pituitary grafting was much greater in C3H/He than in C57BL/6 (*108*) and in SHN than in SLN (*112*). This indicates that the high mammary tumor strains of mice have greater mammary responsiveness to pituitary mammotropin than do the low mammary tumor strains. Since no distinct differences in the pituitary and placental mammotropin levels in the circulation were generally found between high and low mammary tumor strains, it is conceivable that mammary sensitivity to pituitary mammotropin may be more important in the development and growth of normal and neoplastic mammary glands than is the amount of hormones acting on the glands.

c) Role of mammary tumor virus (MTV) on mammary response to pituitary mammotropin

Following a report which suggested the participation of MTV in the increase in mammary response to prolactin (*6*), mammary lobulo-alveolar growth was studied in MTV-susceptible (C3HeB/FeJax) and -insusceptible (C57BL/6) strains of female mice infected with or without MTV (*98*).

Since both strains originally had no MTV, it was introduced to newborn pups of each strain by foster nursing with C3H/He mice with MTV within 24 hr after birth. Mammary growth was evaluated at 90, 130, and 180 days of age and after 40 days of isologous pituitary grafting at 90 days of age (130 days old). In C3HeB/FeJax strain, mammary rating for lobulo-alveolar development was significantly higher in mice with MTV than in mice without MTV not only at 130 and 180 days of age but also after 40 days of pituitary grafting. In C57BL/6 strain, no difference in mammary lobulo-alveolar rating was found between mice with and without MTV at any age examined, all glands being restricted only to a duct system. However, mammary growth in C57BL/6 mice with MTV was significantly promoted by pituitary grafting when compared to mice without MTV. These results provide evidence that MTV has an ability to increase mammary sensitivity to prolactin not only in mice susceptible to MTV but also in mice resistant to it.

3) Changes in mammary DNA synthesis during different reproductive states and effects of pituitary grafting

While little differences in DNA content and histological structures were found between different stages of the estrous cycle, mammary DNA synthesis as an indicator of the dynamic aspects of mammary glands changed cyclically during the estrous cycles in mice and rats. In C3H/He mice aged 3–4 months showing consecutive regular 4 day estrous cycles, mammary DNA synthesis was significantly higher at proestrus (PE) than at estrus (E) and diestrus (D) (*159*). On the other hand, in 50-day-old rats, DNA synthesis increased from the 2nd day of diestrus (D2) toward PE and showed peak activity at E followed by a decrease. This pattern in DNA synthesis was similar in 90-day-old rats except that no significant difference existed between D2 and PE (*72*). The species differences in the changes in DNA synthesis during the estrous cycle may be attributable to the differences in changes of pituitary prolactin secretion, upon which mammary DNA synthesis is largely dependent (*99*, *100*). While plasma prolactin level peaks on the afternoon of D2 in C3H/He mice (*157*), it shows peak on the afternoon of PE in rats (*65*).

Distinct species-differences in mammary gland DNA synthesis are also observed after pituitary grafting and during the latter half of pregnancy, whereas synthesis during lactation is very low in both species. In C3H/He mice, DNA synthesis is much higher, even after 60 days or more of pituitary grafting (*100*, *159*) and at the end of pregnancy (*86*) than at E. In rats, DNA synthesis declines to less than one-half at PE or one-fifth at E after 20 days of pituitary grafting (*83*) and at the end of pregnancy (*72*). There were no species differences in the changes of mammary DNA content and histological structures; in both species, DNA content increased and development of lobulo-alveolar system became conspicuous by pituitary grafting and with the advance of pregnancy (*72*, *150*). Furthermore, prolactin levels in the circulation are high under these conditions in both species. The causes of the species differences in mammary DNA synthesis are obscure at present.

4) Role of estrogen in normal mammary growth

While pituitary and ovarian hormones are the most important regulators of normal mammary growth, prolactin may be the primary growth stimulator in this process (*65*). Gonadal steroids appear to participate in mammary growth both directly and indirectly. Estrogen, acting directly, alters mammary response to pituitary mammotropins, while its indirect effect is to stimulate pituitary prolactin secretion.

a) Local effect of small amount of estrogen (*75*)

Pellets of estradiol benzoate (EB), mixed with cholesterol at several ratios, were implanted into the fat pads of the right third thoracic mammary glands of ovx, 3-month-old female rats. The contralateral glands served as the controls. Rats implanted with EB at the ratio of 1: 5,000 showed constant diestrous vaginal smears preceded by E for several days. Seven to 10 days after the onset of D, some rats were killed by decapitation. The remaining rats were further grafted with 1 or 2 isologous pituitaries under the kidney capsule and killed after 20 days. Mammary DNA content and lobulo-alveolar formation were stimulated only around the implanted pellet in rats bearing both EB pellet at the ratio of 1:5,000 and grafts of 2 pituitaries. On the other hand, at all dose levels examined, EB implants alone did not induce mammary growth. These results suggest that EB increases the mammary response to pituitary mammotropins. The amount of EB which was effective did not, by itself, promote mammary growth. Thus, one of the actions of estrogen on mammary growth appears to be a sensitization of the mammary glands to pituitary mammotropins.

b) Effect of large amount of estrogen on normal mammary growth

Mammary gland was markedly involuted in C3H/He female mice given a single subcutaneous injection of 100 μg hexestrol dicaprilate, a long-acting estrogen. Meanwhile, this treatment increased pituitary prolactin levels. This mammary degeneration, however, was completely counteracted by the simultaneous isografting of 4 pituitaries, indicating that an additional supply of prolactin from the grafts can overcome the inhibitory action of estrogen on mammary growth (*79*). These results demonstrate further the existence of an antagonistic effect between prolactin and high levels of estrogen on mammary growth in mice. A similar antagonism between high doses of estrogen and prolactin has been observed in carcinogen-induced mammary tumors in rats (*77*, *84*).

5) Normal mammary growth of female athymic nude mice

The importance of an immune mechanism in the etiology of both human and experimental mammary tumors has recently been emphasized (*10*, *33*, *56*). Athymic nude mice may be an important model for research in this field. It was of interest, therefore, to assess normal mammary growth in female nude mice (nu/nu) and to compare this growth to that of normal females (nu/+) with the same genetical background (BALB/c) (*87*).

Both at virginal stages and on day 1 of lactation (approximately 3 months of age), synthesis and content of mammary DNA were significantly lower in nu/nu mice than in nu/+ mice. On the other hand, there were little differences between these groups of mice in pituitary prolactin secretion, weight and histological structure of the ovaries and pattern of estrous cycles. From these results, it can be inferred that a thymus deficiency has suppressing effects on mammary growth and function. This effect, however, may be independent on changes in pituitary and ovarian mammotropin secretion.

3. Abnormal (Preneoplastic and Neoplastic) Mammary Growth

The concept and priniciple of mammary tumor growth or "progression" have elaborately been described by Medina (*60–63*).

It is widely recognized that mammary tumorigenesis is generally controlled by the following factors: (a) hormones, (b) MTV, (c) genetical predisposition, and (d) immunological factors. Most recently, increased information pertaining to human breast cancer (*19*) has been accumulated because of the development of assay methods for hormones and MTV and epidemiological analysis. Furthermore, several types of human breast cancer have been successfully maintained in culture systems (*55*, *118*, *138*) and human breast displasias suspected of being preneoplastic have been transplanted into athymic nude mice (*46*). These techniques are expected to be of widespread use for further research in this field.

In this section, research pertaining to this subject performed in our laboratory will be discussed briefly.

1) Hormonal control of mammary tumorigenesis

Among several hormones, pituitary and ovarian hormones play major roles in the development and growth of mammary tumors, as in normal mammary growth, and numerous reviews pertaining to experimental animals (*20*, *29*, *30*, *35*, *36*, *51*, *63*, *113*, *119*, *127*, *140*, *142–145*) and to humans (*11*, *12*, *15*, *26*, *28*, *34*, *37*, *40*, *48*, *49*, *59*, *66*, *124*, *129*, *131–133*, *135*, *136*) are available. Recently, receptors or binding proteins for prolactin, estrogen and progesterone in normal and neoplastic mammary glands and interrelationships between these hormones and their receptors have been intensively studied for the purpose of assessing the responsiveness of a particular tissue to either steroid hormones (*5*, *9*, *58*, *146*) or to prolactin (*52*). However, up to the present time, receptor estimates for certain hormones do not always evaluate quantitatively responsiveness to the specific hormone. It is important that simultaneous assays of receptors to more than one hormone is accomplished in order to evaluate adequately the hormone responsiveness of a given tissue.

a) Mice

Abnormal outgrowth of the mammary lobulo-alveolar system is often observed in mammary glands of aged mice with MTV. They are called mammary hyperplastic alveolar nodules (HAN) (*62*, *141*) and are known to represent the preneoplastic state in this species. Prolactin has been considered to be important in the formation and growth of HAN. Thus, the effects of ergocornine and 2-bromo-α-ergocryptine (CB-154),* prominent suppressors of pituitary prolactin secretion, on HAN were studied (*148*, *149*). Daily subcutaneous injections with either drug to multiparous C3H/He female mice, free of palpable mammary tumors, resulted in a significant decrease in the number and size of HAN and an increase in the number of "ghosts" (remnants of regressed HAN) when compared to controls (Fig. 2a *vs*. b, c). The suppressive effects were much more prominent in CB-154 than were those of ergocornine. Associated with these effects, pituitary content and concentration of prolactin were significantly reduced and mammary lobulo-alveoli were conspicuously absent in these mice. On the other hand, pituitary growth hormone (GH) levels of treated mice were not altered at all and the ovaries were histologically normal and the estrous cycles were regular. These results suggest that HAN depend largely upon prolactin for formation and growth. This view has been supported by subsequent experiments in our laboratory (*152*).

Adreno-ovariectomy (adx-ovx) induced a significant decrease in size and number of HAN and an increase in the number of ghosts in multiparous, 7–8-month-old C3H/He mice. On the other hand, adx-ovx mice receiving 1.5 or 3 isologous pituitaries under the kidney capsules had numbers of HAN and ghosts similar to intact controls 40 days after pituitary grafting. There was a linear relationship between the number of pituitaries grafted and the number of HAN or ghosts. The average size of HAN was larger in mice with 3 pituitary grafts (Fig. 2e) than in the intact control (Fig. 2a). These results provide evidence that prolactin can promote the maintenance and growth of mammary HAN in mice free of steroid hormones. Daily injections of mice with human placental lactogen (HPL) has also prevented the involution of HAN by ovx (Fig. 2f) (*155*).

* The reader can refer to several articles pertaining to the mechanism of action of ergocornine, CB-154 and related alkaloids (*4*, *13*, *23*, *24*, *123*). These drugs are effective not only on *in situ* pitutitaries, but also on pituitaries grafted to sites distant from the central nervous system (*73*). The drugs appear to inhibit the release, but not the synthesis, of prolactin (*156*). They were found to compete with the release-promoting action of dibutyryl adenosine 3′,5′-monophosphate (*80*) at pituitary cell level (*95*).

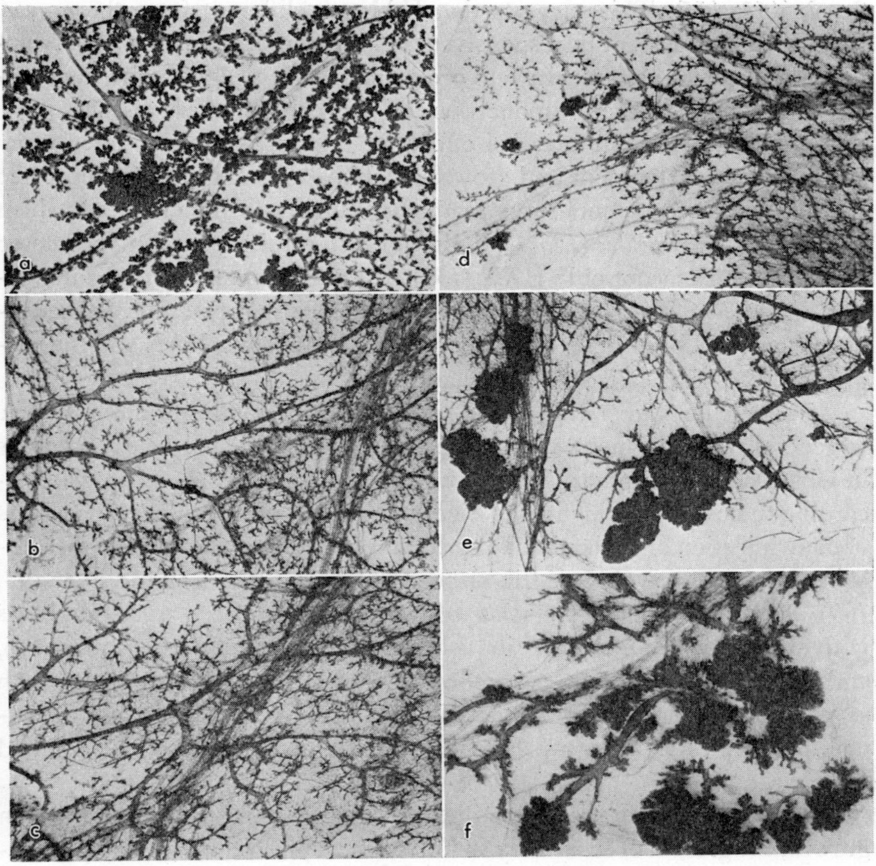

FIG. 2. Representative wholemount preparations of the third thoracic mammary glands of multiparous C3H/He strain of female mice stained with hematoxylin (×5)

(a) Intact control (8 months old); moderate lobulo-alveolar system with several HAN. (b) Mice given 0.2 mg ergocornine for 40 days (8 months old); lobulo-alveoli are scarce and there are no HAN. (c) Mice given 0.2 mg CB-154 for 40 days (8 months old); similar to b. (d) Ovx mice (10 months old); mammary glands are completely regressed. (e) Adx-ovx mice grafted with 3 pituitaries (8 months old); numerous HAN are seen, while normal glands remain regressed. (f) Ovx mice given twice daily injections of 0.5 mg HPL for 20 days (10 months old); similar to e.

While such replacement therapies as pituitary grafting and hormone injections were stimulatory to HAN, they did not always prevent the involution of the normal lobulo-alveolar system in ovx or adx-ovx mice (Fig.

2e, f) (*152*, *155*). This suggests that HAN are different from the normal lobulo-alveolar system in responsiveness to mammotropins, *i.e.*, HAN appear to be much more sensitive to prolactin or have a higher growth potential in response to the hormone than do normal mammary tissues.

Because of the suppressive effects of ergocornine and related ergot alkaloids on development and growth of HAN, these drugs also depressed the appearance of spontaneous mammary tumors in intact mice with or without pituitary grafts (*153*, *154*). By contrast, pituitary grafting promoted the appearance of not only HAN (*152*), but also mammary tumors in adx-ovx mice (*154*). These findings provide evidence that prolactin is the primary hormone for both the development of precancerous HAN and the progression of these lesions to malignancy.

Meanwhile, the *growth* of the spontaneous mammary tumors in mice is generally not hormone responsive, *i.e.*, is autonomous. In experiments in which paired mammary tumors were matched as closely as possible according to host body weight, site, size, and growth rate of tumors, no effects of daily injection of prolactin or of pituitary grafting on the growth of established tumors were observed in either C3H/He or Swiss albino mice (*93*, *109*). Mammary tumors transplanted from SHN and SLN mice into hosts with different hormonal conditions showed the same pattern of growth (*94*), and DNA synthesis of these tumors was not affected by treatments with several hormones (*158*). Differences in the metabolic characteristics of normal, preneoplastic, and neoplastic mammae in mice have also been studied (*1*).

While most spontaneous mammary tumors in mice are autonomous in growth, the growth of mammary tumors which appear during the reproductive periods in some strains of mice, mostly those originating in Europe (GR/A, RIII, BR6, *etc.*), is pregnancy-dependent. The tumors grow rapidly during the latter half of pregnancy, peak in size at the end of pregnancy and abruptly involute after parturition. Lactation affects little the growth pattern of this type of tumors. These tumors regrow during subsequent pregnancies and eventually some become autonomous. The specific hormones important in this process had not been known. Force-bred female mice of GR/A strain bearing palpable mammary tumors were given subcutaneous injections with several hormones singly or in combination from one day before till one day after parturition. One group of mice received grafts of 3 isologous pituitaries during days 12 and 14 of pregnancy. One day after parturition, DNA synthesis of normal and neoplastic mammary glands was examined. EB or pituitary grafts alone had no effects on the synthesis of either normal mammary glands or tumors, despite an increase in plasma prolactin levels. Progesterone significantly increased DNA synthesis of both normal and neoplastic glands when compared to the controls, while plasma prolactin levels remained low. The administration of progesterone and HPL in combination stimulated DNA synthesis of tumors more than progesterone alone, but not progesterone plus EB (*158*). Moreover, in ovx mice, progesterone was effective on mammary tumors, but had little effect on normal mammary glands during pregnancy (*160*). Correlations in DNA synthesis between normal mammary glands and pregnancy-dependent mammary tumors were statistically significant in mice treated with progesterone, either alone or in combination with EB or HPL (*158*). These results have demonstrated that pregnancy-dependent mammary tumors of GR/A mice are primarily progesterone responsive, although a synergistic enhancing action of estrogen or placental lactogen does appear to exist. They further suggest that pregnancy-dependent mammary tumors still retain the intrinsic biological characteristics of normal mammary glands, while there are some differences in hormone responsiveness between normal and neoplastic glands.

More than 74% of pregnancy-dependent mammary tumors in GR/A mice are diagnosed as mammary tumor type p, or plaques, about 13% as adenoacantoma or pale cell carcinoma and the remaining 13% as adenocarcinoma (*102*). When these tumors were transplanted into normal female athymic nude mice or females with subcutaneous pellet implants of progesterone, 30–40% of tumors were palpable in both groups by 30 weeks after transplantation and all were diagnosed as adenocarcinoma (Nagasawa, Yanai, and Morii, unpublished).

b) *Rats*

It has been established that anterior pituitary hormones are essential for mammary tumorigenesis. Regression of 7, 12-dimethylbenz [a] anthracene (DMBA)*-induced mammary tumors can be prevented by the administration of estrogen to adx-ovx rats, but not in hypophysectomized rats. Hypophysectomy has also been shown to prevent the induction of DMBA-induced mammary tumors by estrogen (*29*, *64*, *65*, *144*). These studies provided the impetus to determine the importance of prolactin or GH on the

* A single intragastric or intravenous administration of this carcinogen to about 50-day-old female rats (Sprague-Dawley rats are most effective) can induce mammary tumors at a high rate within 2–3 months after treatment. Most of the tumors induced are adenocarcinoma and are highly hormone responsive. This type of tumor is one of the most widely used as an animal model for human breast cancer.

development and growth of DMBA-induced mammary tumors in rats under the conditions of apparent absence of steroid hormones. Regression of mammary tumors by adx-ovx was completely prevented by daily injections with prolactin beginning on the day of adx-ovx. Moreover, a higher dose (2.5 mg×2/day) recovered the growth of tumors which had regressed most completely on 20 days after adx-ovx. On the other hand, GH had no effect on mammary tumors even at the dose which accelerated the growth of normal mammary glands and increased the body weight.

Depression by ergocornine of pituitary prolactin secretion also completely suppressed DMBA-induced mammary tumor growth and prevented the development of new tumors (*70*). In contrast, stimulation of pituitary prolactin secretion by an estrogen implant into the median eminence (*88*) or by hypothalamic lesions (*145*) resulted in the promotion of DMBA-induced (*71*) and spontaneous (*145*) mammary tumorigenesis. These results provide substantial evidence that prolactin is the principal hormone responsible for the development and growth of both carcinogen-induced and spontaneous mammary tumors in rats. In addition, HPL was found to stimulate DMBA-induced mammary tumors in a manner similar to prolactin (*81*). Acceleration of appearance and growth of mammary tumors during pregnancy may partly be ascribed to placental lactogen, acting both directly and indirectly through its promotion of progesterone secretion from the ovaries.

c) *Role of estrogen in mammary tumorigenesis*

The relation between prolactin and estrogen action on mammary tumors appears to be similar to that on normal mammary glands. An *optimal* amount of estrogen stimulates pituitary prolactin secretion and increases the response of mammary tumor cells to prolactin. The administration of prolactin or HPL prevents regression by adx-ovx of DMBA-induced mammary tumors, at least for a period of time. This was followed by tumor regression again, if the dose of the hormone had been small (*74*, *81*). Furthermore, DNA synthesis of DMBA-induced mammary tumors was more apparent after injection of estrogen than after pituitary grafting in adx-ovx rats, whereas there was little difference between these two treatments in their effects on serum prolactin level (*84*).

Large amounts of estrogen act antagonistically to prolactin and inhibit the growth-promoting effect of prolactin on mammary tumors despite the fact that large doses of the steroid stimulates pituitary prolactin secretion. Treatment with large doses of estrogen suppressed both growth and DNA synthesis of DMBA-induced mammary tumors, whereas circulating levels of prolactin were as high as those observed in treatment with smaller doses of the hormone. A further increase in blood prolactin by pituitary grafting, however, resulted in a counteraction of the inhibitory effects of large amounts of estrogen on mammary tumor growth (*77*, *84*).

d) *Pattern of estrous cycles in relation to mammary tumorigenesis*

The pattern of estrous cycles was examined in 3–4-month-old SHN and SLN female mice. SHN mice had much longer diestrous periods than SLN mice, while there were little differences in the length of the other stages of the cycle (*96*). Moreover, a distinct alteration in the pattern of estrous cycles from SHN-type to SLN-type was observed in highly inbred C3H/He females maintained by brother×sister mating without selection for mammary tumorigenesis. This was associated with a decrease in mammary tumor incidence (mammary tumor incidence in breeders were more than 90% until the 70th generation, but 0% at the 110th generation) (*90*, *96*). While the causality between the pattern of estrous cycles and mammary tumorigenesis is not clearly understood, it is plausible that the hormonal conditions which induce long diestrous periods may also be favorable for mammary tumorigenesis.

2) *Relation between growth of mammary tumors and prolactin in the circulation*

In view of the importance of prolactin in growth of mammary tumors in rats, the relation of serum prolactin levels to growth of DMBA-induced mammary tumors was studied (*89*). Beginning about 45 days DMBA injection and approximately at monthly intervals thereafter for a total of 165 days, serum prolactin levels were measured in rats. Although the average number and the size of mammary tumors increased with the advance of age, serum prolactin levels remained within normal ranges and did not change significantly from month to month, as observed in mice; there were no distinct differences between high and low mammary tumor strains of mice in pituitary prolactin secretion (Section 2–2–a). While athymic nu/nu female mice were inferior to controls (nu/+) with the same genetical background (BALB/c) in normal mammary growth, there were no significant differences between these groups in pituitary and plasma levels of prolactin (*87*).

In humans, although far from being conclusive, there does not appear to be a positive correlation between blood prolactin levels and the risk of developing breast cancers (*27*, *39*, *54*, *59*). There is an diurnal change as well as change with the menstrual cycle in pituitary prolactin secretion, so that studies based on measurement of one-time prolactin levels may reflect only one side of the situation.

3) Mammary tumor virus (MTV) and mammary tumorigenesis

General problems in this subject have been detailed in mice (*113*, *114*), monkeys (*16*) and humans (*21*, *22*, *126*).

We have established two strains of mice with different mammary tumorigenesis (SHN and SLN) from the same basal stock of Swiss albino. These mice are unrelated in origin to other strains with mammary tumors (*112*). F_1 females of (SHN×SLN) and (SLN×SHN) crosses were maintained as virgins and checked for palpable mammary tumors every 7 days. Mammary tumor incidences by 10 months of age were 58 and 7% in (SHN ×SLN) F_1 nursed by SHN and in (SLN×SHN) F_1 nursed by SLN, respectively. Because of the genetic identity and the same environmental conditions, the difference in mammary tumor incidence between the groups may be caused by a greater activity of MTV in SHN than in SLN; in other words, selection for mammary tumorigenesis resulted in a distinct difference in MTV activity. In this respect, genetic control of MTV transmission has recently been discussed (*38*).

4) Genetical predisposition and mammary tumorigenesis

The fact that many inbred strains of mice with different mammary tumorigenic potential have been established reflects clearly the significant influence of genetics in mammary tumorigenesis. Recently, the importance of the family history on human breast cancerogenesis has been stressed (*3*).

Two new strains of mice, SHN and SLN were established by selecting a Swiss albino stock to two ways. Currently, tumor incidence and age in multiparous SHN mice have been 100% and 6.6 months, respectively, and in SLN were 55.7% and 10.1 months, respectively. The number of tumors per mouse and growth potential of the tumors are also significantly higher in SHN than in SLN (*78*, *112*). SHN are different from SLN with regard to several characteristics related to mammary tumorigenesis, *e.g.*, normal and preneoplastic mammary growth, reproductivity, lactational performance, mammary sensitivity to pituitary mammotropin, activity of MTV (*112*) and the pattern of estrous cycles (*96*). Therefore, selection for mammary tumorigenic potential would be, in essence, selection of one or more of these related characteristics.

5) Relative importance of genotype and type of MTV on mammary tumorigenesis in mice

It is generally accepted that mammary tumorigenesis in mice is mainly controlled by factors such as hormones, genetic predisposition, MTV, immunity, *etc.*, and that these factors act synergistically or compensatorily rather than independently. However, the mechanism of their interrelations or their relative importance has been quite obscure. As one step to elucidate the relative importance of genotype and type of MTV in determining the biological and morphological characteristics of mammary tumors during reproductive states, mammary tumorigenesis was studied in force-bred mice of the following six groups, *i.e.*: GR/A, SHN, (GR×SHN) F_1, (SHN×GR) F_1, GR/A foster-nursed by SHN [GR/fSHN] and SHN foster-nursed by GR/A [SHN/fGR] (*102*) (Fig. 3). In GR/A, both F_1 hybrids and GR/fSHN, mammary tumor incidence by the 3rd pregnancy was 88–100%. All of these tumors were pregnancy-dependent, almost all were diagnosed as plaques or mammary tumor type p and they showed a similar hormone responsiveness (*158*). On the other hand, in SHN and SHN/fGR, mammary tumor incidence and percentage of pregnancy-dependent tumors were very low and most of these tumors were adenocar-

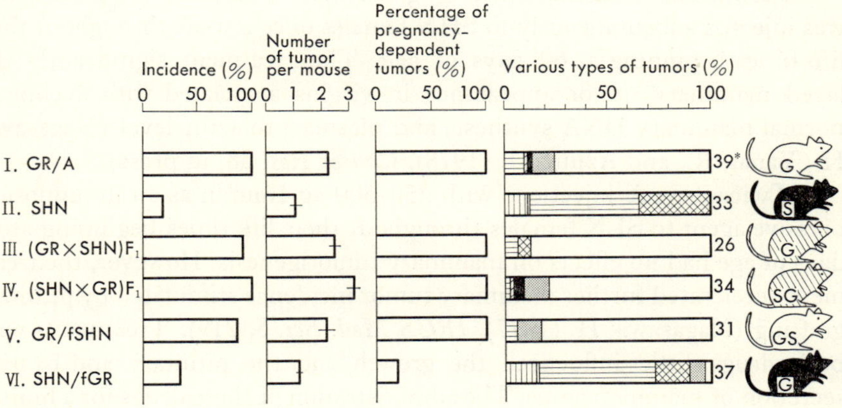

FIG. 3. Relation between genotype and type of mammary tumor virus (MTV) on incidence and number of mammary tumors, percentage of pregnancy-dependent tumors, and histological types of tumors at the third pregnancy in mice

▥ adenocarcinoma type A; ⊟ adenocarcinoma type B; ⊞ mixed type of A and B; ▨ adenocarcinoma type C; ■ adenoacantoma; ▒ pale cell carcinoma; □ mammary tumor type p and plaques. Genotype: GR/A; SHN; F_1 between SHN and GR/A. Type of MTV: G, GR/A; S, SHN. * Number of tumors examined.

cinomas. Numbers of tumors per mouse were 2.2–3.2 in GR/A, both F_1 hybrids and GR/fSHN mice and about 1 in SHN and SHN/fGR mice. Taking into consideration of the genotype(s) and type(s) of MTV of each group of mice (Fig. 3), it can be concluded that the relative importance of these factors for determining the biological and morphological characteristics of mammary tumors during the reproductive period in mice is in the order of GR/A genotype, SHN genotype, GR/A type of MTV and SHN type of MTV.

Recently, we found that introduction of SHN-MTV to SLN females and SLN-MTV to SHN females by foster-nursing pups immediately after birth had little influence on mammary tumorigenesis in virgins. The result would indicate again greater importance of genotype than MTV in mammary tumorigenesis (Nagasawa and Nakajima, unpublished).

6) Immuno-potentiation or -suppression and mammary tumorigenesis

Based on the recent emphasis of the importance of the immune mechanism on mammary tumorigenesis both experimental and clinical (*10*, *33*, *56*), the effects of immuno-potentiation or -suppression on spontaneous mammary tumorigenesis in mice have been studied.

For immunopotentiation, 100 μg cell wall skeleton of *Nocardia rubra* was injected subcutaneously to SHN females once a week throughout their life times beginning at 60 days of age. The treatment significantly delayed mammary tumor appearance in virgins associated with decline in normal mammary DNA synthesis and plasma prolactin level (Nagasawa, H., Yanai, R., and Azuma, I. (1978). *Cancer Res.* **38**, in press).

Twice-a-week injections with 250–500 μg Imuran as an immunosuppressive agent to SLN females throughout their life times beginning at 60 days of age had no effects on mammary tumorigenesis. However, the treatment accelerated further mammary tumor incidence stimulated by pituitary grafting (Nagasawa, H. (1977). *IRCS Med. Sci.* **5**, 219). Treatments with both drugs little influenced the growth and the pituitary and ovarian secretion of mammotropins. The administration of these drugs for a limited period of 2–5 months of age had no effect on mammary tumorigenesis.

7) Number and growth of autonomous and spontaneous mammary tumors in mice

In both breeders and virgins of C3H/He strain, nearly 90% of mice had only one tumor in their lifetimes (*78*). While 4 was the maximal number of tumors in breeders of both SHN and SLN strains, more than 70% of

SHN breeders had multiple tumors and about 60% of SLN breeders had only a single tumor. In virgin females, more than 40% of SHN had 3 or 4 tumors, but all SLN had only 1 or 2 tumors (*112*).

In SHN virgins, spontaneous mammary tumors which appeared first increased in size linearly until 4–6 weeks after appearance. Average tumor sizes were about 10 and 20 mm by weeks 2 and 6, respectively. The tumors which appeared later showed the same pattern of growth. The growth of the first tumors was retarded by the appearance of the second tumors in breeders, but not in virgins in either C3H/He or SHN strain (*78*, *112*).

No difference was observed between SHN and SLN in the growth of spontaneous mammary tumors. Mammary tumors transplanted into hosts from the respective strains showed also the same growth patterns in both strains. However, SHN tumors became palpable one week after transplantation, two weeks earlier than SLN tumors, indicating a strain-difference in "take" of the transplanted tumors (*94*). Furthermore, SHN tumors were superior to SLN tumors in both "take" and growth when transplanted into common hosts, athymic female nude mice (Nagasawa, Yanai, and Morii, unpublished). These findings show the intrinsic higher growth potential of mammary tumors in SHN than in SLN.

As detailed in Section 3–1–a, mammary tumors of GR/A mice which appear during the reproductive periods are generally benign and pregnancy-dependent. On the other hand, tumors which develop after retirement or in virgins are malignant and autonomous in growth. The patterns of development and growth of these different types of tumors in GR/A mice and their interrelationships were studied (*161*). Female GR/A mice were mated at 60–70 days of age and were subjected to concurrent pregnancy until the 3rd pregnancy. Mammary tumor incidences were 58% and 100% at the 1st and the 2nd pregnancies, respectively, all of which were pregnancy-dependent for growth. Meanwhile, after the 3rd parturition, 3.9% of the pregnancy-dependent mammary tumors progressed to autonomy. All tumors which developed after cessation of breeding were autonomous and the incidence and the onset age of these tumors were more than 90% and about 11 months, respectively. Approximately 30% of tumors which appeared and regressed during the reproductive periods recurred once again after retirement. These tumors were autonomous and represented 37% of the total number of tumors which developed after retirement. Incidence and age of mammary tumors in virgin females of GR/A strain were 100% and 13.8 months, respectively, and these tumors were also completely autonomous in growth. Whereas 74% of pregnancy-dependent mammary tumors

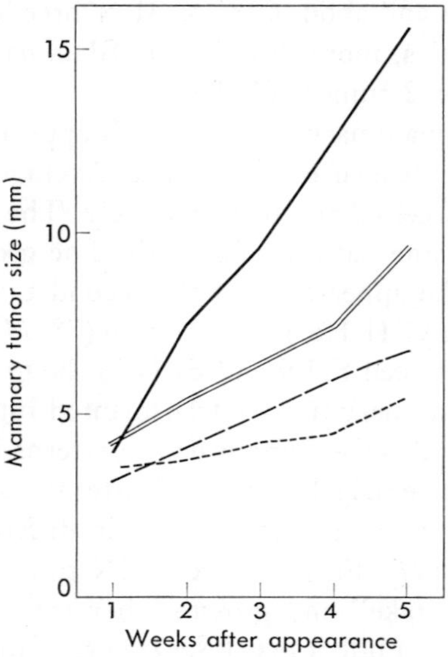

FIG. 4. Growth curves of several types of autonomous mammary tumors in mice

—— SHN (breeding) (35); ═══ GR (retired) (19); - - - GR (virgins) (19); ······ GR (recurred after retirement). Numerals in parentheses show number of tumors examined.

were histologically classified as plaques and mammary tumor type p, 88 and 100% of the autonomous tumors in retired and virgin females were diagnosed as carcinomas similar to those of SHN. On the other hand, the growth rates of these autonomous tumors in GR/A mice were much slower than those in SHN (Fig. 4), suggesting the no parallelism between the structure and the biological characteristics of mammary tumors.

8) Importance of primiparous age and litter number on mammary tumor age in mice

In mice spontaneous mammary tumors generally develop earlier and more frequently in breeders than in virgins. This is attributable to a more conspicuous multiplication of MTV, stimulated secretion of pituitary and ovarian mammotropins and resultant marked growth of the mammary glands, especially of the lobulo-alveolar system, during repetition of pregnancy. On the other hand, even during virginal periods, MTV and mammotropins may continuously influence mammary growth and, in its turn, mammary tumorigenesis. The relative importance of the primiparous age (the virginal period) and the litter number on mammary age (the onset age of mammary tumors) were, therefore, studied (*69*, *91*). A partial correlation coefficient between the primiparous age and mammary tumor age when the litter number was fixed and that between litter number and tumor age when primiparous age was fixed were both positive and statistically highly significant. These results indicate the significant role of both primiparous age and litter number in determining mammary tumor age. The relative importances of these two factors and the rest factors were calculated according to the principle of path coefficient (*130*). The relative importances of primiparous age, litter number and the rest factors were 27.4, 45.8, and 26.8%, respectively in C3H/He and 17.2, 43.8, and 39.1%, respectively in Swiss albino. This shows that litter number is the most important factor for determining the tumor age and that more than 60% of the variations of tumor age is dependent upon both the primiparous age and litter number. In this study, litter number means only the number of deliveries, and other reproductive factors such as litter size, rearing and/or lactational performance of mothers and the accompanying mammary gland functions, *etc.*, are all involved in the other factors. The rest factors also include individual differences in the multiplication of MTV, in genetic predisposition and further in all other intangible factors. Nevertheless, the rest factors play a less important role in determining mammary tumor age than do the other two factors, *i.e.*, the primiparous age and litter number (number of deliveries). The importance of the number of deliveries may partly reflect the importance of mammary DNA synthesis, which is very conspicuous during pregnancy in mice, in mammary tumorigenesis. This problem will be discussed in Section 5.

4. *Longterm effects of perinatal treatments with hormones and drugs on normal and abnormal mammary growth*

It has been recognized that, when certain hormones are administered to pregnant mothers, an abnormality of the hypothalamus-pituitary-gonadal system occurs in their offspring, which brings about irreversible and deleterious changes in their target organs. An example in humans is an increased incidence and an earlier onset of malignant as well as benign lesions of the vagina and uterine cervix in women whose mothers received diethylstilbestrol (DES) during pregnancy, especially during its early stages (*31*). This clinical phenomenon is in accordance with a number of earlier studies on experimental animals (*7*, *8*, *134*).

Quite similarly, neonatal treatments with estradiol-17β (*47*, *67*, *107*), progesterone (*47*) or testosterone (*67*, *107*) resulted in the stimulation of normal, preneoplastic and neoplastic mammary growth in BALB/cfC3H female mice with MTV. The experimental animals showed constant estrous vaginal smears and their ovaries consisted only of anovulatory follicles. Plasma prolactin levels in these mice were generally higher than those in the controls (*107*). Even 5β-dihydrotestosterone, which is biologically inactive in the adult, was also found to induce similar abnormalities at advanced ages in SHN female mice, if administered prenatally or neonatally (*162*). On the other hand, such treatments in mice without MTV (BALB/c and C57BL) stimulated normal mammary growth, but not preneoplastic and neoplastic mammary growth at all (*67*, *107*), indicating the necessity of MTV for neoplastic mammary response to neonatal steroid hormone treatment. Neonatal administration of prolactin altered little either mammary growth or pituitary prolactin secretion in mice (*67*, *107*).

In contrast, neonatal treatments of rats with estradiol-17β, testosterone, or prolactin suppressed DMBA-induced mammary tumorigenesis, despite the observation that these treatments induced a constant vaginal estrus, an anovulatory syndrome and further increased secretion of prolactin, luteinizing hormone (LH) (*103*, *104*), and estrogen (*111*).

Neonatal administration of ethamoxytriphetol (MER-25), an antiestrogen, resulted in an increased incidence of HAN and mammary tumors and stimulated pituitary prolactin secretion in SHN female mice. Conversely, the administration of CB-154 to pregnant mothers (prenatal treatment) delayed mammary tumor appearance in their female offspring. (Nagasawa, H. and Yanai, R. (1978). *J. Endocr. Invest.* **1**, in press). Prenatal MER-25 treatment or neonatal CB-154 treatment had little affect on mammary growth.

The administration of monosodium glutamate (MSG) and related substances has been shown to induce acute degeneration of hypothalamic neurons in neonatal and fetal rodents (*116*) and infant monkeys (*115*) and sometime induces obesity at advanced ages. A single subcutaneous injection of 4 mg MSG to 1-day-old female mice resulted in marked and irreversible suppression of normal and preneoplastic mammary growth and a decrease in the pituitary contents of prolactin and GH (*97*). Pregnancy-dependent mammary tumorigenesis in GR/A mice was also inhibited by the same treatment associated with no alteration in reproductive ability (Nagasawa, H. and Yanai, R. (1978). *Proc. Soc. Exp. Biol. Med.* **158**, 128–129).

Perinatal hypothyroidism induced by 6-propyl-2-thiouracil feeding also persistently depressed the pituitary secretion of prolactin and GH in female and male rats (*50*).

The long-term effects of these hormones and drugs on normal and neoplastic mammary growth will vary according to dosage, age of the treated subjects and duration of treatment. Clinically, care and concern should be exercised over needless or excessive use of hormones and drugs during pregnancy, particularly at stages when the development of the central nervous system is maximal.

5. Mammary DNA Synthesis as an Important Factor for Mammary Tumorigenesis

The relationship between frequency of cell division and tumorigenesis has been inferred experimentally and clinically. However, little systematic information is available on this problem. In this section, experimental results on the rate of mammary DNA synthesis under different environmental conditions will briefly be reviewed and the dependency of mammary tumorigenesis on DNA synthesis will be discussed. The reader can refer to a more detailed account of this problem in Ref. *68*.

The age of the animal is critical for the induction of mammary tumors in rats by polycyclic aromatic hydrocarbons such as DMBA and 3-methylcholanthrene. Mammary tumors in rats can be induced by the administration of a carcinogen at 23 days of age. Tumor incidence reaches a maximum if the carcinogen is administered at 50–60 days of age, after which tumor incidence abruptly declines. The cause of this age-dependency of carcinogen-induced mammary tumorigenesis in rats was quite obscure. We have examined the changes with age in: (a) normal mammary development by wholemount preparations; (b) plasma prolactin levels on the afternoon of proestrus by radioimmunoassay, and (c) mammary DNA synthesis by the *in vitro* incorporation of [^{3}H] thymidine into mammary DNA (*83*). While mammary gland rating and plasma prolactin levels were significantly lower in 30-day-old rats when compared to 70-, 90-, and 110-day-old rats, mammary DNA synthesis increased from 30 to 50 days of age, then abruptly decreased. These changes correlated very well with the changes in carcinogen-induced mammary tumorigenesis; mammary tumor incidence was the greatest when the carcinogen was administered at 50 days of age, the time when mammary DNA synthesis is maximal.

Carcinogen-induced mammary tumorigenesis in rats is inhibited if prolactin secretion is increased prior to carcinogen treatment (*144*). An explanation has been proposed by studies showing that mammary DNA synthesis was lowered by several treatments which stimulate pituitary prolactin secretion or increase prolactin levels in the circulation. For instance, mammary DNA synthesis of rats grafted with pituitaries was less than half that of the controls after 20 days of grafting, while these rats showed plasma prolactin levels similar to those at PE, and greater mammary growth than the control (*83*). This is attributable to the differentiation, hypertrophy and mitotic rest of mammary cells following proliferation stimulated by prolactin from the grafts. All emphasize that mammary DNA synthesis at the time of carcinogen action on the glands may be a limiting factor for the induction of mammary tumors by a carcinogen.

In order to elucidate further the relationship between mammary DNA synthesis and mammary tumorigenesis, the effects of factors which promote or inhibit spontaneous mammary tumorigenesis, *i.e.*, pituitary grafts and CB-154, on mammary DNA synthesis in mice have been studied (*159*). The administration of CB-154 to C3H/He female mice resulted in an inhibition of the rise of mammary DNA synthesis which is normally seen at PE. In contrast, mammary DNA synthesis was significantly increased by pituitary grafting when compared with that of the control at PE. These results again show the close relationship of mammary DNA synthesis to not only carcinogen-induced but also spontaneous mammary tumorigenesis.

These results imply that one role of prolactin in mammary tumorigenesis is, *via* its stimulation of mammary DNA synthesis, to create mammary gland conditions favorable for the action of carcinogenic factors. To test this hypothesis, mammary DNA synthesis and mammary tumorigenesis were examined in a high mammary tumor strain of SHN female mice given 2 isologous pituitaries each at 20–23 days of age (*100*). While there were no significant differences in mammary tumor incidence between mice with pituitary grafts and the controls (96 and 89%, respectively), mammary tumor age was significantly reduced in the former when compared with the latter (5.9 and 8.9 months, respectively). Moreover, the variation of mammary tumor age was reduced to about one-half by the pituitary grafts. Mammary DNA synthesis at 70 days of age varied between 120 and 400 dpm/μg DNA and between 13 and 710 dpm/μg DNA, mostly less than 120 dpm/μg DNA, in the experimental and control groups, respectively. It can be concluded from these findings that marked reduction in both mammary tumor age and its variability by pituitary grafting is ascribed to the continuous promotion of mammary DNA synthesis by prolactin from the grafts.

Our next study was to determine the relationship, if any, between mammary DNA synthesis and protection by pregnancy and lactation of mammary tumorigenesis (*72*). Mammary tumorigenesis in rats is facilitated when the administration of carcinogen precedes pregnancy, however, it decreases when the carcinogen exposure occurs during pregnancy. In virgin rats at 55–60 days of age, mammary DNA synthesis increases from D2 and shows peak activity on the afternoon of E followed by a gradual decrease. This pattern also occurs in 80–90-day-old rats except that no difference exists in DNA synthesis between PE and D2. This cyclic mammary DNA synthesis pattern appears to persist throughout the fertile life of female rats. In contrast, mammary DNA synthesis during pregnancy peaks on day 6 and abruptly decreases thereafter, exceeding that observed at E only during the first one-third of pregnancy. The average values on days 18 and 22 of pregnancy are less than 1/3 and 1/5 of the value at E, respectively. Thus, if the carcinogen is administered after the first one-third of pregnancy, the incidence of mammary tumors would be expected to decrease sharply when compared with incidence from administration during the virginal period, based on the hypothesis which predicts a positive relationship between mammary DNA synthesis and mammary tumorigenesis.

Normal or prolonged lactation in mice and rats is also recognized to result in a decrease in the incidence of spontaneous or carcinogen-induced mammary tumors and an increase in tumor age when compared with forced breeding without subsequent lactation. In accordance, mammary DNA synthesis is at a very low level during lactation in mice (*86*) and rats (*72*). These observations in experimental animals showing protection by pregnancy and lactation against mammary tumorigenesis and its relationship to mammary DNA synthesis may have some bearing on the etiology of human breast cancer (*72*).

Early pregnancy followed by full-term birth in humans reduces the risk of breast cancer; the risk of women who experience pregnancy while younger than 18 years of age is about one-third of that of women who first deliver at 35 years or older (*17*, *32*, *57*). A reduced risk of breast cancer has also been observed in lactating women, although recent reports have provided evidence to the contrary (*17*, *57*). A similarity may exist between rats and humans in mammary growth pattern (DNA synthesis) and subsequent mammary tumorigenesis. Under the influence of follicular estrogen, breast parenchymal growth and DNA synthesis in humans are stimulated, reaching a peak at midcycle. Breast proliferative mitotic activity is reduced to baseline values toward the end of the cycle. Only during the first trimester of pregnancy, breast parenchymal growth and DNA synthesis are pronounced. The latter half of pregnancy is the period of proliferative and mitotic rest and breast parenchyma shows only minor DNA synthesis.

Both animals and humans are constantly exposed to carcinogenic agents during their life times. It is conceivable, therefore, that the longer the total period of low mammary DNA synthesis, *i.e.*, proliferative mitotic rest, owing to pregnancy, lactation, *etc.*, the smaller is the risk of mammary malignancy. In contrast, when malignant mammary foci exist before pregnancy, their growth may be accelerated during subsequent pregnancy, resulting in earlier and more frequent appearance of tumors. An analogous condition is observed in women in late pregnancy in whom the risk of breast cancer is greater than in nulliparous women of similar age (*17*, *57*). It is probable that decreased risk in early pregnancy is involved in tumor *initiation* and the increased risk in late pregnancy is related to *promotion* of the growth of transformed cells.

Experimental results showing a close relationship between DNA synthesis and mammary tumorigenesis provide the impetus to explore the possibility of preventing or inhibiting mammary tumorigenesis by suppressing mammary DNA synthesis. To examine this possibility, mammary tumorigenesis in rats with different rates of mammary DNA synthesis at the time of carcinogen administration was studied (*99*). At 50 days of age, mammary DNA synthesis is significantly higher at PE than D2. In accordance, mammary tumorigenesis was greater in animals given the carcinogen at PE than in the animals given it at D2. Inhibition by CB-154 of the rise in mammary DNA synthesis at PE also suppressed carcinogen-induced mammary tumorigenesis. Meanwhile, at 90 days of age, when little difference was found in mammary DNA synthesis between PE and D2, there were no significant differences in mammary tumorigenesis between animals receiving the carcinogen at PE and D2. Intravenous injection with the carcinogen 24 hr after a single injection of prolactin, when mammary DNA synthesis peaked, resulted in a stimulation of mammary tumorigenesis. All results have demonstrated a dependency of carcinogen-induced mammary tumorigenesis upon optimal mammary DNA synthesis. They also suggest that inhibition or prophylaxis of mammary tumorigenesis could be possible by reducing mammary DNA synthesis for only limited periods during the lifetime. Most recently, experimental results supporting this hypothesis have been obtained in our laboratory (Yanai and Nagasawa, unpublished). The incidence of pregnancy-dependent mammary tumors in GR/A female mice mated at 60 days of age, after receiving daily injections with 0.2 mg CB-154 for 10 days between 35 and 45 days of age, was 0% at first pregnancy, whereas that of the untreated control was 40%.

SUMMARY

The reliance of several methods for evaluating mammary growth was described and the importance of mammary DNA synthesis, which represents the dynamic aspect of mammary proliferation, was stressed (Section 1).

Growth pattern of normal mammary glands and the factors concerned were discussed from the view point that normal mammary growth is a preceding and a essential step for mammary tumorigenesis (Section 2).

Kinetics of development and growth of spontaneous and carcinogen-induced mammary tumors and factors concerned were discussed (Section 3).

Irreversible alteration in pituitary and ovarian hormone secretion and in mammary growth induced by perinatal treatment with hormones and drugs were discussed and the caution against the use of them during pregnancy has again been claimed (Section 4).

Finally the significance of mammary DNA synthesis in mammary tumorigenesis was studied and the possibility of protection of mammary tumorigenesis by reducing mammary DNA synthesis has been inferred (Section 5).

Acknowledgments

This paper is dedicated to the memory of the late Dr. Waro Nakahara, the former President of the National Cancer Center, Tokyo, in recognition of his constant encouragement and support.

We thank Dr. Clifford W. Welsch, Department of Anatomy, Michigan State University, East Lansing, Michigan, USA, for reading the original manuscript and for valuable comments.

Research done in our laboratory was partly supported by grants-in-aid for Cancer Research from the Ministry of Health and Welfare, the Ministry of Education, Science and Culture, and the Society for Promotion of Cancer Research, Japan.

A portion of this research was done during the tenures of Dr. H. Nagasawa as a Postdoctoral Research Training Fellow, International Agency for Research on Cancer (IARC), World Health Organization (WHO) (R.215, 1968–1969) at Department of Physiology, Michigan State University, East Lansing, Michigan,

USA (Prof. J. Meites) and as a Travel Fellow, IARC, WHO (T. 885, 1974) at Cancer Research Laboratory, University of California, Berkeley, California, USA (Prof. H. A. Bern and Prof. S. Nandi).

REFERENCES

1. Abraham, S. and Bartley, J. C. (1974). Comparison among the metabolic characteristics of normal, preneoplastic, and neoplastic mammary tissue. In *Hormones and Cancer*, ed. McKerns, K. W., pp. 29–74. New York, London: Academic Press.
2. Anderson, R. R. (1974). Endocrinological control. In *Lactation: A Comprehensive Treatise*, vol. I, ed. Larson, B. L. and Smith, V. R., pp. 97–140. New York, London: Academic Press.
3. Anderson, D. E. (1976). Genetic predisposition to breast cancer. In *Breast Cancer: A Multidisciplinary Approach*, ed. St-Arneault, G., Band, P., and Israël, L., pp. 10–20. Berlin, Heiderberg, New York: Springer-Verlag.
4. Barfknecht, C. F., Rusterholz, D. B., and Parsons, J. A. (1974). Inhibition of prolactin by ergoline congeners. *J. Med. Chem.* **17**, 308–312.
5. Baulieu, Etienne-Emile (1976). Steroid receptors and hormone receptibility: New approaches in pharmacology and therapeutics. In *Breast Cancer: Trends in Research and Treatment*, ed. Heuson, J. C., Mattheiem, W. H., and Rosencweig, M., pp. 165–176. New York: Raven Press.
6. Ben-David, M. and Heston, W. E. (1969). Mammary tumor virus potentiation of endogenous prolactin effect on mammary gland differentiation. *J. Natl. Cancer Inst.* **42**, 207–218.
7. Bern, H. A., Jones, L. A., Mori, T., and Young, P. N. (1975). Exposure of neonatal mice to steroids: Longterm effects on the mammary gland and other reproductive structures. *J. Steroid Biochem.* **6**, 673–676.
8. Bern, H. A., Jones, L. A., Mills, K. T., Kohrman, A., and Mori, T. (1976). Use of the neonatal mouse in studying longterm effects of early exposure to hormones and other agents. *J. Toxicol. Environ. Health* Suppl. **1**, 103–116.
9. Bruchovsky, N. and Van Doorn, E. (1976). Steroid receptor proteins and regulation of growth in mammary tumors. In *Breast Cancer: A Multidisciplinary Approach*, ed. St-Arneault, G., Band, P., and Israël, L., pp. 121–142. Berlin, Heiderberg, New York: Springer-Verlag.
10. Brennan, M. J. (1976). Murine and rat mammary tumors as models for the immunological study of human breast cancer. *Cancer Res.* **36**, 728–733.
11. Bulbrook, R. D. (1974). Hormonal factors in mammary carcinogenesis. In *Characterization of Human Tumors*, vol. 1, ed. Davis, W. and Maltoni, C., pp. 178–187. Amsterdam: Excerpta Medica.
12. Bulbrook, R. D., Wang, D. Y., and Swain, M. C. (1972). Prolactin and

breast cancer. In *Prolactin and Carcinogenesis*, ed. Boyns, A. R. and Griffiths, K., pp. 143–153. Cardiff: Alpha Omega Alpha.

13. Cassady, J. M., Li, G. S., Spitzner, E. B., Floss, H. G., and Clemens, J. A. (1973). Ergot alkaloids. Ergolines and related compounds as inhibitors of prolactin release. *J. Med. Chem.* **17**, 300–301.
14. Ceriani, R. L. (1974). Hormone and other factors controlling growth in the mammary gland: A review. *J. Invest. Dermatol.* **63**, 93–108.
15. Chemama, R., Jayle, M. F., and Ennuyer, A. (1974). Treatment by progestin-oestrogen-corticosteroid combination. In *Mammary Cancer and Neuroendocrine Therapy*, ed. Stoll, B. A., pp. 265–282. London: Butterworths.
16. Chopra, H. C. (1976). An oncorna-type virus from monkey breast tumor. *Prog. Med. Virol.* **22**, 104–122.
17. Cole, P. (1974). Epidemiology of human breast cancer. *J. Invest. Dermatol.* **63**, 133–137.
18. Cowie, A. T. (1974). Hormonal factors in mammary development and lactation. In *Mammary Cancer and Neuroendocrine Therapy*, ed. Stoll, B. A., pp. 3–24. London: Butterworths.
19. Cutler, S. J., Devesa, S. S., and Barclay, T.H.C. (1976). The magnitude of the breast cancer. In *Breast Cancer: A Multidisciplinary Approach*, ed. St-Arneault, G., Band, P., and Israël, L., pp. 1–9. Berlin, Heiderberg, New York: Springer-Verlag.
20. Dao, T. L. and Sinha, D. (1972). Oestrogen and prolactin in mammary carcinogenesis *in vivo* and *in vitro* studies. In *Prolactin and Carcinogenesis*, ed. Boyns, A. R. and Griffiths, K., pp. 189–199. Cardiff: Alpha Omega Alpha.
21. Dmochowski, L. (1973). The viral factor in the genesis of breast cancer: Present evidence. *Triangle* **12**, 37–47.
22. Dmochowski, L. (1973). Studies on the interrelationship of type B and type C virus particles in breast cancer and in leukemia. *Unifying Concepts of Leukemia. Bibliotheca Haematologica* No. 39, 45–60.
23. Floss, H. G., Cassady, J. M., and Robbers, J. E. (1973). Influence of ergot alkaloids on pituitary prolactin and prolactin-dependent process. *J. Pharmacol. Sci.* **62**, 699–715.
24. Flückiger, E. W. (1978). Lactation inhibition by ergot drugs. This volume, pp. 71–82.
25. Forsyth, I. A. (1974). The comparative study of placental lactogenic hormones: A review. In *Lactogenic Hormones, Fetal Nutrition and Lactation*, ed. Josimovich, J. B., pp. 49–67. New York, London, Sydney, Toronto: John Willey and Sons.
26. Fotherby, K. (1974). Pituitary gonadotrophin production and breast cancer. In *Mammary Cancer and Neuroendocrine Therapy*, ed. Stoll, B. A., pp. 123–135. London: Butterworths.
27. Franks, S., Ralphs, D.N.L., Seagroatt, V., and Jacobs, H. S. (1974). Prolactin

concentrations in patients with breast cancer. *Br. Med. J.* **4**, 320–321.

28. Friesen, H. G. (1976). The role of prolactin in breast cancer. In *Breast Cancer: A Multidisciplinary Approach*, ed. St-Arneault, G., Band, P., and Israël, L., pp. 143–149. Berlin, Heiderberg, New York: Springer-Verlag.
29. Furth, J. (1973). The role of prolactin in mammary carcinogenesis. In *Human Prolactin*, ed. Pasteels, J. L. and Robyn, C., pp. 233–248. Amsterdam: Excerpta Medica.
30. Furth, J. (1975). Hormones as etiological agents in neoplasia. In *Cancer*, vol. 1, ed. Becker, F. F., pp. 75–120. New York: Plenum.
31. Herbst, A. L., Poskanzer, D. C., Robboy, S. J., Friedlander, L., and Scully, R. E. (1975). Prenatal exposure to stilbestrol: A prospective comparison of exposed female offsprings with unexposed controls. *New Engl. J. Med.* **292**, 334–339.
32. Henderson, B. E., Powell, D., Rosario, I., Keys, C., Hanisch, R., Young, M., Casagrande, J., Gerkins, V., and Pike, M. C. (1974). An epidemiologic study of breast cancer. *J. Natl. Cancer Inst.* **53**, 609–614.
33. Heppner, G. H. (1976). Immunology: Breast cancer. In *Breast Cancer: A Multidisciplinary Approach*, ed. St-Arneault, G., Band, P., and Israël, L., pp. 95–108. Berlin, Heiderberg, New York: Springer-Verlag.
34. Heuson, J. C. (1974). The role of prolactin inhibition in treatment. In *Mammary Cancer and Neuroendocrine Therapy*, ed. Stoll, B. A., pp. 349–368. London: Butterworths.
35. Heuson, J. C., Legros, N., Heuson-Stiennon, J. A., Leclercq, G., and Pasteels, J. L. (1976). Hormone dependency of rat mammary tumors. In *Breast Cancer: Trends in Research and Treatment*, ed. Heuson, J. C., Mattheiem, W. H., and Rozencweig, M., pp. 81–93. New York: Raven Press.
36. Hilf, R. (1972). Mammary tumor growth and biochemistry as influenced by prolactin. In *Prolactin and Carcinogenesis*, ed. Boyns, A. R. and Griffiths, K., pp. 181–188. Cardiff: Alpha Omega Alpha.
37. Hilf, R. and Wittliff, J. L. (1974). Characterizations of human breast cancer by examination of cytoplasmic activities and estrogen receptors. In *Hormones and Cancer*, ed. McKerns, K. W., pp. 103–130. New York, London: Academic Press.
38. Hilgers, J. and Bentvelzen, P. (1976). Interaction between viral and genetic factors in murine mammary cancer: Possible implication for human disease. In *Breast Cancer: Trends in Research and Treatment*, ed. Heuson, J. C., Mattheiem, W. H., and Rozencweig, M., pp. 3–9. New York: Raven Press.
39. Hill, P., Wyder, E. L., Kuwar, H., Helman, P., Rona, G., and Kuno, K. (1976). Prolactin levels in population at risk of breast cancer. *Cancer Res.* **36**, 4102–4106.
40. Hobbs, J. R., Barrett, A., De Souza, I., Morgan, L., Raggatt, P., and Salih, H. (1975). Selection of antihormonal therapy of some cancers. In *Host De-*

fence against Cancer and Its Potentiation, ed. Mizuno, D., Chihara, G., Fukuoka, F., Yamamoto, T., and Yamamura, Y., pp. 435–443. Tokyo, Baltimore: Japan Sci. Soc. Press, Univ. Park Press.

41. Hollmann, K. H. (1974). Cytology and fine structure of the mammary gland. In *Lactation. A Comprehensive Treatise*, vol. 1, ed. Larson, B. L., and Smith, V. R., pp. 3–95. New York, London: Academic Press.
42. Horrobin, D. F. (1973). *Prolactin, Physiology and Clinical Siqnificance*. St. Leonardgate: MTP Medical and Technical Publ.
43. Horrobin, D. F. (1974). *Prolactin* 1974. St. Leonardgate: MTP Medical and Technical Publ.
44. Horrobin, D. F. (1975). *Prolactin* 1975. Montreal: Eden Press.
45. Horrobin, D. F. (1976). *Prolactin* 1976. Montreal: Eden Press.
46. Jensen, H. M. and Wellings, S. R. (1976). Preneoplastic lesions of the human mammary gland transplanted into the nude athymic mouse. *Cancer Res.* **36**, 2605–2610.
47. Jones, L. and Bern, H. A. (1977). Long-term effects of neonatal treatment with progesterone, alone and in combination with estrogen, on the mammary gland and reproductive tract of female BALB/cfC3H mice. *Cancer Res.* **37**, 67–75.
48. Juret, P. and Hayem, M. (1974). Pituitary ablation in the treatment of breast cancer. In *Mammary Cancer and Neuroendocrine Therapy*, ed. Stoll, B. A., pp. 283–311. London: Butterworths.
49. Kennedy, B. J. (1974). Hormonal therapies in breast cancer. *Semin. Oncol.* **1**, 119–130.
50. Kikuyama, S., Nagasawa, H., Yanai, R., and Yamanouchi, K. (1974). Effect of perinatal hypothyroidism on pituitary secretion of growth hormone and prolactin in rats. *J. Endocrinol.* **62**, 213–223.
51. Kim, U. and Furth, J. (1976). The role of prolactin in carcinogenesis. *Vitam. Horm.* **34**, 107–136.
52. Kohmoto, K. and Sakai, S. (1978). Prolactin receptors in the mammary gland. This volume, pp. 231–248.
53. Kratochwil, K. (1975). Experimental analysis of the prenatal development of the mammary gland. In *Milk and Lactation*, ed. Kretchmer, N., Bern, E. R., and Milan, F. S., pp. 1–15. Basel, München, Paris, New York, Sydney: S. Karger.
54. Kwa, H. G., Cleton, F., De Jong-Bakker, M., Bulbrook, R. D., Hayward, J. L., and Wang, D. Y. (1976). Plasma prolactin and its relationship to risk factors in human breast cancer. *Int. J. Cancer* **17**, 441–447.
55. Lippman, M. (1976). Hormone-responsive human breast cancer in continuous tissue culture. In *Breast Cancer: Trends in Research and Treatment*, ed. Heuson, J. C., Mattheiem, W. H., and Rozencweig, M., pp. 111–139. New York: Raven Press.

56. Lucas, Z. J. (1976). Immune response to a syngeneic rat mammary adenocarcinoma. In *Breast Cancer: Trends in Research and Treatment*, ed. Heuson, J. C., Mattheiem, W. H., and Rozencweig, M., pp. 59–74. New York: Raven Press.
57. MacMahon, B., Cole, P., and Brown, J. (1973). Etiology of human breast cancer: A review. *J. Natl. Cancer Inst.* **50**, 21–42.
58. McGuire, W. L., Horwitz, K. B., and De La Garza, M. (1976). A biochemical basis for selecting endocrine therapy in human breast cancer. In *Breast Cancer: Trends in Research and Treatment*, ed. Heuson, J. C., Mattheiem, W. H., and Rozencweig, M., pp. 177–184. New York: Raven Press.
59. McGuire, W. L. (1977). Prolactin and breast cancer. In *Prolactin and Human Reproduction*, ed. Crosignani, P. G., and Robyn, C., pp. 143–151. New York, London: Academic Press.
60. Medina, D. (1975). Biologic characteristics of tumor regression in the mouse mammary gland. *Cancer Chemother. Rep.* **5** (Part 2), 127–131.
61. Medina, D. (1975). Tumor progression. In *Cancer*, vol. 3, ed. Becker, F. F., pp. 99–119. New York: Plenum.
62. Medina, D. (1976). Preneoplastic lesions in murine mammary cancer. *Cancer Res.* **36** (Part 2), 2589–2595.
63. Medina, D. (1976). Mammary gland as a morphological end point in carcinogenesis studies. *J. Toxicol. Environ. Health* Suppl. **1**, 551–560.
64. Meites, J. (1972). Relation of prolactin and estrogen to mammary tumorigenesis in the rat. *J. Natl. Cancer Inst.* **48**, 1217–1224.
65. Meites, J., Lu, K. H., Wuttke, W., Welsch, C. W., Nagasawa, H., and Quadri, S. (1972). Recent studies on function and control of prolactin secretion in rats. *Recent Prog. Horm. Res.* **28**, 471–526.
66. Minton, J. P. (1974). Prolactin and human breast cancer. *Am. J. Surg.* **128**, 628–630.
67. Mori, T., Bern, H. A., Mills, K. T., and Young, P. N. (1976). Long-term effects of neonatal steroid exposure on mammary gland development and tumorigenesis in mice. *J. Natl. Cancer Inst.* **57**, 1057–1062.
68. Nagasawa, H. (1977). Mammary gland DNA synthesis as a limiting factor for mammary tumorigenesis. *IRCS J. Med. Sci.* **5**, 405–408.
69. Nagasawa, H. and Kuretani, K. (1966). Influence of primiparous age and litter number on the time of mammary tumor appearance. *Gann* **57**, 491–496.
70. Nagasawa, H. and Meites, J. (1970). Suppression by ergocornine and iproniazid of carcinogen-induced mammary tumors in rats: Effects on serum and pituitary prolactin levels. *Proc. Soc. Exp. Biol. Med.* **135**, 469–472.
71. Nagasawa, H. and Meites, J. (1970). Effects of hypothalamic estrogen implant on growth of carcinogen-induced mammary tumors in rats. *Cancer Res.* **30**, 1327–1329.
72. Nagasawa, H. and Vorherr, H. (1977). Rat mammary deoxyribonucleic acid

synthesis during the estrous cycle, pregnancy and lactation in relation to mammary tumorigenesis: Its implication for human breast cancer. *Am. J. Obstet. Gynecol.* **127**, 590–593.

73. Nagasawa, H. and Yanai, R. (1970). Estrous cycle of mouse with subcutaneous pellet implant of ergocornine and 2-bromo-α-ergokryptin. *Endocrinol. Japon.* **17**, 233–235.

74. Nagasawa, H. and Yanai, R. (1970). Effects of prolactin or growth hormone of carcinogen-induced mammary tumors of adreno-ovariectomized rats. *Int. J. Cancer* **6**, 488–495.

75. Nagasawa, H. and Yanai, R. (1971). Increased mammary response to pituitary mammotropic hormones by estrogen in rats. *Endocrinol. Japon.* **18**, 53–56.

76. Nagasawa, H. and Yanai, R. (1971). Quantitative participation of placental mammotropic hormones in mammary development during pregnancy in mice. *Endocrinol. Japon.* **18**, 507–510.

77. Nagasawa, H. and Yanai, R. (1971). Reduction by pituitary isograft of inhibitory effect of large dose of estrogen on incidence of mammary tumors induced by carcinogen in ovariectomized rats. *Int. J. Cancer* **8**, 463–467.

78. Nagasawa, H. and Yanai, R. (1971). Growth of spontaneous mammary tumors in mice. *Exp. Anim.* **20**, 37–40.

79. Nagasawa, H. and Yanai, R. (1972). Inhibitory effect of estrogen on mammary growth and its counteraction by pituitary isografts in mice. *Endocrinol. Japon.* **19**, 107–110.

80. Nagasawa, H. and Yanai, R. (1972). Promotion of pituitary prolactin release by dibutyryl-adenosine-3′, 5′-monophosphate in rats. *J. Endocrinol.* **55**, 215–216.

81. Nagasawa, H. and Yanai, R. (1973). Effect of human placental lactogen on growth of carcinogen-induced mammary tumors in rats. *Int. J. Cancer* **11**, 131–137.

82. Nagasawa, H. and Yanai, R. (1973). Correlation between some measures as index of mammary tumor size. *Gann* **64**, 405–406.

83. Nagasawa, H. and Yanai, R. (1974). Frequency of mammary cell division in relation to mammary tumors by carcinogen in rats. *J. Natl. Cancer Inst.* **52**, 609–610.

84. Nagasawa, H. and Yanai, R. (1974). Effects of estrogen and/or pituitary graft on nucleic acid synthesis of carcinogen-induced mammary tumors in rats. *J. Natl. Cancer Inst.* **52**, 1219–1222.

85. Nagasawa, H. and Yanai, R. (1975). Some discrepancies between use of DNA synthesis and wholemount preparations as indices of mammary gland response to pituitary mammotrophin. *J. Endocrinol.* **67**, 303–304.

86. Nagasawa, H. and Yanai, R. (1976). Mammary nucleic acids and pituitary

prolactin secretion during prolonged lactation in mice. *J. Endocrinol.* **70**, 389–395.

87. Nagasawa, H. and Yanai, R. (1977). Mammary growth and function and pituitary prolactin secretion in female nude mice. *Acta Endocrinol.* **86**, 794–802.
88. Nagasawa, H., Chen, C. L., and Meites, J. (1969). Effects of estrogen implant in median eminence on serum and pituitary prolactin levels in the rat. *Proc. Soc. Exp. Biol. Med.* **132**, 859–861.
89. Nagasawa, H., Chen, C. L., and Meites, J. (1973). Relation between growth of carcinogen-induced mammary cancers and serum prolactin values. *Proc. Soc. Exp. Biol. Med.* **142**, 625–627.
90. Nagasawa, H., Fujimoto, M., and Kuretani, K. (1967). Normal growth and reproduction of a high and a low mammary tumor strains of mouse. *Gann* **58**, 115–123.
91. Nagasawa, H., Fujimoto, M., and Kuretani, K. (1968). Further study on the influence of primiparous age and litter number on the mammary tumor age in mice. *Gann* **59**, 217–222.
92. Nagasawa, H., Kanzawa, F., and Kuretani, K. (1967). Lactation performance of the high and low mammary tumor strains of mice. *Gann* **58**, 331–336.
93. Nagasawa, H., Kuretani, K., and Kanzawa, F. (1966). Effect of prolactin on the growth of spontaneous mammary tumors in mice. *Gann* **57**, 637–640.
94. Nagasawa, H., Tokuzen, R., and Nakahara, W. (1976). Growth of mammary tumors in a high and a low mammary tumor strains of mice established from the same basal stock of Swiss albino. *Gann* **67**, 913–915.
95. Nagasawa, H., Yanai, R., and Flückiger, E. (1973). Counter-action by 2-Br-α-ergocryptine of pituitary prolactin release promoted by dibutyryl-adenosine 3′, 5′-monophosphate in rats. In *Human Prolactin*, ed. Pasteels, J. L. and Robyn, C., pp. 313–315. Amsterdam: Excerpta Medica.
96. Nagasawa, H., Yanai, R., and Hayashi, S. (1978). Pattern of estrous cycles in relation to mammary tumorigenesis in mice. *Horm. Res.* (in press).
97. Nagasawa, H., Yanai, R., and Kikuyama, S. (1974). Irreversible inhibition of pituitary prolactin and growth hormone secretion and of mammary gland development in mice by monosodium glutamate administered neonatally. *Acta Endocrinol.* **75**, 249–259.
98. Nagasawa, H., Yanai, R., and Miyamoto, M. (1972). Participation of mammary tumor virus in mammary gland sensitivity to prolactin in mice. *Japan. J. Zootech. Sci.* **43**, 519–523.
99. Nagasawa, H., Yanai, R., and Taniguchi, H. (1976). Importance of mammary gland DNA synthesis on carcinogen-induced mammary tumorigenesis in rats. *Cancer Res.* **36**, 2223–2226.
100. Nagasawa, H., Yanai, R., and Taniguchi, H. (1976). Reduction by pituitary grafts of mammary tumor age. Its variability in a high mammary tumor

strain of mice: Effects on mammary DNA synthesis. *Eur. J. Cancer* **12**, 1017–1019.

101. Nagasawa, H., Iwahashi, H., Kuretani, K., and Fujimoto, M. (1966). Relation between area and desoxyribonucleic acid content of the mammary gland in mice. *Endocrinol. Japon.* **13**, 344–348.
102. Nagasawa, H., Morii, S., Tsubura, A., and Yanai, R. (1977). Relative importance of genotype and type of mammary tumor virus on mammary tumorigenesis in mice. *Eur. J. Cancer* **13**, 1119–1123.
103. Nagasawa, H., Yanai, R., Kikuyama, S., and Mori, J. (1973). Effect of neonatal administration of prolactin on pituitary secretion of prolactin and gonadotrophins in adult female rats. *J. Endocrinol.* **59**, 377–378.
104. Nagasawa, H., Yanai, R., Kikuyama, S., and Mori, J. (1973). Pituitary secretion of prolactin, luteinizing hormone and follicle stimulating hormone in adult female rats treated neonatally with oestrogen. *J. Endocrinol.* **59**, 599–604.
105. Nagasawa, H., Iwahashi, H., Kanzawa, F., Fujimoto, M., and Kuretani, K. (1967). A comparative study on the normal mammary gland development in a high and a low mammary tumor strains of virgin mice. *Gann* **58**, 45–53.
106. Nagasawa, H., Iwahashi, H., Kanzawa, F., Fujimoto, M., and Kuretani, K. (1967). Further study on the relation between area and desoxyribonucleic acid content of the mammary gland in mice. *Endocrinol. Japon.* **14**, 23–26.
107. Nagasawa, H., Mori, T., Yanai, R., Bern, H. A., and Karen, T. M. (1978). Longterm effects of neonatal hormone treatments on plasma prolactin levels in female BALB/cfC3H and BALB/c mice. *Cancer Res.* **38**, 942–945.
108. Nagasawa, H., Yanai, R., Iwahashi, H., Fujimoto, M., and Kuretani, K. (1967). Difference in mammary gland susceptibility to prolactin between a high and a low mammary tumor strains of mice. *Endocrinol. Japon.* **14**, 351–356.
109. Nagasawa, H., Yanai, R., Iwahashi, H., Fujimoto, M., and Kuretani, K. (1967). Effect of pituitary isografts on the growth of spontaneous mammary tumors in mice. *Gann* **58**, 337–342.
110. Nagasawa, H., Yanai, R., Kosugiyama, M., Fujimoto, M., and Kuretani, K. (1969). Lactational performance of high (C3H/He) and low (C57BL/6) mammary tumor strains of mice (II). *Exp. Anim.* **18**, 23–27.
111. Nagasawa, H., Yanai, R., Shodono, M., Nakamura, T., and Tanabe, Y. (1974). Effect of neonatally administered estrogen or prolactin on normal and neoplastic mammary growth and serum estradiol-17β level in rats. *Cancer Res.* **34**, 2643–2646.
112. Nagasawa, H., Yanai, R., Taniguchi, H., Tokuzen, R., and Nakahara, W. (1976). Two-way selection of a stock of Swiss albino mice for mammary

tumorigenesis: Establishment of two new strains (SHN and SLN). *J. Natl. Cancer Inst.* **57**, 425–430.

113. Nandi, S. (1974). Mammary tumors in mice. In *Lactation. A Comprehensive Treatise*, vol. II, ed. Larson, B. L. and Smith, V. R., pp. 391–412. New York, London: Academic Press.
114. Nandi, S. and McGrath, C. M. (1973). Mammary neoplasia in mice. *Adv. Cancer Res.* **17**, 353–414.
115. Olney, J. W. and Sharpe, L. G. (1969). Brain lesions in an infant rhesus monkeys treated with monosodium glutamate. *Science* **166**, 386–388.
116. Olney, J. W., Ho Oi-Lan, Rhee, U., and Schainker, B. (1972). Cysteine-induced brain damage in infant and fetal rodents. *Brain Res.* **45**, 309–313.
117. Ozzello, L. (1974). Electron microscopic study of functional and dysfunctional human mammary glands. *J. Invest. Dermatol.* **63**, 19–26.
118. Pasteels, J. L., Heuson-Steinnon, J. A., Legros, N., Leclerg, G., and Heuson, J. C. (1976). Organ culture of human breast cancer. In *Breast Cancer: Trends in Research and Treatment*, ed. Heuson, J. C., Mattheiem, W. H., and Rozencweig, M., pp. 141–153. New York: Raven Press.
119. Pearson, O. H., Murray, R.L.M., Mozaffarian, G., and Pensky, J. (1972). Prolactin and experimental breast cancer. In *Prolactin and Carcinogenesis*, ed. Boyns, A. R. and Griffiths, K., pp. 154–161. Cardiff: Alpha Omega Alpha.
120. Porter, J. C. (1974). Hormonal regulation of breast development and activity. *J. Invest. Dermatol.* **63**, 85–92.
121. Raynaud, A. (1971). Foetal development of the mammary gland and hormonal effects on its morphogenesis. In *Lactation*, ed. Falconer, I. R., pp. 3–29. London: Butterworths.
122. Rivera, E. M. (1974). Hormonal control of cellular events during lactogenesis: Some unsolved problems. In *Lactogenic Hormone, Fetal Nutrition, and Lactation*, ed. Josimovich, J. B., pp. 279–295. New York, London, Sydney, Toronto: John Wiley and Sons.
123. Rusterholz, D. B., Barfknecht, C. F., and Clemens, J. A. (1976). Ergoline congeners as potential inhibitors of prolactin release. *J. Med. Chem.* **19**, 99–102.
124. Saez, S. (1974). Corticotrophin secretion in relation to breast cancer. In *Mammary Cancers and Neuroendocrine Therapy*, ed. Stoll, B. A., pp. 101–122. London: Butterworths.
125. Salazar, H. and Tonbon, H. (1974). Morphologic changes of the mammary gland during development, pregnancy and lactation. In *Lactogenic Hormones, Fetal Nutrition, and Lactation*, ed. Josimovich, J. B., pp. 221–227. New York, London, Sydney, Toronto: John Wiley and Sons.
126. Schochetman, G. and Schlom, J. (1976). RNA tumor virus and breast cancer. In *Breast Cancer: A Multidisciplinary Approach*, ed. St-Arneault, G.,

Band, P., and Israël, L., pp. 21–25. Berlin, Heiderberg, New York: Springer-Verlag.

127. Sinha, D. and Dao, T. (1972). Estrogen and induction of mammary cancer. In *Estrogen Target Tissues and Neoplasia*, ed. Dao, T. L., pp. 307–316. Chicago: Univ. Chicago Press.

128. Sinha, Y. N., Salocks, C. B., and VanderLaan, W. P. (1976). Circulating levels of prolactin and growth hormone and natural incidence of mammary tumors in mice. *J. Toxicol. Environ. Health* Suppl. **1**, 131–160.

129. Smithline, F., Sherman, L., and Kolodny, H. D. (1975). Prolactin and breast carcinoma. *New Engl. J. Med.* **292**, 784–792.

130. Snedecor, G. W. (1966). *Statistical Methods*, 5th ed. Ames: Iowa State Univ. Press.

131. Stoll, B. A. (1974). Tumour regression following ovarian steroid therapy. In *Mammary Cancer and Neuroendocrine Therapy*, ed. Stoll, B. A., pp. 57–81. London: Butterworths.

132. Stoll, B. A. (1974). Psychoendocrine factors and breast cancer growth. In *Mammary Cancer and Neuroendocrine Therapy*, ed. Stoll, B. A., pp. 401–411. London: Butterworths.

133. Tagnon, H. J. (1976). The role of hormones in the modern treatment of advanced breast cancer. In *Breast Cancer: A Multidisciplinary Approach*, ed. St-Arneault, G., Band, P., and Israël, L., pp. 183–195. Berlin, Heiderberg, New York: Springer-Verlag.

134. Takasugi, N. (1976). Cytological basis for permanent vaginal changes in mice treated neonatally with steroid hormones. *Int. Rev. Cytol.* **44**, 193–224.

135. Tchao, R. (1974). Roles of steroid and pituitary hormones in tumor growth. In *Mammary Cancer and Neuroendocrine Therapy*, ed. Stoll, B. A., pp. 249–264. London: Butterworths.

136. Terenius, L. (1974). Anti-oestrogen and their role in mammary cancer. In *Mammary Cancer and Neuroendrocrine Therapy*, ed. Stoll, B. A., pp. 82–100. London: Butterworths.

137. Topper, Y. J. and Oka, T. (1974). Some aspects of mammary gland development in the mature mouse. In *Lactation. A Comprehensive Treatise*, vol. 1, ed. Larson, B. L. and Smith, V. R., pp. 327–348. New York, London: Academic Press.

138. Trempe, G. L. (1976). Human breast cancer in culture. In *Breast Cancer: A Multidisciplinary Approach*, ed. St-Arneault, G., Band, P., and Israël, L., pp. 33–41. Berlin, Heiderberg, New York: Springer-Verlag.

139. Vorherr, H. (1974). *The Breast, Morphology, Physiology, and Lactation.* New York, London: Academic Press.

140. Welsch, C. W. (1975). The role of the neuroendocrine system in murine mammary tumorigenesis. In *Host Defence against Cancer and Its Potensia-*

tion, ed. Mizuno, D., Chihara, G., Fukuoka, F., Yamamoto, T., and Yamamura, Y., pp. 281–301. Tokyo, Baltimore: Japan Sci. Soc. Press, Univ. Park Press.

141. Welsch, C. W. (1976). Prophylaxis of early preneoplastic lesions of the mammary gland. *Cancer Res.* **36**, 2621–2625.
142. Welsch, C. W. (1976). Interaction of estrogen and prolactin in spontaneous mammary tumorigenesis of the mouse. *J. Toxicol. Environ. Health* Suppl. **1**, 161–175.
143. Welsch, C. W. and Meites, J. (1974). Neuroendocrine control of murine mammary carcinoma. In *Mammary Cancer and Neuroendocrine Therapy*, ed. Stoll, B. A., pp. 25–56. London: Butterworths.
144. Welsch, C. W. and Nagasawa, H. (1977). Prolactin and murine mammary tumorigenesis: A review. *Cancer Res.* **37**, 951–963.
145. Welsch, C. W., Nagasawa, H., and Meites, J. (1970). Increased incidence of spontaneous mammary tumors in female rats with induced hypothalamic lesions. *Cancer Res.* **30**, 2310–2313.
146. Wittliff, J. L., Beatty, B. W., Savlov, E. D., Patterson, W. B., and Cooper, R. A., Jr. (1976). Estrogen receptors and hormone dependency in human breast cancer. In *Breast Cancer: A Multidisciplinary Approach*, ed. St-Arneault, G., Band, P., and Israël, L., pp. 59–77. Berlin, Heiderberg, New York: Springer-Verlag.
147. Yanai, R. and Nagasawa, H. (1969). Quantitative analysis of prolactin by disc electrophoresis and its relation to biological activity. *Proc. Soc. Exp. Biol. Med.* **131**, 167–171.
148. Yanai, R. and Nagasawa, H. (1970). Effects of ergocornine and 2-Br-α-ergokryptin (CB-154) on the formation of mammary hyperplastic alveolar nodules and the pituitary prolactin levels in mice. *Experientia* **26**, 649–650.
149. Yanai, R. and Nagasawa, H. (1970). Suppression of mammary hyperplastic nodule formation and pituitary prolactin secretion in mice induced by ergocornine or 2-Br-α-ergocryptine. *J. Natl. Cancer Inst.* **45**, 1105–1112.
150. Yanai, R. and Nagasawa, H. (1971). Mammary growth and placental mammotropin during pregnancy in mice with high or low lactational performance. *J. Dairy Sci.* **54**, 906–910.
151. Yanai, R. and Nagasawa, H. (1971). Pituitary prolactin and growth hormone levels during different reproductive states in mice with a high or a low lactational performance. *Horm. Behav.* **2**, 73–82.
152. Yanai, R. and Nagasawa, H. (1971). Enhancement by pituitary isografts of mammary hyperplastic nodules in adreno-ovariectomized mice. *J. Natl. Cancer Inst.* **46**, 1251–1255.
153. Yanai, R. and Nagasawa, H. (1971). Inhibition by ergocornine and 2-Br-α-ergocryptine of spontaneous mammary tumor appearance in mice. *Experientia* **27**, 934.

154. Yanai, R. and Nagasawa, H. (1972). Inhibition of mammary tumorigenesis by ergot alkaloids and promotion of mammary tumorigenesis by pituitary isografts in adreno-ovariectomized mice. *J. Natl. Cancer Inst.* **48**, 715–719.
155. Yanai, R. and Nagasawa, H. (1973). Enhancement by human placental lactogen of mammary hyperplastic nodules in ovariectomized mice. *Cancer Res.* **33**, 1642–1644.
156. Yanai, R. and Nagasawa, H. (1974). Effect of 2-bromo-α-ergocryptine on pituitary synthesis and release of prolactin and growth hormone in rats. *Horm. Res.* **5**, 1–5.
157. Yanai, R. and Nagasawa, H. (1974). Radioimmunoassay of pituitary and plasma levels of prolactin during oestrous cycles in mice. *J. Endocrinol.* **62**, 685–686.
158. Yanai, R. and Nagasawa, H. (1976). Importance of progesterone in DNA synthesis of pregnancy-dependent mammary tumors in mice. *Int. J. Cancer* **18**, 317–321.
159. Yanai, R. and Nagasawa, H. (1976). Effect of pituitary graft and 2-bromo-α-ergocryptine on mammary DNA synthesis in mice in relation to mammary tumorigenesis. *J. Natl. Cancer Inst.* **56**, 1055–1056.
160. Yanai, R. and Nagasawa, H. (1977). Effects of progesterone and estrogen on growth of pregnancy-dependent mammary tumors in GR/A mice. *Eur. J. Cancer* **13**, 813–816.
161. Yanai, R. and Nagasawa, H. (1978). Development and growth of pregnancy-dependent and -independent mammary tumors in GR/A strain of mice and their relationship. *Gann* **69**, 25–30.
162. Yanai, R., Mori, T., and Nagasawa, H. (1977). Longterm effects of prenatal and neonatal administration of 5β-dihydrotestosterone on normal and neoplastic mammary development in mice. *Cancer Res.* **37**, 4456–4459.
163. Yanai, R., Nagasawa, H., and Kuretani, K. (1968). Disc electrophoretic analysis of growth hormone and prolactin in the anterior pituitary of mouse. *Endocrinol. Japon.* **15**, 365–370.

II – 2

MAMMARY TRANSPLANTATION AND ITS HISTOGENESIS IN MICE

Kazumasa Hoshino

Department of Anatomy, Faculty of Medicine, Kyoto University, Kyoto, Japan

The mammary gland, one of the appendages of the skin, consists developmentally of the parenchyma derived from the ectoderm and the surrounding stroma from the mesenchyme. Therefore, any changes in its structural and functional stages must be considered a result of parenchymal-stromal interactions responding to endogenous environmental stimuli caused mainly by hormonal alterations and the aging phenomena when the mammary gland is undisturbed *in situ*.

Transplantation of mammary glands is a convenient means to separate the parenchyma of the mammary gland from its stroma and make any desirable parenchymal-stromal combinations by varying donor-host matchings. However, until about two decades ago this technique was utilized mainly for the study of mammary carcinogenesis. The etiology of mammary cancer in mice has been related to several factors, including genetic factors, an inherited hormonal sensitivity, the mammary tumor virus, hormonal influences, and dietary and environmental conditions. Thus, mammary transplantation provides not only a means for changing parenchymal-stromal interrelationships but also for combining the other factors listed above when experimental designs are formulated.

In the late 1950's at Yale University, William U. Gardner and I realized that no extensive investigations were available on parenchymal-stromal interactions in relation to the histogenesis of non-cancerous mammary glands. Since then, by full use of the transplantation techniques, studies on regeneration, proliferation, growth, and differentiation of normal mammary glands have been undertaken in our laboratory. The purpose of this article is to review the knowledge of non-cancerous parenchymal-stromal interactions observed from mammary grafts in mice. The fate of transplanted hyperplastic nodules in mice has been reported with and without regard to mammary carcinogenesis since Faulkin and DeOme (*22*) first reported in 1958, but these data will not be discussed here.

1. Genetic Donor-Host Relationships

Various donor-host relationships can be established from their respective genetic backgrounds. Terminology of tissue transplantation has been described as follows (*62*, *69*).

1) Terminology of tissue transplantation

An autograft is a graft in which the donor is also the recipient. An isograft (isogenic or isogeneic graft) is a graft between genetically identical individuals, or more precisely between individuals identical in histocompatibility antigens. An allograft (allogeneic graft) is a graft between genetically disparate individuals of the same species, or more specifically, it is a graft in which the grafted tissue carries a histocompatibility allele or alleles and hence presumably an alloantigen(s) foreign to the recipient. The term homograft has also been used to describe this type of graft, but it is not recommended. A xenograft (xenogeneic graft) is a graft between different species. The term heterograft is also used to describe this type of graft.

2) Five laws of transplantation

Snell and Stimpfling (*69*) summarized a number of studies carried out by previous investigators. They came up with five laws or dicta of transplantation as follows:

1. Grafts within inbred strains are successful; namely, isografts succeed.
2. Grafts between inbred strains are not successful; namely, allografts fail.
3. Grafts from the parent inbred strain to the F_1 hybrid succeed, but the reverse direction fails.
4. Grafts from F_2 or subsequent generations will also grow in all F_1 mice.
5. Grafts from either parental inbred strain are accepted by some members of the F_2 hybrid generation but rejected by others.

3) Sex-linked graft rejection

The sex-linked rejection of skin grafts was first demonstrated by Eichwald and Silmser (*18*). Their experiments revealed that skin isografts from male donors often failed to survive in female host mice. The rate of rejection varied with the strain of mice, the highest being 100% in the C57BL strain. These results were confirmed by Prehn and Main (*59*) and Sachs and Heller (*63*). Hauschka (*30*) suggested two possibilities to explain the results previously reported by Eichwald and Silmser (*18*): either androgen dependence or Y-linked antigenicity. Snell (*68*) supported the latter possibility and postulated that a sex-linked histocompatibility antigen present in the male graft tissue may be located on the non-pairing segment of the Y chromosome and is foreign to the female host.

Thereafter, sex-linked rejection of isografts was reported, in varying degrees, in thymic tissue (*31*), lymph nodes (*23*), lung, salivary gland, blood, spleen and liver (*19*), and pituitary glands (*46*).

Normal mammary gland tissue of the male F_1 CBA or F_1 hybrid mice did not suffer from sex-linked rejection when they were isografted into female siblings (*33*, *38*). Moretti and Blair (*52*) and Erwin (*20*) have observed equal acceptance of mammary gland tissue in C57BL female hosts whether the donor was male or female (Table I). However, a weak sex-linked histocompatibility antigen in the mammary gland tissue of male C57BL mice was immunologically detected by Moretti and Blair (*52*). Blair and Moretti (*4*) further reported that subcutaneous transplantation of either mammary tissue or skin from isologous males into 3-week-old female hosts inhibited the growth of subsequent transplants of male mammary tissue in the gland-free mammary fat pads of the same female hosts, whereas pretreatment by implantation of the same tissue into a mammary fat pad did not evoke this effect. In 1970 these investigators pursued this further and stated that transplants of male mammary tissue survived and grew better in younger hosts than in older hosts. No effect of gonadectomy of the adult male donors upon the survival and growth of mammary tissue transplants was observed. Excision of the local lymph nodes did not affect the partially protected nature of the mammary fat-pad transplantation site (*5*).

Transplantability of normal mammary gland tissue between genetically different donor and host combinations at various transplantation sites reported in the literature has been tabulated (Table I). With a few exceptions, data obtained from mammary glands of the donors with any pretreatments were not included. Likewise, data obtained by skin grafting methods were excluded.

TABLE I. Recovery Rates of Viable Grafts of Normal Mammary Glands

a) Female donor to female host

Donor		Host		Graft site[c]	Recovery rate of successful grafts (%)	Treatment after grafting[d]	Investigators and year (Ref.)
Strain[a]	Age[b]	Strain	Age				
C3H	Multiparous with mammary tumor (MCa)	C3H	8–14w	Sc	154/179 (86)	None	Faulkin and DeOme, 1958 (*21*)
				Sc	152/186 (82)	Estradiol	
				Sc	119/139 (86)	Cortisol acetate	
C3H	Multiparous with MCa	C3H	8–14w	Sc	27/54 (50)	None	DeOme *et al*., 1959 (*17*)
		C3H	59w	Sc	7/12 (58)	None	
		C3H	Multipara	Sc	7/15 (47)	None	
		C3H	3w	4 mgffp	11/19 (58)	Pregnancy	
C3H	Multiparous with MCa	C3H	7 m	4 mgffp	2/4 (50)	None	Faulkin and DeOme, 1960 (*22*)
CBA	38d, 45d	CBA	21–28d	4 mgffp	9/16 (56)	EB, P, PL (14–21d)	Hoshino, 1962 (*32*)
				Retroauricul	9/12 (75)	EB, P, PL (14–21d)	
				Sc	6/12 (50)	EB, P, PL (14–21d)	
				Pararenal fp	5/12 (42)	EB, P, PL (14–21d)	
CBA	48d	CBA	21–28d	Retroauricul	2/3 (67)	EB, P, PL (76d)	
				4 mgffp	3/3 (100)	BE, P, PL (76d)	
				4 mgffp	2/2 (100)	Pregnancy	
CBA	121d	CC	21–28d	4 mgffp	3/6 (50)	EB, P, PL (21d)	
				Retroauricul	4/6 (67)	EB, P, PL (21d)	
				Sc	1/6 (17)	EB, P, PL (21d)	
				Pararenal fp	1/6 (17)	EB, P, PL (21d)	
CBA	48d	CC	21–28d	4 mgffp	1/1 (100)	Pregnancy	
				Retroauricul	1/1 (100)	Pregnancy	

				Sc	1/1 (100)	Pregnancy	
				Pararenal fp	1/1 (100)	Pregnancy	
C57BL	358d	CC	21–28d	4 mgffp	1/1 (100)	Pregnancy	
CC	22–176d	CC	21–28d	4 mgffp	10/11 (91)	EB, P, PL (64–73d)	
				Retroauricul	9/9 (100)	EB, P, PL (64–73d)	
				Sc	9/9 (100)	EB, P, PL (64–73d)	
				Pararenal fp	6/7 (86)	EB, P, PL (64–73d)	
CBA	20–76d	CBA	30–115d	4 mgffp	9/11 (82)	Pregnancy	Hoshino, 1964 (*34*)
				Pararenal fp	9/14 (62)	Pregnancy	
				Sc	17/28 (61)	Pregnancy	
				Mesometrial	2/7 (29)	Pregnancy	
		CC	110–111d	4 mgffp	3/4 (75)	Pregnancy	
				Pararenal fp	4/6 (67)	Pregnancy	
				Sc	4/11 (36)	Pregnancy	
				Mesometrial	2/2 (100)	Pregnancy	
CC	117d	CC	130–186d	4 mgffp	1/3 (33)	Pregnancy	
				Pararenal fp	2/6 (33)	Pregnancy	
				Sc	7/11 (64)	Pregnancy	
				Mesometrial	2/2 (100)	Pregnancy	
CBA	734d	CBA	88–93d	4 mgffp	2/3 (67)	Pregnancy	
CC-1	68d	CC-1	2–8m	4 mgffp	15/21 (71)	Pregnancy	Hoshino, 1965 (*35*)
C57BL	2.5m	CC-2	10m	4 mgffp	7/10 (70)	Pregnancy	Hoshino *et al.*, 1965 (*44*)
				Pararenal fp	5/10 (50)	Pregnancy	
CBA	19m	CC-1	1–4m	4 mgffp	11/20 (55)	Pregnancy	
				Pararenal fp	4/20 (20)	Pregnancy	
C57BL	2.5m	CC-2	9.5m	4 mgffp	6/10 (60)	Pituitary graft	

Continued . . .

TABLE I. Continued.

Donor		Host		Graft site[c]	Recovery rate of successful grafts (%)	Treatment after grafting[d]	Investigators and year (Ref.)
Strain[a]	Age[b]	Strain	Age				
				Pararenal fp	2/10 (20)	Pituitary graft	
CBA	3.5–4.5m	CC-1	10–18m	4 mgffp	12/17 (71)	Pituitary graft	
				Pararenal fp	9/17 (53)	Pituitary graft	
CBA	4m	CC-2	9.5m	4 mgffp	4/4 (100)	Pituitary graft	
				Pararenal fp	3/4 (75)	Pituitary graft	
CBA	19m	CC-1	1–4m	4 mgffp	8/18 (44)	Pituitary graft	
				Pararenal fp	3/18 (17)	Pituitary graft	
C57BL	Pregnant	C57BL	3w	4 mgffp	10/13 (77)	None	Moretti and Blair 1966 (*52*)
		C57BL	10w	4 mgffp	12/15 (80)	None	
		C57BL	3w	4 mgffp	11/13 (85)	E, DOCA pellet	
		C57BL	10w	4 mgffp	11/12 (92)	E, DOCA pellet	
CBA	4m	CBA	3–3.5m	Brown fat	10/16 (63)	EB, P (3w)	Hoshino, 1967 (*37*)
CBA	3m	CC-2	1.5m	Brown fat	13/15 (87)	EB, P (3w)	
CBA	135d	BA-1	Adult	4 mgffp	9/14 (64)	None	Hoshino and Gardner 1967 (*43*)
		BA-2	Adult	4 mgffp	8/14 (57)	None	
C3H	268d	F-1a	Adult	4 mgffp	6/40 (15)	None	Hoshino, 1970 (*38*)
		F-1b	Adult	4 mgffp	1/10 (10)	None	
CC-2	206d	CC-2	Adult	4 mgffp	21/30 (70)	None	
CBA	4m	BA-2	Adult	4 mgffp, Sc	23/96 (24)	None (3–21d)	William and Hoshino 1970 (*75*)
CBA	3m	CC-1	Adult	4 mgffp	42/80 (53)	EB, P (3–21d)	
C3H	Neonate	C3H	Adult	4 mgffp	10/16 (63)	Pregnancy	Currie, Hoshino, and Kim, 1977 (*12*)

A/J	Neonate	A/J	Adult	4 mgffp	12/28	(43)	None	
C3H	Neonate	C3H	Adult	4 mgffp	6/8	(75)	None	
b) Female donor to male host								
CBA	48d	CBA	21–28d	4 mgffp	3/3	(100)	EB, P, PL (12d)	Hoshino, 1962 (*32*)
CBA	44d	CC	21–28d	4 mgffp	1/1	(100)	EB, P, PL (8d)	
				Pararenal fp	1/1	(100)	EB, P, PL (8d)	
				Sc	1/1	(100)	EB, P, PL (8d)	
				Retroauricul	1/1	(100)	EB, P, PL (8d)	
CC	22–107d	CC	21–28d	4 mgffp	3/4	(75)	EB, P, PL (5–12d)	
				Pararenal fp	2/2	(100)	EB, P, PL (5–12d)	
		CC	21–28d	Sc	2/2	(100)	EB, P, PL (5–12d)	
				Retroauricul	1/3	(33)	EB, P, PL (5–12d)	
C57BL	358d	CC	21–28d	4 mgffp	2/3	(67)	EB, P, PL (11d)	
CC	114d	CC	21–28d	4 mgffp	5/12	(42)	EB, P, PL (21d)	
				Sc	1/4	(25)	EB, P, PL (21d)	
				Retroauricul	1/4	(25)	EB, P, PL (21d)	
c) Female donor to castrated male host								
C57BL	4m	CC-2	10.5–13.5m	4 mgffp	8/12	(67)	EB, P pellet (50 mg)	Hoshino *te al.*, 1965 (*44*)
				Pararenal fp	4/12	(33)	EB, P pellet (50 mg)	
CBA	4.5m	CC-1	9–9.5m	4 mgffp	9/14	(62)	EB, P pellet (60 mg)	
				Pararenal fp	1/14	(7)	EB, P pellet (60 mg)	
CBA	19m	CC-1	3.5–4m	4 mgffp	10/20	(50)	EB, P pellet (61 mg)	
				Pararenal fp	3/20	(15)	EB, P pellet (61 mg)	

Continued . . .

TABLE I. Continued.

Donor		Host		Graft site[c]	Recovery rate of successful grafts (%)	Treatment after grafting[d]	Investigators and year (Ref.)
Strain[a]	Age[b]	Strain	Age				
d) Male donor to female host							
CC	129d	CC	54–135d	4 mgffp	15/22 (68)	Pregnancy	Hoshino, 1963 (*33*)
A or	?	F-1c	?	4 mgffp	126/282 (45)	Pregnancy ?	Erwin, 1967 (*20*)
CBA	Adult	CC-1	1–7m	4 mgffp	17/38 (45)	Pregnancy	Hoshino, 1970 (*38*)
		CC-2	1–7m	4 mgffp	49/68 (72)	Pregnancy	
e) Castrated male donor to female host							
C57BL	Adult[e]	C57BL	3w	4 mgffp	10/12 (83)	None	Moretti and Blair, 1966 (*52*)
		C57BL	10w	4 mgffp	12/16 (75)	None	
		C57BL	3w	4 mgffp	12/14 (86)	E, DOCA pellet	
		C57BL	10w	4 mgffp	11/12 (92)	E, DOCA pellet	

[a] Abbreviations for hybrids: CC=reciprocal (CBA×C57BL)F_1; CC-1=(♀C57BL×♂CBA)F_1; CC-2=(♀CBA×♂C57BL)F_1; BA-1=(♀BC_B×♂CBA)F_1; BA-2=(♀CBA×♂BC_B)F_1; F-1a=(♀C57BL×♂C3H)F_1; F-1b=(♀C3H×♂C57BL)F_1; F-1c=(A×C57BL)F_1. The C3H and CBA strains of mice and young of female mice of these strains carry mammary tumor virus (MTV), but the C57BL, BC_B, and A strains and young of females of these strains do not carry MTV.

[b] Ages are expressed as d for days, w for weeks, and m for months.

[c] Abbreviations for the site of transplantation: 4 mgffp=the gland-free 4th mammary fat pad; pararenal fp=the pararenal fat pad; Sc=the subcutaneous tissue; retroauricul=the retroauricular area; brown fat=the interscapular brown fat pad.

[d] Treatments after grafting are abbreviated as follows: EB=estradiol benzoate; P=progesterone; PL=prolactin; E, DOCA=estradiol and desoxycorticosterone acetate.

[e] These C57BL donor mice had been pretreated with pellets containing estradiol and desoxycorticosterone acetate for 1 month. A similar work was reported by Blair and Moretti (*5*), but their data did not state which donors had been gonadectomized prior to the pretreatment with pellets of E, DOCA, therefore the data in their 1970 work are not tabulated in this table.

2. *Methods of Mammary Transplantation in Mice*

Fischer (*24*) was probably the first investigator who used mammary transplantation in experimental carcinogenesis. In his autografting method, he sutured each mammary graft to a 0.5 cm long piece of the bared tail of the same mouse for easy recovery of the grafted mammary tissues. Also in carcinogenesis studies, Shimkin *et al.* (*65*) transplanted subcutaneously a single mammary duct and its terminal branches obtained from a milk-agent-carrying female C3H to a milk agent-free C3H male which was subsequently treated with diethylstilbestrol. In order to study the intrinsic susceptibility or resistance to tumorigenesis of the mammary glands, Prehn (*58*) made a large full-thickness skin graft incorporating one or more mammary glands which remained connected to their own nipple(s). For more detailed mammary carcinogenesis studies, DeOme and his associates in 1958 began an extensive series of transplantation of normal, hyperplastic, and tumorous mammary tissues in mice. Normal mammary tissue was selected from the edge of the gland of multiparous mice (*21*), or the primary lactiferous duct alone was transplanted (*22*). Since 1961 a series of studies on mammary transplantation has been reported from our laboratory. Earlier, we used the so-called blind transplantation method by grafting a piece of mammary fat pad, approximately 2×2 mm, excised from the area adjacent to the nipple, which contained unknown amounts of mammary parenchyma (*32*). In order to transplant a predetermined amount of parenchyma obtained from a known portion of the mammary duct system of the donor's gland, the quantitative transplantation method was developed (*33*, *42*). In 1963, Thompson reported the transplantation of a whole mammary gland, including its own fat pad, nipple, and surrounding skin. One year earlier, Krohn (*49*) described a similar whole mammary gland transplantation technique and observed that the two nipples of the transplanted and lactating mammary gland were actively suckled.

3. *The Quantitative Transplantation of Mammary Ducts*

Hoshino (*33*) described in detail his quantitative transplantation of the mouse mammary duct-segments. The original method consisted of microdissection of the mammary gland of the donor mouse vitally stained with trypan blue, and excision of a predetermined amount of duct-segment(s) from a known portion of its duct system with a desirable amount of its surrounding stromal tissue.

1) Vital staining of mammary glands

An aqueous solution of 0.5 % trypan blue was selected for this purpose. A concentration of more than 0.5 % was often found to be too toxic for the mouse. Seven hours after a single intraperitoneal injection of 0.3 ml into a normal adult mouse, staining conditions usually reached a maximum. Suitable dosages are 0.2, 0.3, or 0.4 ml for a mouse weighing up to 15 g, 15 to 30 g, or over 30 g, respectively. Stainability of mammary glands from individual to individual differs, and sometimes a single intraperitoneal injection results in a very pale blue difficult to microdissect. Routinely in our laboratory, the first injection is given to the donor mouse after 10 p.m. and the second injection is given the next morning before 7 a.m. The vitally stained mammary gland is removed from the donor between 1 and 2 p.m. This double injection procedure usually provides sufficient staining. The time lapse between removal of the vitally stained gland of the donor to completion of the transplantation of all the duct-segments into the host mice should be within 1 hr in order to maintain viability of mammary grafts (*21*, *33*).

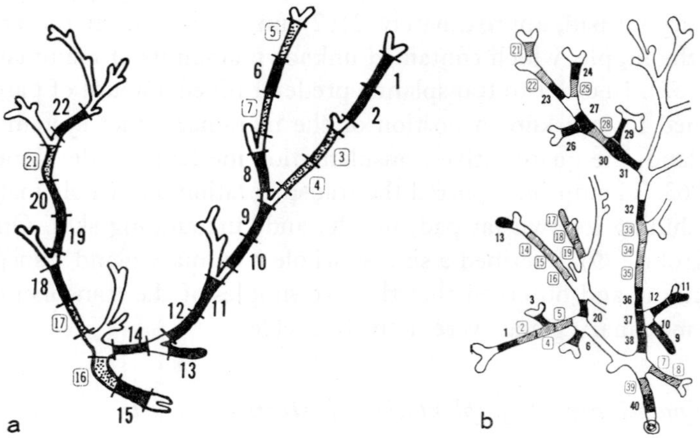

FIG. 1. Sketches of two mammary glands obtained from two donor mice

(a) Twenty-two numbered duct-segments were taken from a male donor mouse and transplanted into 11 female host mice (*33*). (b) Forty duct-segments obtained from a female donor were transplanted into 20 female hosts (*75*). Each segment measured 0.6 mm in length. Successfully transplanted duct-segments are illustrated in black, whereas unsuccessful grafts are illustrated by the shaded areas.

2) Microdissection of vitally stained mammary glands

The vitally stained mammary gland is removed from the donor mouse under Nembutal anesthesia, immediately placed in a Petri dish on filter paper moistened with either Tyrode's solution or Eagle's culture medium, and microdissected from the surrounding adipose stroma with watchmaker forceps under a dissecting microscope. According to the experimental design, a desired amount of stroma (mammary fatty tissue) surrounding each duct-segment should be retained to be transplanted together with the duct-segment. Before excising any duct-segments, sketching or Polaroid photomicrographing of the microdissected mammary duct system usually provides an accurate record of the origin and amount of mammary grafts, as shown in Fig. 1. Each excised duct-segment is placed with watchmaker forceps into the designed site of transplantation, which will be discussed in the next section.

4. *Site of Transplantation*

Several locations have been used as a site of mammary transplantation. These include the skin, the subcutaneous tissue, the retroauricular area, the gland-free 4th mammary fat pad, the pararenal fat pad, the peritoneal cavity, the mesometrial fat layer, the anterior chamber of the eye, the interscapular brown fat pad, and the space under the kidney capsule.

1) Skin

As one means of mammary transplantation, transplantation of the skin accompanied by attached mammary tissue, usually with the nipple, has been undertaken (*49*, *58*, *72*).

2) Subcutaneous tissue

The subcutaneous tissue was the only site of mammary transplantation besides the skin until the gland-free 4th mammary fat pad method was devised by DeOme and Faulkin (*16*). The recovery rates of subcutaneous transplants have been summarized and compared with those attained at other sites (Table I). The retroauricular area used as a transplantation site is a specific location in the subcutaneous tissue with a better blood supply (*32*). The recovery rates of mammary grafts in the subcutaneous area were comparable to those in other sites of transplantation except for a lower recovery rate of grafts in the dorsal subcutaneous tissue in non-castrated male hosts. The ultimate growth extent of the successfully transplanted mammary tissue in the subcutaneous tissue was always smaller than others. In the sites where adipose tissue was present, such as the gland-free 4th mammary fat pad and the pararenal fat pad, the transplanted mammary grafts grew into the host's adipose stroma in addition to the adipose tissue which had been transplanted along with the mammary parenchyma. In sites such as the dorsal subcutaneous area, where almost no adipose tissue of the host is present, the transplanted mammary glands grew only within the adipose tissue originally transplanted, regardless of hormonal treatment. When the fascial connective sheath investing the gland-free 4th mammary fat pad intervened between the transplant and the host's mammary fat tissue, the transplanted mammary glands could not grow through the intervening sheath into the adipose tissue which is enclosed within the sheath. In such a case, the growth extent of the transplanted mammary gland was determined by the original size of the entire graft. The portion of adipose stroma transplanted with the mammary parenchyma apparently did not increase in size, but frequently diminished and was replaced by connective tissue in varying amounts. Therefore, when mammary tissue is transplanted into the gland-free 4th mammary fat pad, such a graft must be inserted into the adipose stroma through a small hole made in the fascial sheath. New vascular structures were usually remarkably well developed around the dorsal subcutaneous grafts and often helped to identify the location of the transplants. From these observations, it was then stressed that adipose tissue is an essential factor controlling the extent of mammary growth (*32*).

TABLE II. Ultimate Size of Successfully Transplanted Mammary Ducts at Different Sites of Transplantation (Greatest Dimension)

Transplantation site	Original length of transplant (mm)		
	<0.2~0.4	0.5~0.9	1.0~3.0
Pararenal fat pad	13.3± 3.5[a] (6.6~17.2)[b]	5.0± 0.8 (3.3~ 5.9)	13.8± 1.2 (11.6~17.3)
4mgffp	12.2± 1.8 (7.4~21.3)	18.2± 1.6 (13.4~22.6)	22.7± 1.2 (21.8~23.5)
Mesometrial fat layer		9.0	4.6± 1.1 (3.0~ 6.7)
Subcutaneous area	1.3± 0.2 (1.0~ 1.8)	1.2± 0.1 (0.8~ 1.8)	1.9± 0.2 (0.3~ 4.0)

[a] Mean±standard error (SE).
[b] Range.
From Ref. *34*.

This was confirmed following the quantitative transplantation of mammary duct-segments (*34*), as shown in Table II.

3) Gland-free 4th mammary fat pad

DeOme and Faulkin (*16*) reported briefly and DeOme *et al.* (*17*) described in detail how to prepare the gland-free 4th mammary fat pad. Their original method was as follows: the anesthesized mouse was pinned, ventral side up, on a cork board and scrubbed with 70% ethanol. An inverted Y-shaped incision was made along the abdominal midline and laterally between the 4th and 5th nipples midway down each hind leg. One at a time the resulting skin flaps, with the 4th mammary gland attached, were carefully separated from the body wall by blunt dissection. The free edge of the skin flap was then pinned to the cork board, exposing the nipple area and most of the 4th mammary fat pad. In a 3-week-old female C3H mouse, the mammary gland elements consist of short branching ducts which extend from the nipple area into the fat pad. The nipple area and the large blood vessels ventral to the lymph node and between the 4th and 5th pads were cauterized. The area containing the growing gland elements, including the adjacent portion of the mammary fat pad and the surrounding loose connective tissue, was then excised with fine scissors. The remaining portion of the fat pad with its circulation intact and without host mammary parenchyma was then ready to receive a transplant, or the skin flap was sutured and the transplantation was carried out at a later date. The surgery described herein did not interfere with the circulation of the remaining fat pad.

A few years later, the original procedure was evaluated from various aspects and compared with the four other surgical approaches (*32*). The results are summarized in Fig. 2. Group A: growth of the remaining portions of the pre-existing mammary glands was not impaired by surgical removal of the primary lactiferous duct or by being amputated from the nipple. Group B: the operation in which the mammary fat pad caudal to the inferior mammary vessels was not removed did not always result in the clearing of the host mammary parenchyma. Group C: only when a part of the primary lactiferous duct adjacent to the nipple was left undisturbed and the 4th mammary fat pad ventral to the ventral inguinal lymph node and the entire 5th mammary fat pad were surgically removed, did the remaining primary lactiferous duct usually not survive. When these lactiferous ducts survived, they grew in a small area of fatty stroma surrounding the retained primary lactiferous duct but did not grow into the cleared fat pad between which there was no connecting fatty stroma retained (Fig. 3). Group D: the opera-

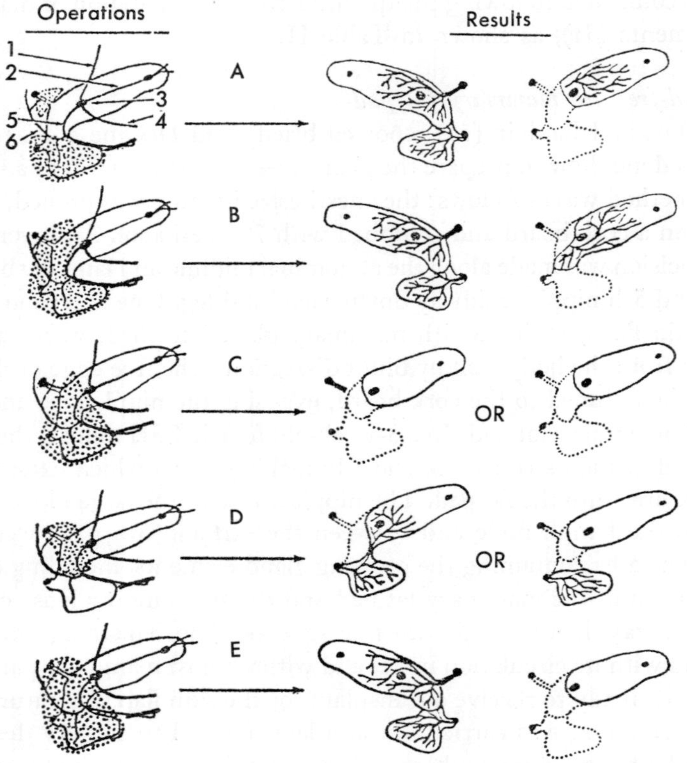

FIG. 2. The five different types of operations (A through E) in relation to their blood supply, in which different amounts and material in different areas of the right 4th and 5th mammary glands and fat pads were removed (shaded areas)

Left side was retained as a control. Mammary growth after these operations is shown. Areas bounded by dotted lines indicate lack of both mammary glands and fat pads. (1) Lateral anastomotic mammary vessels. (2) Dorsal mammary vessels. (3) Ventral inguinal lymph node. (4) Lumbar mammary vessels. (5) Inferior mammary vessels. (6) Branch of these vessels to the 5th mammary glands and the nipple area of the 4th mammary glands.

Operation procedures—Group A: Primary lactiferous duct of 4th, and all parts of 5th mammary glands were removed. Group B: Major parts of 4th mammary gland fat-pad area ventromedial to the ventral inguinal lymph node and the 5th mammary glands and fat pads were removed. Small area laterocaudal to the inferior mammary vessels in 4th mammary fat pad was retained. Group C: Except for a part of the primary lactiferous duct adjacent to nipple, 6 to 10 mm long, 4th mammary fat pad ventral to the ventral inguinal lymph node and 5th mammary glands and fat pad were removed. Group D: Entire area of 4th mammary gland fat pad ventromedial to ventral inguinal lymph node including the primary lactiferous duct was removed. Fifth mammary glands and fat pad were retained intact. Group E: In addition to operation described under Group D, the 5th mammary glands and fat pads were also removed.

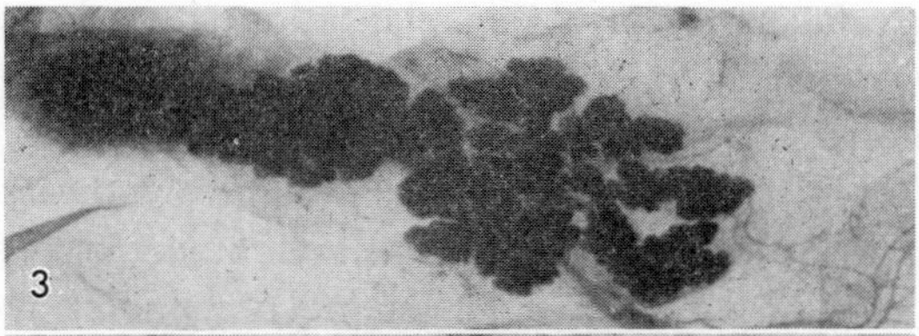

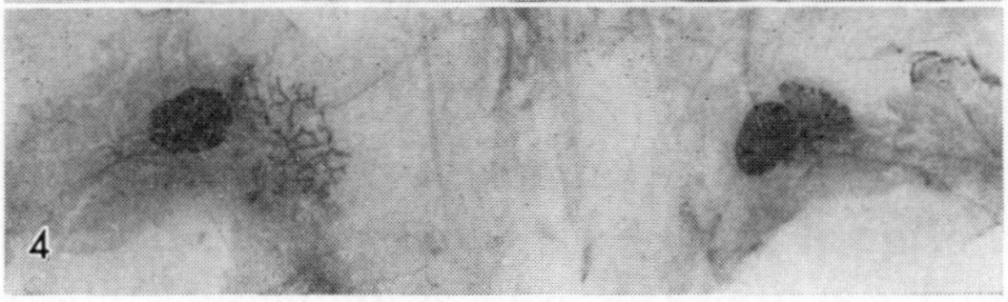

FIG. 3. Mammary gland regenerated from retained small portion of the primary lactiferous duct adjacent to the nipple after excision of mammary parenchyma as shown in Group C, Fig. 2

Growth and lactation in area of the retained fatty stroma are shown. Hemalum. ×10. From Ref. *32*.

FIG. 4. Successful transplant in the gland-free 4th mammary fat pad on the right side of a male host that grew only in area dorsolateral to ventral inguinal lymph node, after treatment with estradiol benzoate, progesterone, and prolactin

Intact control mammary gland of this male donor, which lacked a nipple, is shown on left side. Hemalum. ×2. From Ref. *32*.

tion procedure in this group was the same as the original one. It was found that the mammary parenchyma of the 5th gland would grow into the gland-free 4th mammary fat pad if the fatty tissue between the 4th and 5th glands remained connected. Blair and Moretti (*5*) had to exclude some cases of gland-free fat pads which contained host mammary parenchyma due to incomplete surgical removal of the host's own mammary parenchyma at 3 weeks of age. Group E: when the fat pads of the 4th and 5th mammary glands, sufficient to include all mammary parenchyma and the primary lactiferous ducts, were removed, removal of all mammary parenchyma was assured. Therefore, this type of operation was found to be most satisfactory in preparing the gland-free 4th mammary fat pad as a future site for mammary transplantation. Due to the extent of growth of the host's 4th mammary gland duct system prior to this surgical procedure, as previously reported (*16*, *32*), it is necessary to operate on the proposed host mice while they were less than 25 days of age or weighing 11 g, whichever comes earlier (*32*). The blood supply of the remaining gland-free 4th mammary fat pad was always left undisturbed.

In 1963, the staff of the Cancer Research Genetics Laboratory, University of California, Berkeley, stated that there appears to be nothing special about mammary fat *per se* as a transplantation site other than its great mechanical convenience (*70*).

As shown in Table II, the ultimate growth extent of mammary grafts placed in the gland-free 4th mammary fat pad was always greater than that attained by grafts in other sites such as the subcutaneous tissue, the pararenal fat pad, or the mesometrial fat layer, all of which have much smaller amounts of the adipose stroma (*34*). These results confirmed previously reported findings (*32*).

The ultimate growth extent of mammary grafts in this site was always greater than the original graft size (Table II), but varied in actual size due to experimental conditions as well as individual differences in grafts. Some grafts occupied small areas of the gland-free fat pad (Fig. 4) and the others occupied a considerable area of fat pad (Fig. 5) or the entire fat pad (Fig. 6). Faulkin and DeOme (*22*) estimated the amount of outgrowth produced by a transplant by measuring to the nearest 10% the area of the fat pad occupied by the outgrowth. They claimed that this measure was satisfactory as an actual area measurement, and it avoids error arising from tissue shrinkage in processing and strain and individual variations in the fat pad size.

4) *Pararenal fat pad*

The pararenal fat pad has been used as a retroperitoneal site of mammary transplantation (*34*). The pararenal fat pad provided a satisfactory site for mammary grafts which grew to a much greater extent than that attained by grafts in the subcutaneous area (Fig. 7 and Table II). When the host mice reared young, the surviving mammary grafts in the pararenal fat pads responded to gestational and lactational hormonal stimuli in a manner similar to that exerted by the hosts' own mammary glands and secreted milk. Such milk-secreting mammary grafts often occupied the entire volume of adipose tissue in this site, as shown in Fig. 8 (*34*).

5) *Peritoneal cavity*

Small pieces, approximately 2×2 mm in size, minced from the mammary tissue adjacent to the primary lactiferous ducts were inserted into the peritoneal cavity with fine forceps through a small hole made in the lateral abdominal wall of female isologous host mice. The hosts were subsequently mated and reared young. Mammary grafts which were recovered from the peritoneal cavity floated in it without adhering to the peritoneum and appeared to be spherical. Histologically, these spherical mas-

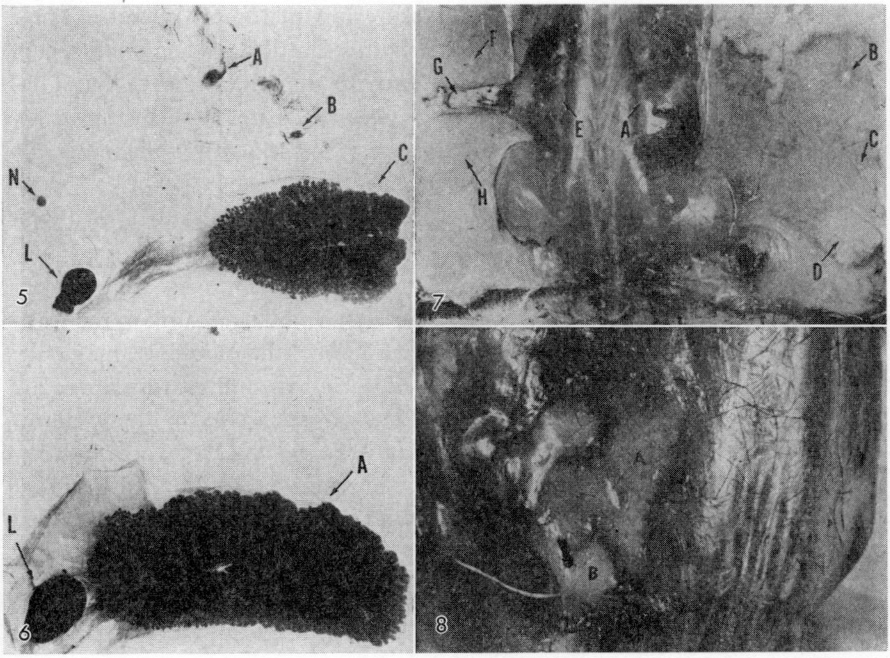

FIG. 5. The whole mounts of two subcutaneous grafts (A and B) and the gland-free mammary fat pad with a successful mammary graft, which occupied almost half of the area and lactated (C)

Hemalum. ×4.5. From Ref. *34*.

FIG. 6. The whole mounts of a successful mammary graft in the gland-free 4th mammary fat pad, which occupied the entire fat pad

Hemalum. ×4.6. From Ref. *34*.

FIG. 7. Photograph of the dorsal view of the host mouse which received eight mammary grafts

Seven grafts were successfully transplanted. The skin was reflected from a mid-dorsal incision to expose the inner surface of the skin body, wall, and subjacent structures. The mesometrial fat layer was surgically fixed extraperitoneally under the subcutaneous tissue through a small fenestra made on the dorsolateral adsominal wall. A and E, grafts in right and left pararenal fat pads; B, C, and F, grafts in the subcutaneous areas; D, a graft in the left gland-free mammary fat pad; H, the left 4th mammary fat pad having its preexisting mammary gland; G, a graft in the mesometrial fat layer ectopically fixed in the subcutaneous area. ×1.4. From Ref. *34*.

FIG. 8. Photograph of the dorsolateral view of the body wall of a female host mouse

(A) a successully transplanted and lactating graft in the left pararenal fat pad. (B) a successfully grafted and lactating mammary transplant in the mesometrial fat layer in the peritoneal cavity. ×3.0. From Ref. *34*.

ses were fully occupied by the milk-secreting mammary glands. Their overall size, however, was not appreciably increased. This again suggested that adipose stroma transplanted together with mammary parenchyma did not increase in size and the surviving adipose stroma was occupied by regenerating mammary parenchymal tissue (Hoshino, unpublished).

6) Mesometrial fat layer

The mesometrium of the mouse contains varying amounts of adipose tissue, and this fat layer has been used as a site of mammary transplantation (*34*). Some of the mesometria were surgically fixed under the subcutaneous tissue between the 3rd (thoracic) and 4th (inguinal) mammary gland areas with silk sutures after being pulled out extraperitoneally through a small fenestra made in the dorso-lateral aspect of the abdominal wall (Fig. 7) and the other mesometria were *in situ* (Fig. 8). Mammary grafts in either situation survived equally on transplantation, grew greater than the original size of grafted duct-segments (Table II), and secreted milk when the host mice lactated (Fig. 9). This experiment again indicated the functional capability of mammary glands is unaffected by the internal environment of the peritoneal cavity.

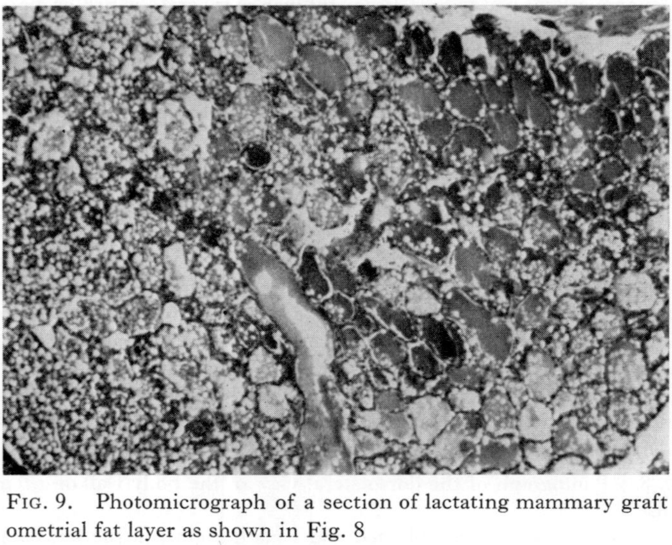

FIG. 9. Photomicrograph of a section of lactating mammary graft in the mesometrial fat layer as shown in Fig. 8
Hematoxylin and eosin. ×70. From Ref. *34*.

7) *Anterior chamber of the eye*

The anterior chamber of the eye has been used as a site of mammary transplantation (*45*).

This site has been utilized for auto-, iso-, allo-, and even xeno-grafting of tissues and has been considered a unique site because of the easy identification and the high successful recovery rate of viable graft tissue since 1947 (*28*). The anterior chamber of the eye is filled with aqueous humor but lacks stromal tissue, thus it was considered an excellent site for the study of parenchymal-stromal interactions in mammary glands during early

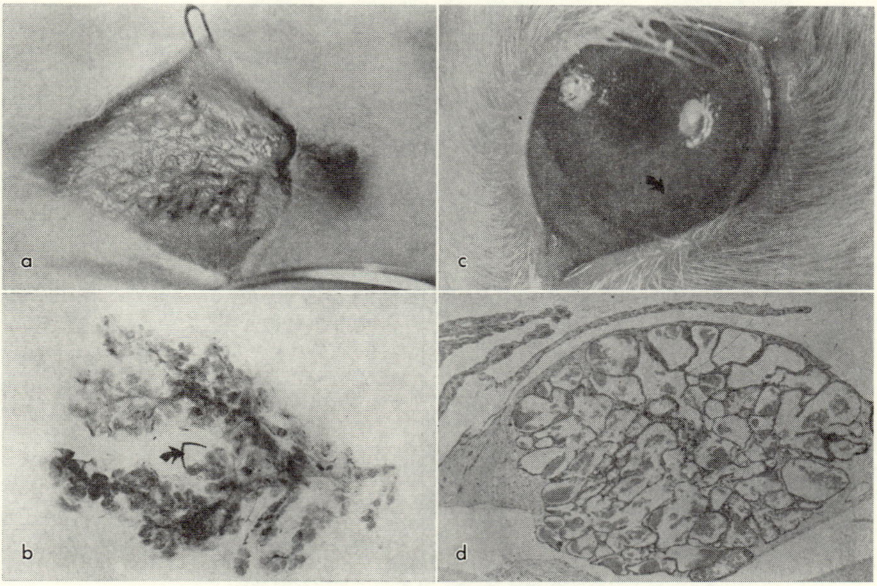

FIG. 10. (a) A donor mammary gland vitally stained with 0.5% aqueous trypan blue solution injected through a tiny lactiferous orifice at the tip of the nipple using a gauge 30 hypodermic needle

(b) A vitally stained lobe of a mammary gland excised and placed in a Petri dish moistened with Eagle culture medium

The known area of the mammary gland as indicated by the arrow was taken and autografted into the anterior chamber of the eye of the rabbit.

(c) A vitally stained mammary segment autografted into the anterior chamber of the eye as indicated by the arrow

(d) Photomicrograph of a milk-secreting mammary graft in the anterior chamber of the eye of the lactating host rabbit

Note its relation to the iris. Hematoxylin and eosin. ×60. Hoshino, unpublished.

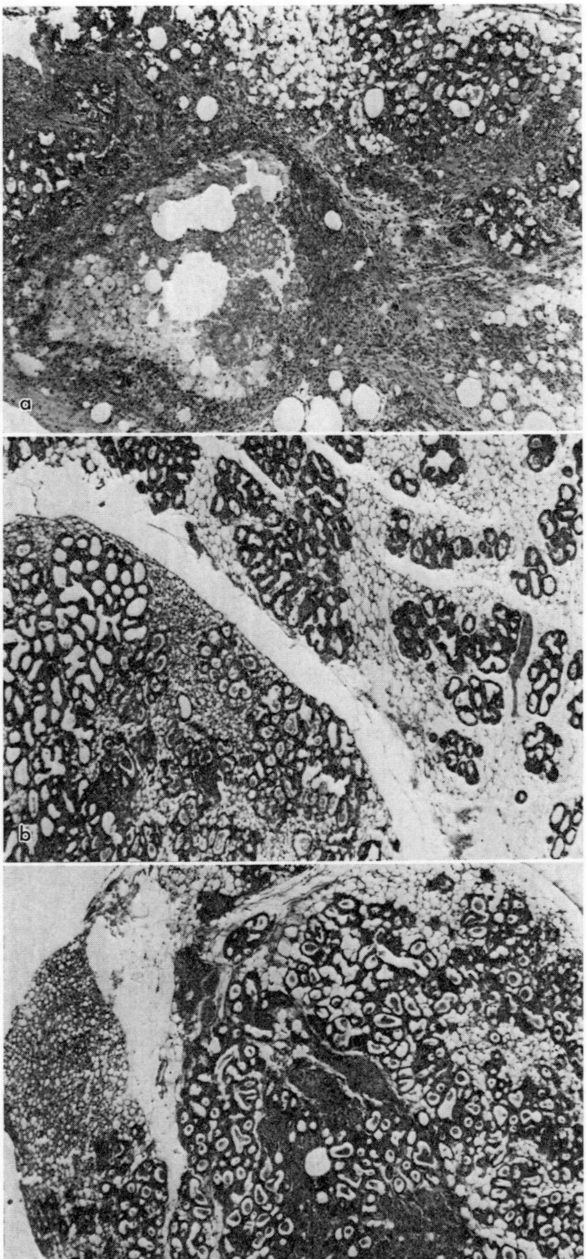
a
b
c

histogenesis of mammary isografts (*45*). The results obtained from this experiment will be described later in Section 11.

In our laboratory, mammary duct-segments of a normal female white rabbit locally obtained were quantitatively autografted into the antrieor chamber of the eye (*40*). These autografts secreted milk in the eye when the rabbit lactated as shown in Fig. 10 (Hoshino, unpublished).

8) *Interscapular brown fat*

Interscapular brown fat was also used as a site of mammary transplantation (*37*).

Interscapular brown fat is morphologically, biochemically, physiologically, and endocrinologically different from white fat (*1*, *47*), but peripherally denervated interscapular brown fat resembles white fat because of an increase in its content of water, glycogen, lipids, and also because of histological changes (*67*). When 3-methylcholanthrene was administered intraperitoneally into the mice, the concentration of this carcinogen was spectrofluorometrically found to be higher in the interscapular brown fat than in the mammary white fat (*41*).

Interscapular brown fat was transplanted from C57BL or CBA mice

←FIG. 11. (a) Photomicrograph of transplanted brown fat and mammary tissue

The main portions of the transplanted brown fat tissue underwent degeneration and necrosis. Tissue surrounding the necrotic mass was replaced by connective tissue. Simultaneously transplanted mammary glands survived severse degenerative changes occurring in the adjacent brown fat, regenerated and grew into the adipose tissue, and responded to the host's endogenous hormonal stimulation during pregnancy. Hematoxylin and eosin. ×40.

(b) Photomicrograph of a part of the brown fat that had been transplanted into the mammary fat pad having its intact mammary parenchyma

On the lower left half, the host's mammary parenchyma grew into the surviving brown fat which retained characteristic multilocular structures, in contrast to the white fat stroma with the host's mammary parenchyma shown on the upper right half. Hematoxylin and eosin. ×40.

(c) Photomicrograph of transplanted brown fat and mammary graft in the gland-free 4th mammary fat pad of a host

The portion on the left side retained typical multilocular brown fat structures after transplantation, whereas the portion on the right side resembled white fat tissue. The center portion of the transplanted brown fat underwent necrosis and was replaced with connective tissue. Transplanted mammary gland regenerated and grew into the adjacent brown fat graft tissue. Mammary graft tissue grew better in the tissue which resembled white adipose tissue than in the graft retaining its characteristics of brown fat. Hematoxylin and eosin. ×40. Hoshino, unpublished.

into female F_1 reciprocal hybrids at (1) gland-free 4th mammary fat pads, (2) mammary fat pads with the pre-existing hosts' mammary glands, or (3) gland-free 4th mammary fat pads accompanied by mammary tissue of the same donor mice. When grafts were examined after normal pregnancy and parturition of the hosts, some grafts became necrotic fibrotic, and others entirely or partially lost their multilocular characteristics of brown fat and resembled white fat, as shown in Fig. 11 (Hoshino, unpublished). Some surviving brown fat retained the characteristics of brown fat on transplantation. Both the hosts' and donors' mammary glands grew into the transplanted brown fat, and responded to endogenous hormones normally and secreted milk (Fig. 11). When brown fat grafts were encapsulated, mammary ducts were unable to penetrate the fibrous capsule (*35*).

When immature brown fat tissue was cultured in synthetic media, they differentiated and retained an appearance typical of brown fat, but when they were cultured with serum, the cells progressively accumulated cytoplasmic lipid and resembled white fat cells (*66*).

Mammary duct-segments, each 0.6 mm long, transplanted by the quantitative transplantation method into the denervated and sham-operated interscapular brown fat pads for 3 weeks, were found to survive equally well in both sites (Table III). Successfully transplanted mammary grafts in either site actively regenerated and responded equally well to exogenously administered progesterone and estradiol benzoate as shown in Fig. 12 (*37*).

The reasons why mammary glands of the second (axillary) or 3rd (thoracic) pairs of non-lactating mice usually would not grow into and occupy the whole body of the interscapular brown fat pads which are

TABLE III. Rates of Recovery of Regenerating Mammary Grafts from Either Sham-operated or Peripherally Denervated Interscapular Brown Fat Pads

Experimental group	Site of transplantation	
	Sham-operated brown fat pads	Denervated brown fat pads
Series I: female CBA donor to female host CBA mice	10/16[a] (62.5%)	14/16 (87.5%)
Series II: female CBA donor to female (female CBA×male C57BL) F_1 hybrid host mice	13/15 (86.7%)	(12/15 80.0%)

[a] Number of successful mammary grafts/number of mammary transplants. Differences in rates of recovery are not statistically significant.
From Ref. *37*.

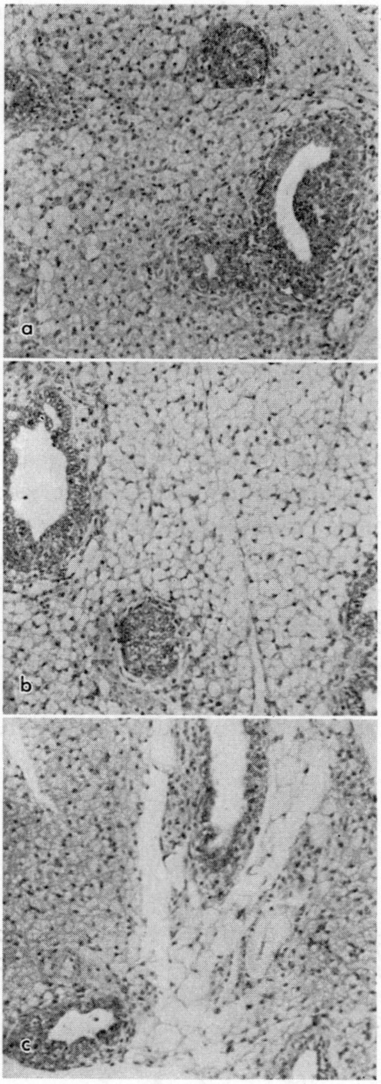

FIG. 12. Photomicrographs of mammary grafts regenerating in the interscapular brown fat (a) showing multilocular characterisctic histological features, in the denervated interscapular brown fat (b) which resembled histological features of white fat, and in the sham-operated interscapular brown fat (c) where enlarged monolocular fat cells surrounded the regenerating mammary graft tissue

Hematoxylin and eosin. ×120. From Ref. *37*.

ventrally continuous with white fat stroma of those mammary glands are unknown. However, lactating glands often grew into the adjacent brown fat pad (Hoshino, unpublished).

9) Space under the kidney capsule

The space under the kidney capsule was used as a site of transplantation for isolated embryonic mammary epithelium together with isolated mesenchyme derived from either mammary anlagen or salivary glands (*64*). Details of this work will be discussed later in Section 12.

5. *Transplantability in Relation to the Origin of Duct-segments*

It was necessary to find out from which portion of the mammary duct-segment the process of regeneration of surviving mammary grafts begins. For this purpose the following experiments were undertaken (*34*).

The original portions of mammary duct-segments were for descriptive purposes designated as shown in Fig. 13. Recovery rates of mammary grafts derived from various ductal portions indicated that the original portion of the duct-segments transplanted or the original size of the grafts did not influence the overall transplantability (Tables IV–VI), except the nipples. The nipples transplanted with the primary lactiferous ducts were absorbed, or when they persisted, were encapsulated and were never vi-

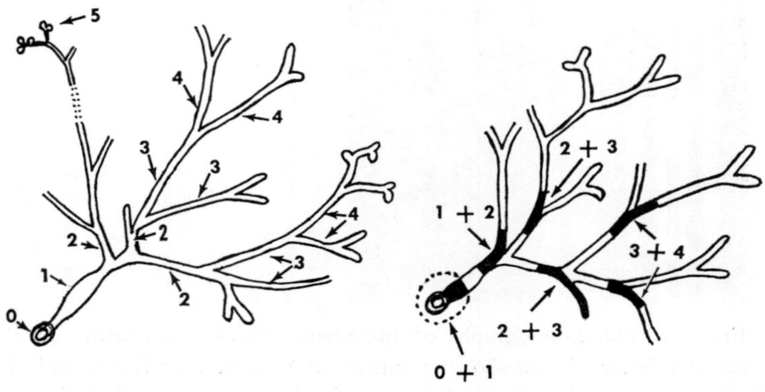

FIG. 13. The designated portions of the original mammary graft duct-segments are shown

0, nipple; 1, primary lactiferous duct; 2, secondary lactiferous duct; 3, tertiary lactiferous duct; 4, quaternary lactiferous duct; 5, end bud. From Ref. *34*.

TABLE IV. Recovery Rate of Grafts that Consisted of Segments of Different Lengths from Different Portions of Donors' Mammary Ducts

Portion[a]	Original length of transplant (mm)					Total (%)
	<0.2~0.5	0.6	0.7~1.0	1.2~1.4	1.5~3.0	
0+1	5/12[b]	5/5[(a)]	2/6	0/4[(b)]	0/1	12/28 (43)
1 or 1+2	4/7	2/4	7/8	3/5	3/10	19/34 (56)
2 or 2+3	1/4	6/11	6/10	5/10	7/15	25/50 (50)
3 or 3+4	4/5	6/7	8/14	8/15	15/29	41/70 (59)
4 or 5	9/20	5/6	6/9	4/6	1/2	25/43 (58)
Total (%)	23/48[(c)] (48)	24/33[(d)] (73)	29/47 (62)	20/40 (50)	26/57[(e)] (46)	122/225 (54.2)

[a] Portions are designated in Fig. 13.

[b] Number of successful grafts/number of transplants. Statistical differences: (*b*)<(*a*), (*c*) <(*d*), and (*e*)<(*d*).

From Ref. *34*.

TABLE V. Recovery Rate of Grafts that Were Obtained from Different Portions of Donors' Mammary Ducts and Transplanted at Different Sites in Hosts

Portion[a]	Transplantation site				Total (%)
	Pararenal fat pad	Dorsal subcutis	4mgffp	Mesometrial fat pad	
0+1	1/2[b]	1/11[(a)]	9/13[(g)]	1/2	12/28[(h)] (43)
1 or 1+2	4/9	8/16[(b)]	6/8	1/1	19/34 (56)
2 or 2+3	4/11	18/31[(c)]	2/4	1/4	25/50 (50)
3 or 3+4	9/18	22/39[(d)]	7/9	3/4	41/70 (59)
4 or 5	10/18	10/17[(e)]	5/8		25/43 (58)
Total (%)	28/58[(i)] (48)	59/114[(f)] (52)	29/42[(j)] (69)	6/11 (55)	122/225 (54.2)

[a] Portions are designated in Fig. 13.

[b] Number of successful grafts/number of transplants. Statistical differences: (*a*) is smaller than any of (*b*)***, (*c*), (*d*), (*e*), (*f*), (*g*), and (*h*). (*i*)<(*j*). ***(*a*)<(*b*), however, is not significant when Yates' correction (Croxton, '59) is applied.

From Ref. *34*.

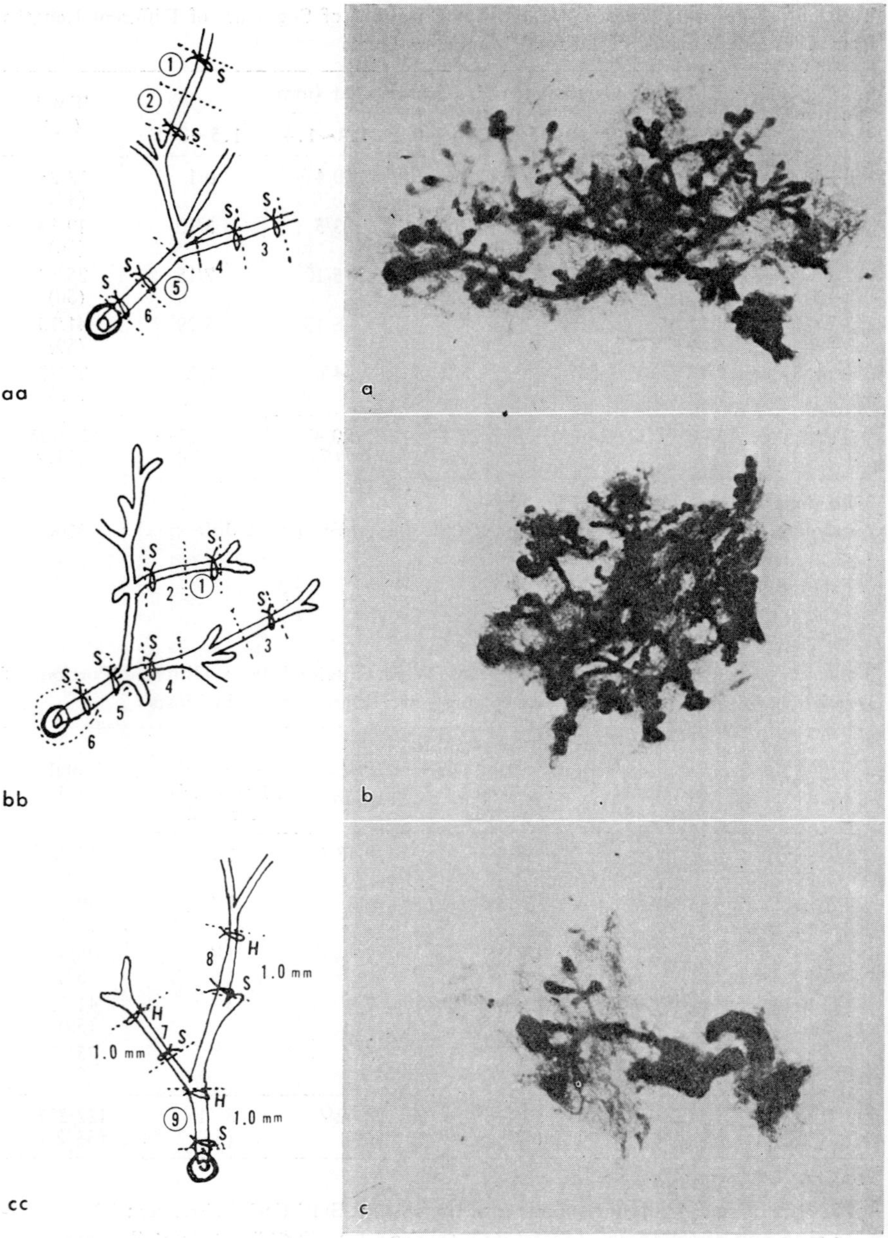
aa
a
bb
b
cc
c
1.0 mm
1.0 mm
1.0 mm

TABLE VI. Recovery Rate of Grafts that Were Obtained from Different Portions of Mammary Ducts of CBA and Hybrid Female Donors of Different Ages and Transplanted into Hosts of Different Ages and Sex

Donor (age)[b]	Host (age)	Portion of donors' mammary duct[a]					Total (%)
		0+1	1 or 1+2	2 or 2+3	3 or 3+4	4 or 5	
♀ CBA (20–76)	♀ CBA (30–115)	6/16[c]	7/9	9/13	9/15	6/7	37/60$^{(h)}$ (62)
♀ CBA (72–76)	♀ CC-F_1 (110–111)	2/2	0/1	4/4$^{(a)}$	6/11	1/5	13/23$^{(i)}$ (57)
♀ CC-F_1 (117)	♀ CC-F_1 (130–186)	1/1	1/1	1/2	4/4$^{(c)}$	5/14	12/22$^{(j)}$ (55)
♀ CBA (734)	♀ CBA (88–93)		1/3	4/6	5/9	2/3	12/21$^{(k)}$ (57)
♀ CBA (20–84)	♂ CBA (24–46)	2/4	5/7	4/10	11/13$^{(d)}$	3/5	25/39$^{(l)}$ (64)
♀ CBA (734)	♂ CC-F_1 (41)		1/1	0/2	1/2	2/2	4/7 (57)
♀ CBA (20–84)	♂ CBA (28–46)	1/5	4/11	3/12$^{(b)}$	5/11	6/7$^{(g)}$	19/46$^{(m)}$ (41)
♀ CBA (734)	♂ CBA (168)		0/1	0/1	0/5$^{(e)}$		0/7$^{(n)}$ (0)
Total (%)		12/28 (43)	19/34 (56)	25/50 (50)	41/70$^{(f)}$ (59)	25/43 (58)	122/225$^{(o)}$ (54.2)

[a] Portions are designated in Fig. 13.
[b] Day of age at the time of transplantation.
[c] Number of successful grafts/number of transplants. Statistical differences: $(b)<(a)$, $(b)<(g)$, $(e)<(c)$, $(e)<(d)$, $(e)<(f)$, $(m)<(h)$, $(m)<(l)$, and (n) is smaller than any of (h), (i), (j), (k), (l), (m), and (o).
From Ref. *34*.

←FIG. 14. On the left side, the sketches of the three donors' mammary glands from which duct-segments were excised after being ligated with 7–0 silk surgical suture (S) or human hair (H) at either proximal or distal ends are illustrated The locations of excision of segments are shown by dotted lines across mammary ducts. The length of each grafted duct-segment illustrated in aa and bb was 0.6 mm. The numbers beside each segment indicate the numerical order of excision of segments. Segments with numbers circled were successfully grafted and regenerated apparently normal mammary glands as shown on the right side. On the right side, the whole mounts of three successfully grafted and regenerating mammary transplants are illustrated.

(a) This mammary graft regenerated from the duct-segment with a silk suture at the end proximal to the nipple as shown in aa, 1. (b) This mammary graft regenerated from the duct-segment with a silk ligature at the end distal to the nipple as shown in bb, 1. (c) This mammary graft regenerated from the duct-segment with double ligatures at the both ends as shown in cc, 9. M in c indicates a non-viable portion of the transplanted duct-segment that had been replaced by connective tissue and still retained the shape of the original graft. Hemalum. ×20. From Ref. *34*.

able or at least partially replaced by connective tissue. Regardless of the origin of the duct-segments transplanted and the original size of the grafts, the ultimate extent of regenerating mammary grafts were determined by the amounts of adipose tissues available for grafts to proliferate (Table II).

6. *Directional Preference of Mammary Duct-segments in Regeneration*

In the previous section, it was concluded that mammary glands could regenerate from any portion of the duct. However, it was not known if mammary duct-segments would have preference in their growth direction in reference to their nipples. In order to clarify this question, the following experiments were carried out (*34*).

Forty-two mammary duct-segments were ligated by a single knot of either 7–0 surgical silk suture or contrasting human hair, which had been soaked in 70% ethanol and rinsed with Tyrode's solution. Ligatures were placed proximal to or distal to the nipples after the donors' mammary glands were vitally stained, removed, microdissected, and sketched (Fig. 14). All duct-segments measured 0.6 mm, except for three segments having two ligatures each. The amounts of mammary parenchyma remaining outside of the ligature were minimal, providing the ligature had not slipped off. The gland-free mammary fat pads were used as a site of transplantation. The results are illustrated in Fig. 14.

Five out of 42 duct-segments with ligatures were recovered viable and had regenerated mammary ducts. All ligatures including those with rejected duct-segments were recovered at the transplantation site encapsulated with thickened connective tissue. Newly regenerating mammary glands were found in grafts taken from the portion of the duct distal to the nipple, from the portion of the duct proximal to the nipple and also the duct-segment between the two ligatures (Fig. 14). Thus, this experiment revealed that mammary ducts do not have any directional preference in reference to their nipples and could regenerate from any portion. However, dense fibrous connective tissue encapsulating the mammary grafts reduced mammary transplantability to an unusually low rate of 12% (*34*).

7. *Sexual Differences in Mammary Transplantability*

Different combinations of donors and hosts can be made using males and females. The most common type is the female donor-female host combination. As far as transplantability of mammaıy isografts is concerned, both the male donor-female host combination and the female donor-castrated male host combination yielded recovery rates of viable grafts comparable to those attained by the female donor-female host combination (Table I). However, the functional fate of viable grafts in the different types of host mice depended on the hormonal environment in the hosts and the periods of transplantation. Non-castrated hosts provided mammary grafts with the least favorable hormonal environment, and transplantability was the poorest (Tables VII and VIII).

Mammary glands of the female mouse masculinized by prenatal administration of androgen were tested for their functional capability following transplantation (*36*). Development of both the nipples and the mammary anlagen of the female fetuses exposed *in utero* to 5 mg of testoste-

TABLE VII. Recovery Rate of Grafts Transplanted from CBA and Hybrid Female Donors of Different Ages into Hosts of Different Ages and Sex at Four Different Sites

Donor (age)[a]	Host (age)	Site of transplantation				Total (%)
		Pararenal fat pad	Dorsal subcutis	4mgffp	Mesometrial fat pad	
♀ CBA (20-76)	♀ CBA (30-115)	9/14[b]	17/28[(a)]	9/11	2/7	37/60[(h)] (60)
♀ CBA (72-76)	♀ $CC\text{-}F_1$ (110-111)	4/6	4/11	3/4	2/2	13/23[(i)] (57)
♀ $CC\text{-}F_1$ (117)	♀ $CC\text{-}F_1$ (130-186)	2/6	7/11	1/3	2/2	12/22[(j)] (55)
♀ CBA (734)	♀ CBA (88-93)	1/6	9/12[(b)]	2/3		12/21[(k)] (57)
♀ CBA (20-84)	♂̸ CBA (24-46)	6/10	13/20[(c)]	6/9		25/39[(l)] (64)
♀ CBA (734)	♂̸ $CC\text{-}F_1$ (41)	2/2	2/4	0/1		4/7 (57)
♀ CBA (20-84)	♂ CBA (28-46)	4/12	7/24[(d)]	8/10[(g)]		19/46[(m)] (41)
♀ CBA (734)	♂ CBA (168)	0/2	0/4[(e)]	0/1		0/7[(n)] (0)
Total (%)		28/58[(q)] (48)	59/114[(f)] (52)	29/42[(r)] (69)	6/11 (55)	122/225[(o)] (54.2)

[a] Day of age at the time of transplantation.

[b] Number of successful grafts/number of transplants. Statistical differences: (*d*) is smaller than any of (*a*), (*b*), (*c*), (*e*), (*f*), and (*g*). (*e*) is smaller than any of (*a*), (*b*), and (*f*). (*n*) is smaller than any of (*h*), (*i*), (*j*), (*k*), (*l*), (*m*), and (*o*). (*m*)<(*h*), (*m*)<(*l*), and (*q*)<(*r*).

From Ref. *34*.

TABLE VIII. Recovery Rate of Grafts of Different Lengths that Were Transplanted from Female Donors to Female Hosts, Castrated Male Hosts of Non-castrated Male Hosts at Different Sites

Transplantation site	Original length of transplant (mm)					Total
	<0.2∼0.5	0.6	0.7∼1.0	1.2∼1.4	1.5∼3.0	
Female donor to female host						
Pararenal fat pad	4/8[a]	4/5[(a)]	5/6[(b)]	3/4[(c)]	0/9[(d)]	16/32[(e)]
Dorsal subcutis	3/10[(f)]	10/12[(g)]	8/13	6/12	10/15[(h)]	37/62[(i)]
4mgffp	7/11	4/4	1/2	1/1	2/3	15/21
Mesometrial fat	1/2	1/1	2/4	1/2	1/2	6/11
Subtotal	15/31[(j)]	19/22[(k)]	16/25	11/19[(l)]	13/29[(m)]	74/126[(n)]
Female donor to castrated male host						
Pararenal fat pad	1/3	1/2	2/3	1/1	3/3	8/12
Dorsal subcutis			5/5	4/9	6/10	15/24[(o)]
4mgffp	1/2	2/3	2/2		1/3	6/10
Subtotal	2/5	3/5	9/10	5/10	10/16	29/46
Female donor to non-castrated male host						
Pararenal fat pad	1/3	0/2	1/4	0/1	2/4	4/14[(p)]
Dorsal subcutis	0/3	0/2	3/7	3/8	1/8	7/28[(q)]
4mgffp	5/6	2/2	0/1	1/2		8/11[(r)]
Subtotal	6/12	2/6	4/12	4/11	3/12	19/53
Total (%)	23/48[(t)] (48)	24/33[(u)] (73)	29/47 (62)	20/40[(v)] (50)	26/57[(w)] (46)	122/225[(s)] (54.2)

[a] Number of successful grafts/number of transplants. Statistical differences: (*d*) is smaller than any of (*a*), (*b*), (*c*), (*e*), and (*h*). (*f*)<(*g*). (*k*) is greater than any of (*j*), (*l*), (*m*), and (*n*). (*q*) is smaller than any of (*i*), (*o*), (*r*), and (*s*). (*p*)<(*r*). (*u*) is greater than any of (*t*), (*v*), (*w*), and (*s*).
From Ref. *34*.

rone propionate injected in their mothers on day 12 of pregnancy was remarkably inhibited. These female young were masculinized and also had vaginal atresia and retention of serous fluids in the uterine horns. Mammary duct-segments from those masculinized glands were isografted in the left side of the gland-free 4th mammary fat pad, and grafts from control donors into the opposite side. Following isografting, the hosts were mated and both grafts were examined at parturition. Both masculinized and control mammary grafts regenerated and responded to endogenous gestational hormones and secreted milk (Fig. 15). The recovery rates of viable grafts from the androgen-treated group (17/21; 81%) and from the untreated control group (15/21; 71%) were also comparable.

FIG. 15. Whole mount of the stained milk-secreting transplanted mammary glands in the gland-free 4th mammary fat pads

A graft regenerating in the fat pad on the left side derived from an untreated control donor, and the one on the left side derived from a prenatally androgen treated donor. Alum carmine. ×2.2. From Ref. *36*.

The results indicated that parenchymal cells of morphologically masculinized female mammary glands were not functionally impaired during prenatal masculinization (*36*).

8. *Heterochronic Donor-Host Relationship*

Apart from autografting, various ages of donors and hosts could be matched to make a specific donor-host combination in order to study the influence of age upon mammary glands of the donor and also upon physiological conditions (internal environment) of the host animals in conjunction with the transplantability and functional fate of mammary isografts.

To the best of my knowledge, the oldest donor mouse whose mammary glands were isografted was 26 months of age (*76*) and the next was a 734-day-old CBA virgin female mouse (*34*). The youngest donor was a neonate which donated mammary glands within 16 hr after birth (*12*). The youngest host mice were 21-day-old females of either the C3H or CBA strain, or those of (CBA×C57BL) F_1 hybrids (*17*, *32*). The oldest host mice were 18-month-old (♀C57BL×♂CBA) F_1 hybrid virgins (*44*). Transplantability of mammary grafts in these donor-host combinations is summarized in Table I. Mammary grafts even from a quiescent gland of the 734-day-old virgin mouse secreted milk when the host mice lactated (*34*). Isografts of neonatal mammary glands in adult female hosts which were mated 1 day after transplantation exhibited a midpregnant functional stage only 19 days after birth and milk-secretion at 30 days after birth (Fig. 16, Currie, Hoshino, and Kim, unpublished). These mammary graft tissues apparently are the youngest glands that reached

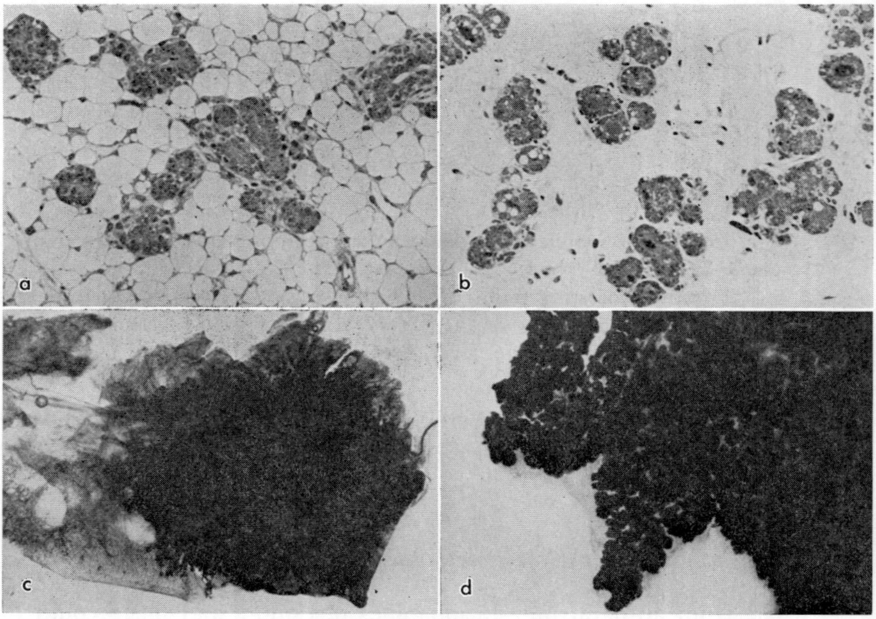

FIG. 16. Photomicrograph of a mammary graft (a) which was successfully isografted from a neonate into the gland-free 4th mammary fat pad of an adult virgin C3H female host

It regenerated and responded to endogenous hormonal stimuli in a manner similar to that of the host's mammary gland (b) when examined on day 12 of pregnancy. This graft was recovered from the host, 19 days after isografting, at only 19 days of age of the donor's mammary gland. It is apparently the youngest mammary gland which reached a mid-pregnant functional stage *in vivo*. Hematoxylin and eosin staining after plastic embedding. ×600.

Whole mounts of a mammary graft (c) and of a host's mammary gland (d) which were obtained from the C3H host mouse at day 0 postpartum are shown. This graft was isografted from a neonate into the gland-free 4th mammary fat pad of a virgin female C3H mouse that was subsequently mated and had normal parturition. This mammary graft (c) derived from a neonate not only survived on transplantation but also secreted milk, 30 days after birth, comparable to the lactating host's mammary gland (d). Alum carmine. ×9. Currie, Hoshino, and Kim, unpublished.

such functional stages *in vivo*. Histological features of those grafts as well as non-secreting grafts in unmated host mice were indistinguishable from those exhibited by mammary glands of the host mice (*12*). The results indicated that the age of the donor mice was not the determining factor in the success of transplantation. The mammary parenchyma of all ages had the capability of regeneration and growth in a new environment as long as the environment was favorable, even in the older host mice.

According to the experiments by Mori, Mills, and Bern (unpublished), and cited by Ref. *3*, when mammary glands of neonatally estrogen-exposed Balb/cfC3H female mice were transplanted into the gland-free mammary fat pads of normal mice on the day after completion of neonatal treatment for 5 days, the transplanted glands at 3 months following transplantation were indistinguishable from the host glands.

9. *Life Span of Mammary Parenchyma*

In the preceding section, it was concluded that mammary parenchyma of all ages exhibited the capability of regeneration and growth in a new environment as long as the environment was favorable. However, it was not known how long mammary parenchyma would be capable of regenerating when the *in vivo* environment was renewed repeatedly. In order to determine whether the life span of the mammary gland would be limited to the life span of the mouse, a serial transplantation of mammary duct-segments derived from the original donor's gland was carried out for several generations (*14*, *39*, *43*, *76*).

In the first experiment (*43*), mammary duct-segments, 0.6 mm long with a small amount of surrounding adipose tissue, were transplanted from the 3rd mammary gland of a 135-day-old CBA female mouse into the gland-free 4th mammary fat pads of young adult female host mice as the T_1 generation for serial transplantation. The hosts were (♀ BC_B ×♂ CBA) F_1 hybrid (designated as BA-1) and (♀ CBA×♂ BC_B) F_1 hybrid (designated as BA-2) mice. Serial transplantations were made approximately every 3 months. Some host mice were mated soon after they received mammary grafts (parous line). Others were not mated until serial transplantations were performed from them to the succeeding generations (virgin line). The recovery rates of regenerating mammary grafts are summarized in Table IX. The data showed that selected and surviving mammary graft tissue can regenerate and grow the normal structures of mammary glands when placed in younger animals. At the T_6 or T_7 generation, transplantability remained reasonably high. However, it was not known whether the reduced transplantability of mammary grafts after three or four generations of serial transplantation was due to the lack of transplantability of the adipose tissue and connective tissue closely attached to the duct-segments or to that of the mammary parenchyma.

TABLE IX. Incidence of Successful Mammary Transplants at Different Generations of Serial Transplantation

Transplantation generation	Virgin line: No. of successful grafts	Virgin line: No. of transplants	Virgin line: %	Virgin line: No. of host mice	Parous line: No. of successful grafts	Parous line: No. of transplants	Parous line: %	Parous line: No. of host mice
BA_1 host line								
T_1	9	14	64.3	7				
T_2	33	66	50.0	33				
T_3	4	38	10.5	19	11	26	42.3	13
T_4	11	20	55.0	10	1	34	2.9	17
T_5	12	18	66.7	9	6	16	37.5	8
T_6	26	36	72.2	18	23	36	63.9	18
Total T_3-T_6	53	112	47.3	56	41	112	36.6	56
T_1-T_6	95	192	49.5	96				
BA_2 host line								
T_1	8	14	57.1	7				
T_2	18	34	52.9	17				
T_3	19	34	55.9	17	26	36	72.2	18
T_4	18	32	56.3	16	3	36	8.3	18
T_5	3	40	7.5	20	19	40	47.5	20
T_6	20	42	47.6	21	25	40	62.5	20
T_7	11	38	28.4	19	2	14	14.3	7
Total T_3-T_7	71	186	38.2	93	75	166	45.2	83
T_1-T_7	97	234	41.5	117				

From Ref. *42*.

White fat tissue has been reported to be not readily transplantable (*32*, *57*). The longest life span of the mammary gland tissue of the original donor CBA mouse in this experiment was 1,379 days and at the end of the experiment this mammary gland was found to have be capable of responding to endogenous hormonal stimuli in a manner similar to that of the mammary glands of the hosts. This result suggests that the capability of the mammary parenchymal tissue to survive *in vivo* was much longer than the life span of the mouse, providing the environmental conditions were favorable.

Contrarily, in the following year, Daniel *et al.* (*14*) stated that their results, in which transplantability is measured by growth rate, were interpreted as indicating a relatively short life span even under optimum conditions. Their results showed that the maximum time that any normal transplant series could be carried was 24 months, a period within the life span of a mouse. Further, they oddly stated that it is possible that normal glands could be maintained for far longer periods if the interval between transplantations was lengthened, which seemed to contradict their preceeding statement. They transplanted approximately 0.5 mm long duct segments into the gland-free 4th mammary fat pads using the C57BL, Balb/c, and C3H strains of mice. The methods of evaluation of the results were as follows:

At the close of each transplant generation all the 4th mammary fat pads and a portion of the hosts' thoracic mammary glands were removed, fixed, extracted in acetone, stained with hematoxylin, and stored in methyl salicylate. The amount of outgrowth was recorded as follows: 0% fat pad filled indicated that no recognizable gland could be located with the dissecting microscope. 1–5% indicated that identifiable mammary tissue was present but had grown only 1–5 times the size of the original transplant. Where more development had occurred, growth was estimated by determining to the nearest 10% the amount of the available fat pad occupied by the gland.

At each generation the per cent of successful transplants and the mean per cent of fat pad filled were calculated. The latter figure, which is a measure of growth, was calculated on the basis of successful trans-

TABLE X. Serial Transplantation of Mouse Mammary Gland

	Mice				Transplants			
Exp.	Strain	Age at transplantation (wks)	Reproductive state of host[a]	Trypan blue used[b]	Tissue	Growth rate of donor outgrowth	Total time carried	Total generations carried
1	Balb/c	12–20	LP	No	Lobule	Average	6 m	4
2	C57	3	LP	Yes	Lobule	Average	11 m	4
3	C57	3	V	Yes	Duct	Average	11 m	4
4	Balb/c	3	V	Yes	Duct	Fast	24 m	7
5	C3H	3	LP	No	Lobule	Fast	12 m	6
6	C3H	3	V	No	Nodule	Fast	8.5 yr	34
7	C3H	3	V	No	Nodule	Fast	8 yr	32

[a] V, virgin; LP, lactating or pregnant.
[b] See the text.
From Ref. *14*.

plants only (1–100% fat pad filled). Fat pads which showed no evidence of mammary outgrowths were not included in this calculation because these failures reflected technical difficulties—problems associated with locating the donor tissues due to opacity of fat and imperfect vital staining with trypan blue, or difficulties experienced in removing transplants from very small outgrowths. The results are summarized in Table X. There were no statements in their paper concerning the ages of the original donors, thus the total life span of the original mammary gland in each serial transplantation line could not be calculated. In their experiment the longest period of serial transplantation was found to be 24 months, thus, the life span of the original mammary gland, including the age of the donor mouse at the time of grafting, obviously exceeded 24 months.

In 1970, Hoshino reported additional cases which confirmed the previous results (*43*). He concluded that the capability of serially transplanted mammary parenchyma to regenerate in a series of new and favorable environments was not age-dependent. The longest life span reported in this paper was 1,414 days after 6 generations in Line 1 with the survival rate of 26/36 (72%) and 1,379 days after 7 generations in Line 2 with a survival rate of 11/38 (29%). Mammary tissues in these lines could have been maintained much longer if the experiments did not have to be terminated.

In 1971, Young and associates extended the work previously reported by Daniel *et al.* in 1968, and concluded that the aging of mouse mammary tissue, as measured by a reduced capacity for ductal elongation during serial transplantation, is not consistently influenced by the age of mice used as original tissue donors. They observed that mammary grafts from young and old females showed similar growth characteristics when grown in a young environment and, within a given experiment, both had a similar life span. Old hosts, on the other hand, did not support comparably active growth of tissue regardless of the age of the donors from which initial transplants were obtained. They considered their results in view of the fact that mammary growth is an endocrine-dependent process, and particularly, elongation of ducts in virgin females requires stimulation by mammogenic hormones released during regular estrous cycling (*55*). Slow growth of the glands carried in old hosts could therefore be due to irregular or infrequent estrus. Thus the old hosts lacked, or had in reduced amount, hormonal factors required for mammary gland growth. The transplants were not permanently affected by these conditions however, for rapid growth commenced again when retransplanted into young animals. They speculated that the ability of grafts from old donors to proliferate rapidly in young hosts suggested that the life span of the mammary gland is influenced primarily by the number of cell divisions rather than by the passage of chronological or metabolic time. The mammary gland of a 26-month-old donor mouse was serially transplanted for 5 generations (10 months), the age (life span) of this mammary gland being 36 months of age (*76*).

It was observed that at the time of serial transplantation, surviving and regenerating mammary graft tissues sometimes consisted of small glands with a few small and fragile duct systems. Stainability of these regressing grafts with trypan blue was usually poor. This type of weakly regenerating graft was found irrespective of either the age of the tissue or the number of transplantation generations (Hoshino, *39*). Similar phenomena were experienced by Daniel *et al.* (*14*) and they suggested the possibility of a heterogenous population of mammary epithelial cells with respect to their proliferative potential. Bern *et al.* (*2*) observed that mammary tissue of C3H mice cultivated for 15 days in 199 media with or without cortisone, although exhibiting general necrosis histologically, maintained enough viable cells *in vitro* to sustain outgrowth development *in vivo*. Daniel and DeOme (*13*) succeeded in producing normal mammary outgrowth by implanting monolayer cultured mouse mammary cells into the gland-free 4th mammary fat pads. Hoshino and his associates (*9* and *45*) reported that small mammary duct isografts dissociated in the gland-free 4th mammary fat pads in 24 hr following transplantation but eventually regenerated into single mammary glands at each site of transplantation.

10. Pretreatment of Donor Mice

Prior to mammary transplantation, the donor mice can be conditioned according to the experimental designs by various means. Female donors may be mated and mammary tissues may be obtained from them during pregnancy (*52*), at parturition, during lactation, or during involution. Donors can be virgin as used most widely, or multiparous (*21*). Male donor mice can be castrated (*52*). In order to hormonally stimulate the donors' mammary glands, the donors may be injected with hormones or implanted with pellets containing hormones. Moretti and Blair (*52*) implanted pellets containing estradiol and desoxycorticosterone acetate into castrated male donors 1 month prior to transplantation. Pituitary isografts have been placed in the donor mice for 3 weeks prior to mammary transplantation to enhance growth (*45*). In order to study the immediate effects of 3-methylcholanthrene, a carcinogen, upon mammary glands, donors were pretreated with 3-methylcholanthrene intraperitoneally 9 hr prior to mammary isografting. Transplantability of these pretreated glands was not altered by 3-methylcholanthrene (*75*). The 3-methylcholanthrene was found to have a greater affinity for the mammary parenchyma than for the mammary fat (*41*). The pretreatment of the donors by intraperitoneal injections of tritiated thymidine was used as a tracer of the donors' mammary cells in order to differentiate them from the hosts' cells (*9*).

11. Parenchymal-stromal Interactions in Mammary Grafts

The ultimate size of the regenerating mammary grafts is determined by the amount of adipose tissue at the site of transplantation available for growth of the transplants, the period of transplantation, and the hormonal environment, but neither by the original size of the transplants nor the age of the donors (*34*). Mammary parenchyma was found to be capable of surviving and regenerating *in vivo* indefinitely through serial transplantation as long as favorable environmental conditions were continually provided (*39*, *43*). Until Williams and Hoshino (*75*) undertook the study of early histogenesis of transplanted mammary glands, the earliest recovery of transplanted normal mammary tissue recorded in the literature was 11 days after transplantation (*32*), and there were no reports concerning earlier histogenesis during regeneration of normal mammary isografts. In order to study detailed aspects of parenchymal-stromal interactions in mammary glands during the early process of regeneration of

TABLE XI. Successful Mammary Transplants Recovered from Host Mice

Experimental group	Days			
	3	4	5	6
I. No treatment[a]	3/9[b]	5/9	0/9	1/9
II-A. Estrogen-progesterone treatment to hosts	6/10	5/10	5/10	7/10
II-B. 3-Methylcholanthrene pretreatment to donors and estrogen-progesterone treatment to hosts	7/10	—	—	—

[a] In this group, none of the 18 grafts were recovered 24 or 48 hr after transplantation. From Ref. *76*.

mammary grafts, a series of experiments were carried out and reported (*9*, *45*, *75*).

The first part of this series of experiments was concerned with the fate of mammary grafts within 21 days after isografting in the gland-free 4th mammary fat pad (*75*). Mammary duct-segments, each 0.6 mm long, from virgin female CBA mice at 3 to 4 months of age, with and without pretreatment with 3-methylcholanthrene, were isografted into adult virign female F_1 hybrid mice, (CBA$\times$BC$_B$) F_1 or (C57BL$\times$CBA) F_1. Some of the host mice were treated daily with estradiol and progesterone injections. The grafts were examined at various intervals between 24 hr and 21 days after transplantation. The recovery rates of mammary grafts are summarized in Table XI. No mammary tissue was recovered from the transplantation sites at 24 and 48 hr following transplantation even after histological examinations. Three days after transplantation, varying degrees of organization of duct-like structures was observed (Fig. 17a). With estrogen-progesterone treatment to the hosts, rather well-organized duct-like structures were observed. At 21 days following transplantation only one mammary gland with extensive organization of the mammary duct system was recovered at each site of transplantation (Fig. 17b). Also at 3 days after transplantation from a donor pretreated with 3-methylcholanthrene and a host mouse treated with estrogen and progesterone before and after mammary transplantation, the size and complexity of the regenerating duct-like structures were comparable to those shown in Fig. 17a, the only striking difference being the large number of lymphocytic cells present in the adjacent stroma (Fig. 17c). However, at 7 days after transplantation, the evidence of such lymphocytic infiltration was much less and some cytoplasmic vacuoles and the basement membrane were present (Fig. 17d).

after mammary transplantation							Recovery rate (%)
7	8	9	10	12	14	21	
4/9	2/9	1/6	3/9	2/9	1/9	1/9	23/96 (23.95)
3/10	—	—	4/10	—	6/10	6/10	42/80 (52.5)
5/10	—	—	—	—	5/10	6/12	23/42 (54.8)

[b] Number of successful grafts/total number of mammary transplants.

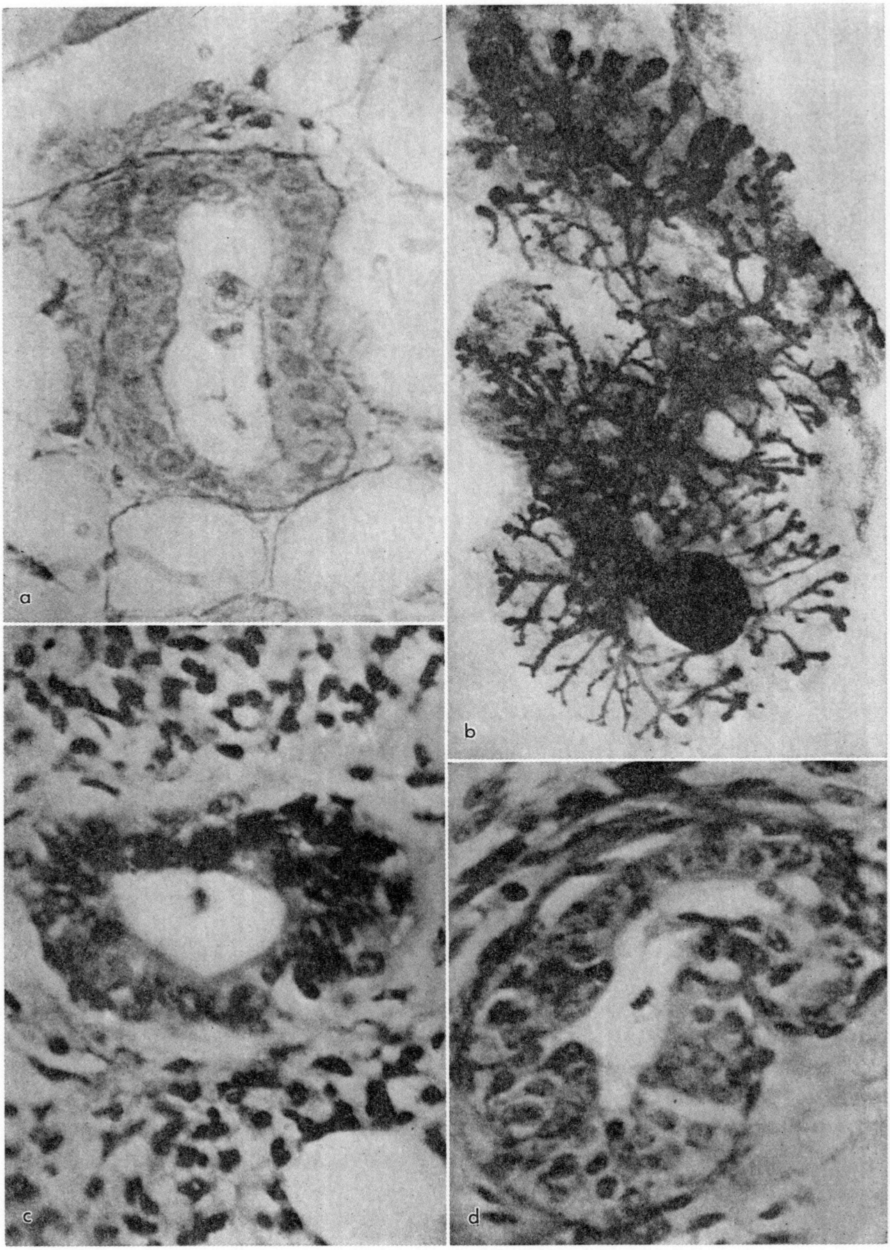
a
b
c
d

The second part of this series of experiments was undertaken (*9*), because in the previous experiments no transplanted mammary tissue was recovered at 24 and 48 hr following transplantation. In order to trace the fate of the mammary grafts during the very early stages of transplantation, the mammary glands of the donor mice were prelabeled with [^{3}H] thymidine. Two 6-week-old virgin female (CBA×C57BL) F_1 mice were pretreated with four intraperitoneal injections of 50 μg [^{3}H] thymidine every 12 hr. Three hours after the last injection, single mammary duct-segments, each 0.6 mm long without appreciable amounts of surrounding stromal tissue, were transplanted into the gland-free 4th mammary fat pads of 3.5- to 5-month-old virgin females of the same hybrid mice by the quantitative transplantation method. The host mice were killed at 24, 48, 72, and 96 hr following transplantation. The tissue at the transplantation site was removed, fixed, embedded in paraffin, and cut serially. The serial sections were in turn processed for autoradiography with Kodak NTB 11 liquid emulsion, using the dipping technique (*51*). After three weeks exposure at 4°C, the emulsion covering the tissue sections was developed with Kodak D-19 developer. The tissues obtained from the left side were stained with the Heidenhain's iron hematoxylin and eosin, and the tissues obtained from the right side were stained with periodic acid-Schiff reagent. Six host mice were killed 21 days after transplantation and

←FIG. 17. (a) Photomicrograph of a mammary duct-like structure recovered 3 days after transplantation which was surrounded by two apparently membrane-like sheets at its outer and lumenal surfaces

Note the presence of cells in its central space. Periodic acid-Schiff reaction and hematoxylin. ×400.

(b) Photomicrograph of a whole mount of a mammary graft recovered 21 days after transplantation from an untreated donor into a host treated with estrogen and progesterone before and after mammary isografting

Alum carmine. ×15.

(c) Photomicrograph of a mammary duct-like structure recovered 3 days after transplantation from a donor pretreated with 3-methylcholanthrene into a host mouse treated with estrogen and progesterone before and after mammary transplantation

Note lymphocytic stromal reaction. Hematoxylin and eosin. ×400.

(d) Photomicrograph of a regenerating mammary graft recovered 7 days after transplantation in a host mouse of the same group as in C

Note fibroblastic stroma with minimal lymphocytic infiltration. Also note the presence of basement membrane and suggestion of vacuoles in the epithelial cells. Periodic acid-Schiff reaction and hematoxylin. ×400. From Ref. *75*.

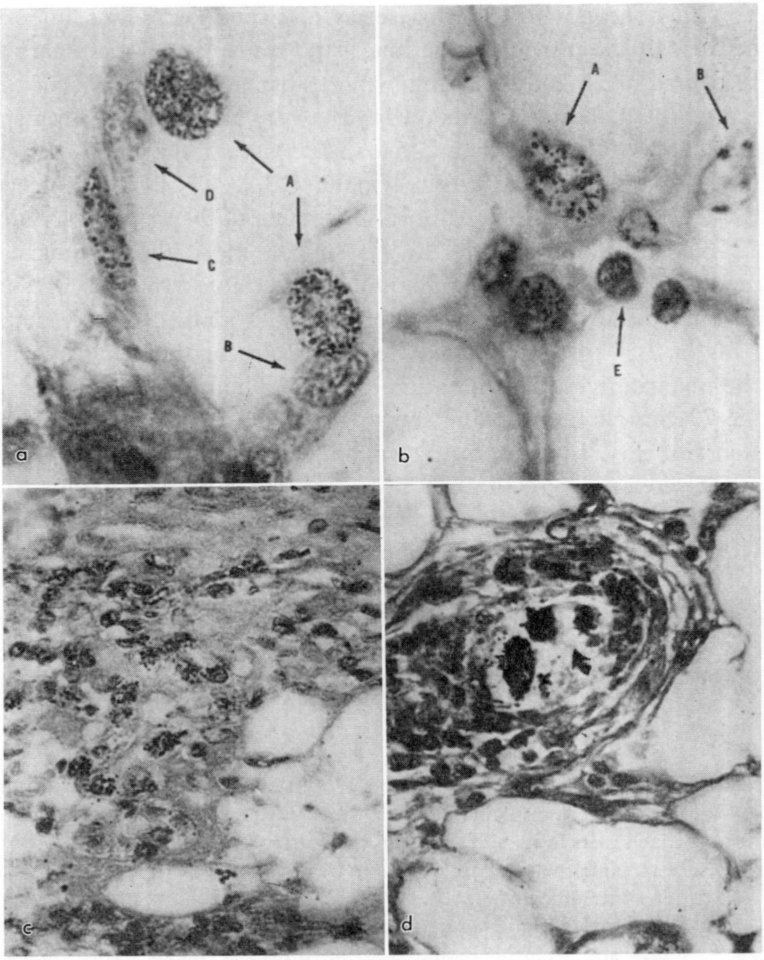

FIG. 18. (a, b, and c) Autoradiographic photomicrographs of 3 different mammary grafts examined 24 hr after transplantation

They showed labeled and unlabeled mammary epithelial cells which were scattered in the adipose tissue of the host mice at the site of transplantation. Iron-hematoxylin and eosin. a and b, ×1,500; c, ×800. A, labeled mammary epithelial cell; B, unlabeled mammary epithelial cell; C, labeled fibroblast; D, unlabeled fibroblast; E, labeled leukocyte

(d) Autoradiographic photomicrograph of a regenerating mammary graft examined 72 hr after transplantation

Note the aggregation of labeled cells in the central space, one of which (with an arrow) was undergoing mitosis. Iron-hematoxylin and eosin. ×800. From Ref. *9*.

their mammary glands including the surviving grafts were prepared as whole mounts after staining with alum carmine.

Labelled cells were recovered in varying intensities at the sites of transplantation throughout the 96 hr following transplantation. In some cases, fibroblasts and leukocytes were also labeled, but the labeled and non-labeled mammary epithelial cells were easily identified in the gland-free pads (Fig. 18a, b). Although at the time of transplantation the mammary duct-segments were tubular, neither the tubular form of the duct-segments nor the glandular forms of mammary structures was recovered. At 24 hr following transplantation, many labeled and non-labeled epithelial cells were seen scattered in the adipose stroma at the site of transplantation (Fig. 18c). This indicated dissociation of the 0.6 mm long mammary duct-segments within 24 hr following transplantation. At 48 hr following transplantation, the general findings were similar to those described at 24 hr. At 72 and occasionally 48 hr following transplantation, the once scattered, labeled cells formed aggregations of varying sizes, which often contained non-labeled epithelial cells. Located in irregular spaces in some aggregations of epithelial cells were seen heavily labeled cells frequently undergoing mitosis (Fig. 18d). In some cases, the central space was expanded to resemble the lumen of a mammary duct surrounded by a better organized epithelial lining. At this stage, the basement membrane was usually not present or was incomplete. Moreover, a few labeled epithelial cells were still scattered in the surrounding stromal tissues (Fig. 19a). At 96 hr following transplantation, the mammary ducts had a predominantly multilayered epithelium but some were monolayered (Fig. 19b). Only after 72 hr following transplantation did the regenerating basement membrane appear to be complete with the newly formed mammary ducts in their most advanced stage (Fig. 19c). All stages of regeneration of transplanted mammary tissue described above were observed at 96 hr after transplantation. At 21 days following transplantation, all isolated aggregations of mammary epithelial cells were somehow integrated into a common duct system and only single mammary glands were recovered at each site of transplantation (Fig. 19d). The present experiment revealed that from scattered mammary epithelial cells a single mammary gland could be completely regenerated. Now it is not difficult to accept the previously observed data that a new mammary gland could be regenerated from any portion of the duct system, with the exception of the nipple, regardless of the age of donors, the size of grafts, the direction of a duct in reference to its nipple, and also the life span of the host mice.

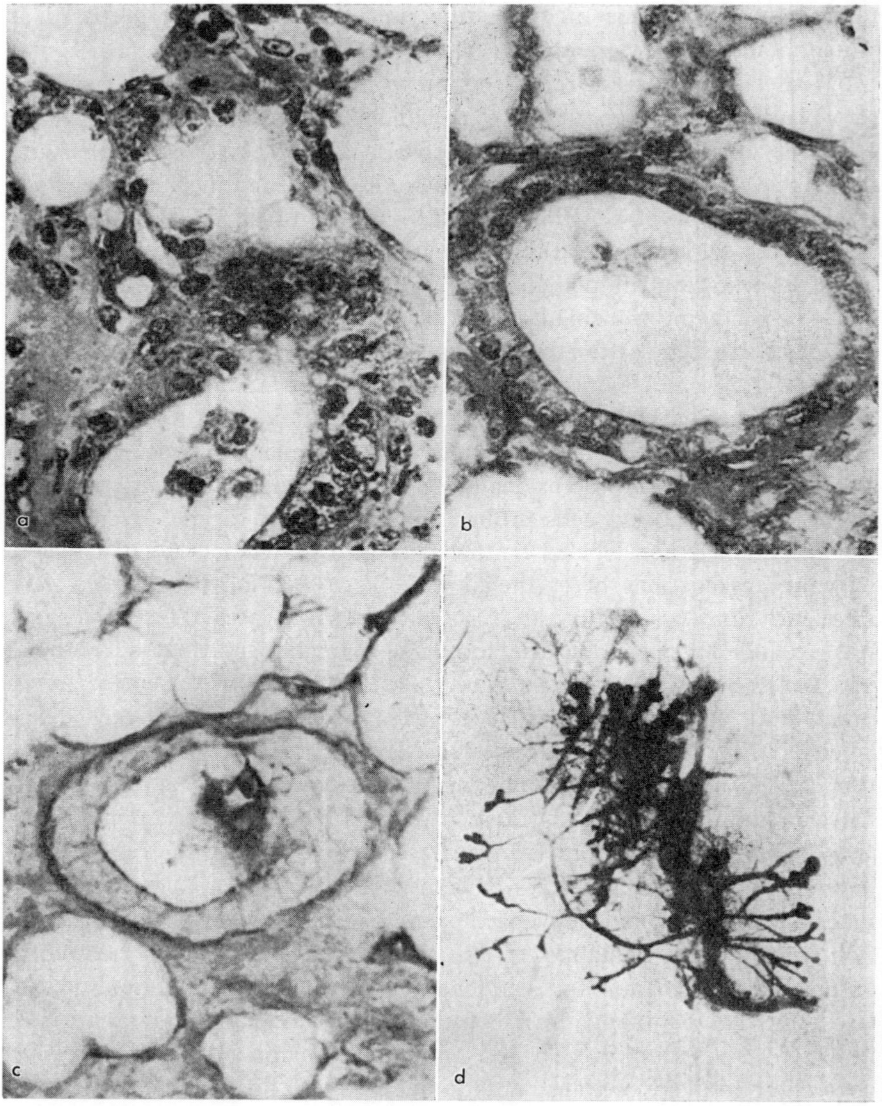

FIG. 19. (a) Photomicrograph of regenerating mammary structures having a duct-like appearance observed 72 hr after transplantation

Note that the epithelial lining is partially monolayerd and also multilayered. The cells were still present in the central space. Some scattered epithelial cells were seen in the surrounding stromal tissue. Iron-hematoxylin and eosin. ×800.

(b) Photomicrograph of a well-established mammary duct structure with monolayered epithelial lining observed 96 hr after transplantation

The present experimental results are compatible with the findings reported by Daniel and DeOme (*13*) that normal mammary outgrowth was produced following implantation of approximately 5×10^5 cells obtained from monolayer culture of mouse mammary gland cells into the gland-free 4th mammary fat pads (Fig. 20), and also with the observations made by Bern *et al.* (*2*) that although the explants exhibited general necrosis after organ culture, histological features did not reflect on the growth capability after transplantation into the gland-free fat pad. In any of these works, only one mammary gland was reproduced at each transplantation site despite the fact that it was reconstructed from many scattered dissociated cells. Some mechanism must be present to identify cells of one kind and to establish a union of all dissociated components in order to form the single mammary gland structure. Moscona's hypothesis (*53*) is worthy of consideration.

The 3rd part of this series of experiments was undertaken to determine how mammary transplants behave when transplanted into a site lacking adipose stroma (*45*). For this purpose, the anterior chamber of the eye was selected as the site for mammary transplantation. As previously described in Section 4, the anterior chamber of the eye provides transplanted tissues with a unique environment. Small mammary duct-segments, approximately 0.6 mm long carrying a very small amount of surrounding adipose stromal tissue, were isografted from normal adult female CBA mice to 4-to 6-month-old (CBA×C57BL) F_1 hybrid mice by the quantitative transplantation method. The mammary graft donors received double pituitary isografts subcutaneously several weeks prior to mammary transplantation, to enhance transplantability and regeneration of the mammary grafts (Hoshino, unpublished). Single mammary duct-segments were isografted into each gland-free mammary fat pad, and four duct-segments were transplanted into each anterior chamber of the eye. No further treatment was given to the host mice. Tissue at the sites of transplantation in the gland-free 4th mammary fat pads were removed at 1, 2, 3, 5, 6, 9, 12,

The cells in the central space were still present. Iron-hematoxylin and eosin. ×800.

(c) Photomicrograph of a regnerating mammary duct structure observed 72 hr after transplantation

Note complete re-establishment of the basement membrane. Periodic acid-Schiff reaction without nuclear staining. ×800.

(d) Photomicrograph of a mammary gland which has regnerated from a graft in 3 weeks

Whole mount preparation stained with alum carmine. ×12. From Ref. *9*.

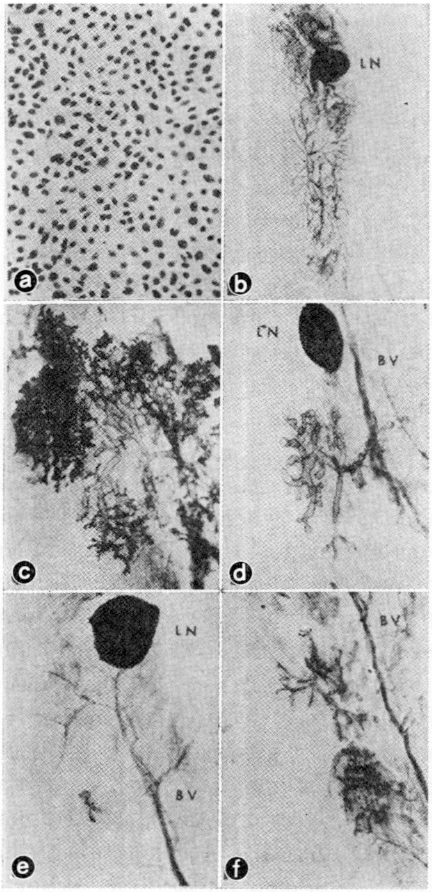

FIG. 20. All photographs of glands (a through f) show the 4th mammary fat pads containing mammary gland outgrowths. All fat pads were removed from host mice 3 months after transplantation of cultured cells and stained with hematoxylin. Non-mammary structures present in the fat pads are lymph nodes (LN) and blood vessels (BV).

(a) Representative area from 7-day culture of mouse mammary epithelium. Hematoxylin-eosin. ×90. (b) Normal mammary outgrowth from cells 4 weeks in culture. ×2 2/3. (c) Mammary outgrowth containing a dense hyperplastic area. Transplanted from a 2-week culture. ×4.5. (d) Mammary outgrowth from a 4-week culture. The ducts are dilated and lack normal end buds. ×4.5. (e) Outgrowth from cells cultured for 5 weeks. Outgrowth organized into mammary epithelium but failed to fill a significant amount of the fat pad. ×4.5. (f) Fat pad containing two focuses of glandular outgrowth. Although both outgrowths arose from the same 2-week culture they apear to have different patterns of growth. ×4.5. From Ref. *13*.

24, 48, and 72 hr and at 5, 7, and 21 days following transplantation. The isografted tissue was removed from the anterior chamber of the eye at 1, 2, 3, 4, 5, 7, 14, and 21 days following transplantation. One-third of the grafts recovered from the anterior chamber of the eye were prepared for electron microscopic investigations. All other grafts were examined following staining with Gomori and Grocotts' methenamine silver, and hematoxylin and eosin. In another series of experiments, 96 duct-segments from an adult female Balb/c mouse pretreated with double pituitary isografts for 3 weeks were isografted into both sides of the anterior chambers of the eyes of 12 untreated adult female mice.

The findings from mammary isografts recovered from the gland-free 4th mammary fat pads confirmed previously reported results concerning the fate of mammary grafts recovered 24 hr or later following transplantation. The present experiment included the data obtained from the mammary grafts recovered earlier than 24 hr which had never been reported before.

Soon after isografting, mammary isografts began to lose their original architecture and the basement membranes irregularly followed the disorganized mammary epithelial lining and were also partially damaged. These degenerative changes continued steadily (Fig. 21a). Even 3 hr after transplantation, a peculiar type of mass appeared either in the stromal tissue of the recipient mammary fat pads close to the degenerating mammary graft tissue or in the lumens surrounded by grafted mammary cells (Fig. 21b). These peculiar masses were colorless and laminated, resembling the so-called hyalin body often observed in injured tissues or cysts. However, they were neither stained with eosin nor aldehyde fuchsin nor with Congo red. After 6 hr, mammary epithelial cells began to migrate out of the dissociated epithelial lining through the damaged basement membranes into the surrounding stromal tissue of the recipient fat pads (Fig. 21c). At 24 hr many grafted duct-segments had already lost their original tubular architecture (Fig. 21a). After 72 hr following isografting, reorganizing and regenerating ductal structures were often encountered. Whenever such regenerating structures were found, well-developed capillaries were discovered adjacent to these structures and the basement membranes surrounded almost completely the regenerating mammary epithelial lining. On the other hand, in the tissues adjacent to these well-regenerating structures, there were still a number of mammary epithelial cells scattered in the stromal tissue (Fig. 22a). Mitoses were found in regenerating mammary epithelial cell aggregates at 48 hr after transplantation, but

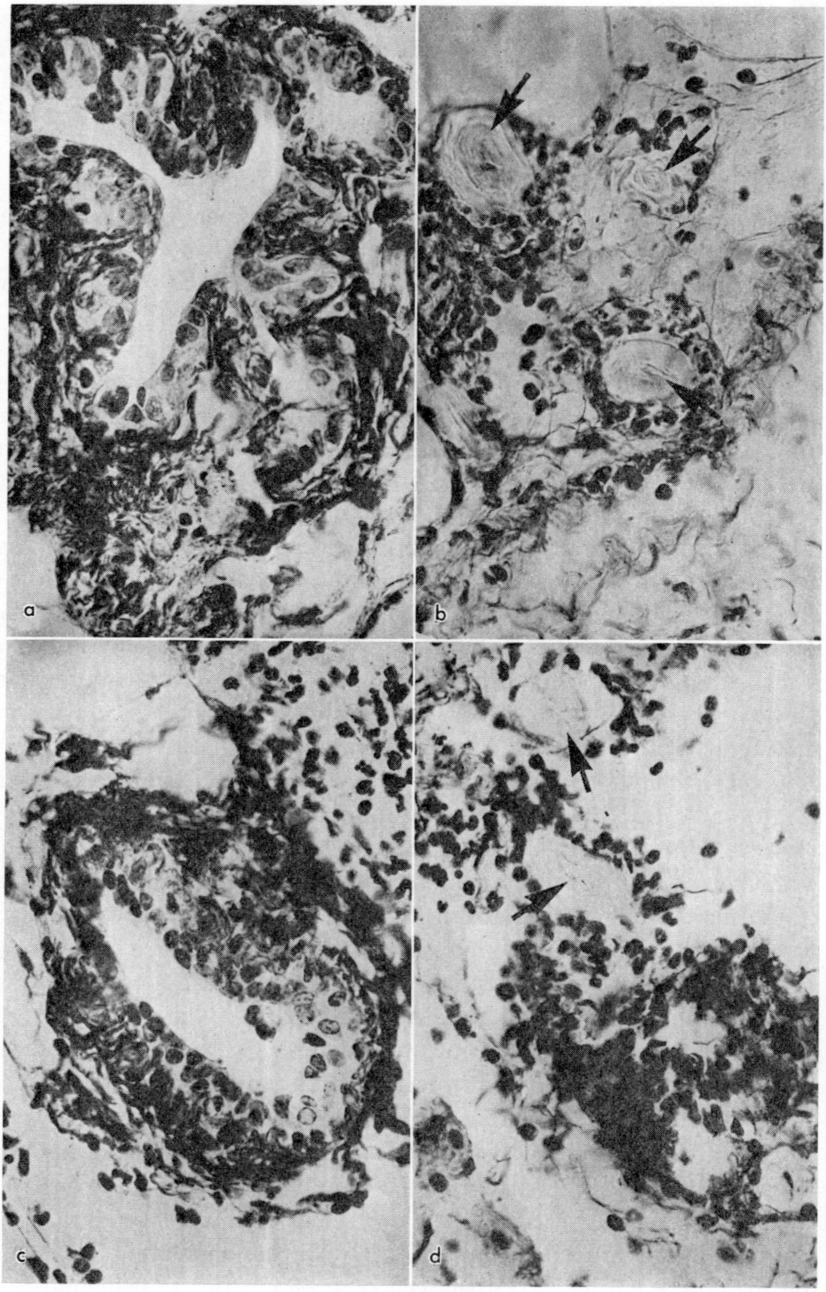
a
b
c
d

more often at later times. Even 7 days after grafting, when many well reorganized tubular structures were recovered from the transplantation sites, scattered mammary epithelial cells remained in the recipient's stromal tissue (Fig. 22b). However, at 21 days following transplantation, only single mammary glands were dicovered at each transplantation site.

In contrast to the findings observed from the mammary grafts recovered from gland-free fat pads, some striking differences were observed in the grafts in the anterior chamber of the eye.

Light microscopically, the most significant changes appeared in mammary isografts which were recovered at 2, 5, 14, and 21 days following transplantation into the anterior chamber of the eyes.

At 2 days after isografting, partially preserved mammary ducts had a multi-layered epithelial lining which was surrounded by a corrugated and a partially disrupted basement membrane (Fig. 22c, d). Some mammary epithelial cells appeared outside the disrupted basement membrane in the surrounding adipose stromal tissue where leucocytic infiltration was often observed. Some epithelial cells appeared to be moving along the edge of the mammary isograft. Some fibrous connective tissue surrounded the mammary ducts (Fig. 23a). The peculiar masses resembling the so-called hyalin body also appeared (Fig. 23b). At this time, the grafts were not affixed to the iris surface.

←FIG. 21. (a) Photomicrograph of a 3-hr isograft in the 4th mammary gland-free fat pad showing the irregularly infolding and disorganized mammary epithelial lining and surrounding basement membrane

Gomori and Grocott's methenamine silver. ×1,400.

(b) Photomicrograph of a 9-hr isograft in the 4th mammary gland-free fat pad having several peculiar masses, as indicated by the arrow, resembling the so-called hyalin body

Gomori and Grocott's methenamine silver. ×1,400.

(c) Photomicrograph of a 12-hr isograft in the 4th mammary gland-free fat pad

Note mammary epithelial cells which migrated out of the dissociated epithelial lining through the disrupted basement membrane and scattered into the adjacent stromal tissue of the recipient's fat pad. Gomori and Grocott's methenamine silver. ×1,400.

(d) Photomicrograph of a 24-hr isograft in the 4th mammary gland-free fat pad

Note the dissociated grafted duct-segments which have lost their original tubular architecture. Arrow indicates the presence of the peculiar masses resembling the so-called hyalin body. Gomori and Grocott's methenamine silver. ×1,400.

From Ref. *45*.

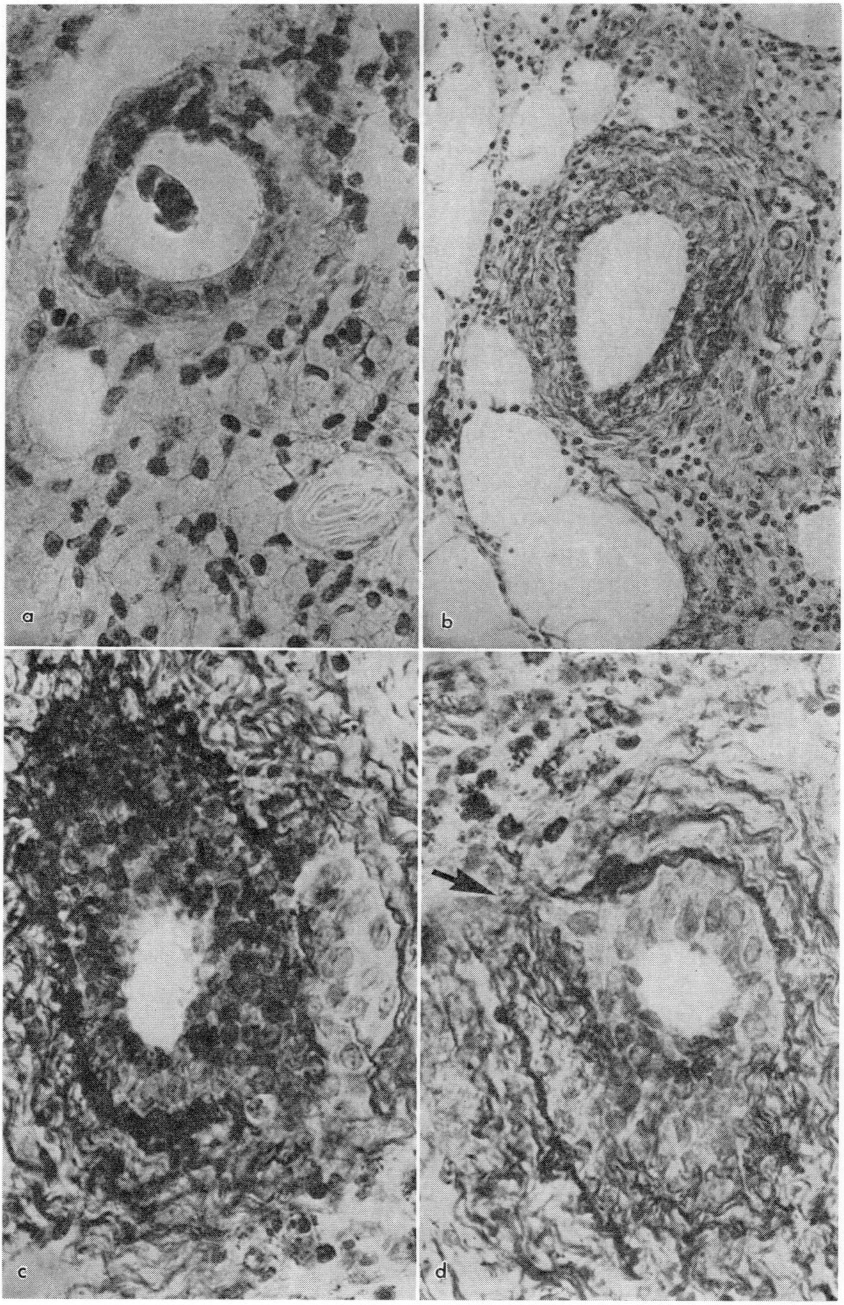
a
b
c
d

At 5 days after transplantation, the most organized ductal structures were observed in the grafts. The mammary epithelial cell lining consisted of a single layer of cells surrounded by a much less corrugated and more distinct basement membrane which was, in turn, surrounded by denser fibrous connective tissue as compared with those observed in earlier grafts (Fig. 23c). At this stage, the grafted tissues adhered to the surface of the iris and were revascularized. The amount of surrounding fibrous connective tissue increased at the expense of the adipose tissue which was originally transplanted with the mammary duct-segment. In some grafts, new mammary ducts branched from the transplanted duct-segments. The lumens of the surviving ducts often contained eosinophilic fluid.

At 14 days after transplantation, the amount of adipose tissue retained in the grafted tissue remarkably diminished and was mainly replaced by fibrous connective tissue. Some of the surviving ducts appeared well-preserved, but others lacked a discernible basement membrane. In the latter, mammary epithelial cells were disorganized, vacuolated and occupied the ductal lumen (Fig. 23d).

At 21 days after transplantation, the adipose tissue was now almost completely replaced by fibrous connective tissue which was thick and dense. Mammary epithelial cells of some ducts were lined in a single layer and surrounded by a tightly woven basement membrane distinctly different from mammary ducts observed earlier.

Electron microscopically, in the mammary graft tissue throughout

←FIG. 22. (a) Photomicrograph of a 5-day isograft in the 4th mammary gland-free fat pad which re-established its tubular structure

Note that there were still a number of mammary epithelial cells scattered in the adjacent stromal tissue. Hematoxylin and eosin. ×1,400.

(b) Photomicrograph of a 7-day isograft in the 4th mammary gland-free fat pad having re-established a better organized mammary epithelial lining which was completely surrounded by the re-established basement membrane

However, scattered mammary epithelial cells remained in the recipient's stromal tissue. Gomori and Grocott's methenamine silver. ×600.

(c) Photomicrograph of a 2-day isograft in the anterior chamber of the eye showing corrugated basement membrane

Gomori and Grocott's methenamine silver. ×1,400.

(d) Photomicrograph of a 2-day isograft in the anterior chamber of the mouse eye

Arrow demonstrates disrupted basement membrane. Note mammary epithelial cells adjacent to this area. Gomori and Grocott's methenamine silver. ×1,400.

From Ref. *45*.

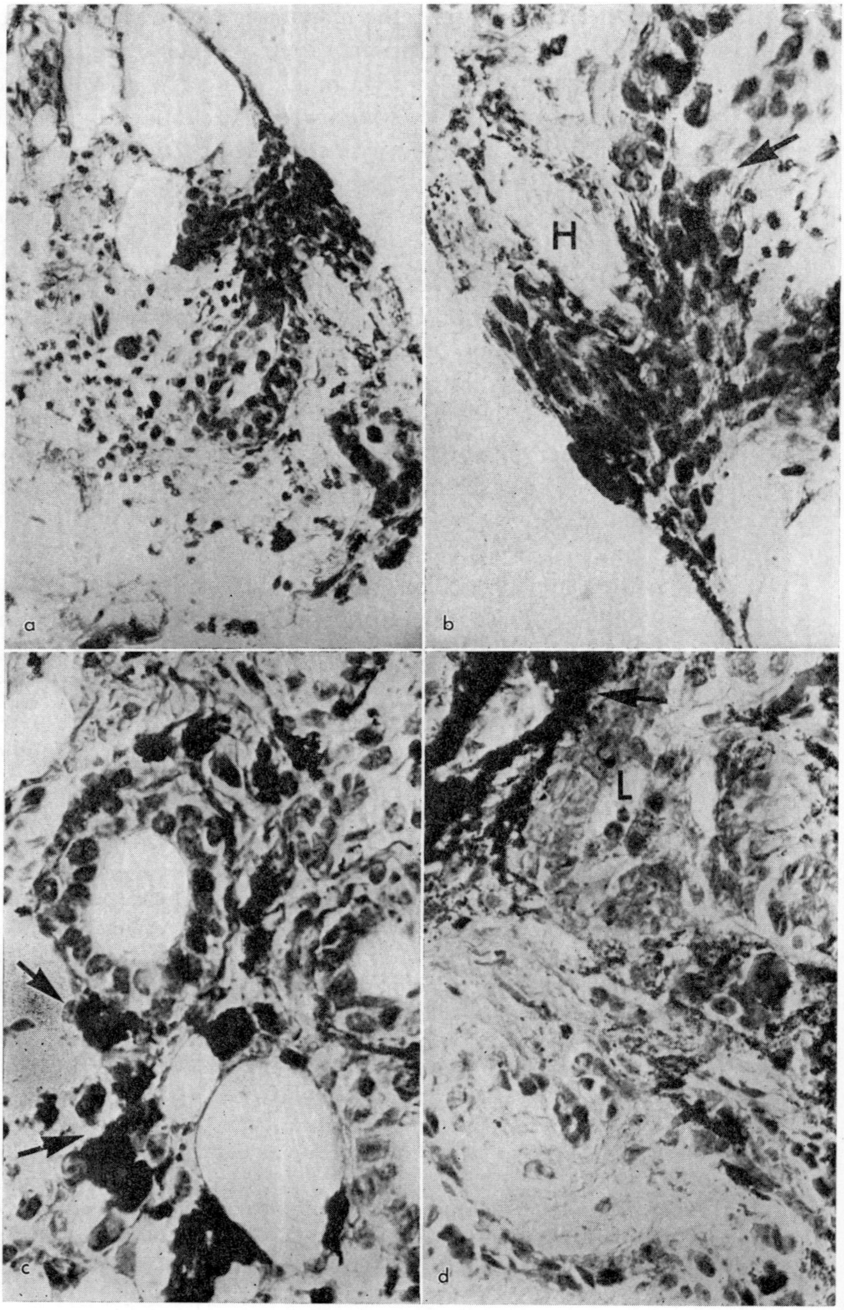
a
H
b
c
L
d

the investigations, the basal lamina, in contrast to its smooth linear appearance in the controls (Fig. 24a) always showed irregular configurations or at least partial disappearance.

At 2 days after transplantation, the basal lamina at the basal surface of the epithelial cells or myoepithelial cells revealed infoldings into the interstitial spaces and a scalloped or whirl-like appearance (Fig. 24b, c). At 5 days after isografting, these changes became less distinct (Fig. 24d).

At 14 days after transplantation, the basal lamina revealed discontinuity and fragmentation of its structure, and irregular densities in the detached pieces and necrotic cellular debris appeared in the interstitial spaces (Fig. 25a).

At 21 days after isografting, the basal lamina remained along the basal surface of the epithelial cells even when overgrown connective tissue cells were situated close to the epithelial cells. The basal lamina showed interruptions in continuity, irregular thickness and multilaminations in areas near degenerative epithelial changes (Fig. 25b).

In another series of experiments with Balb/c mice, mammary grafts were removed from the anterior chamber of the eye 21 days after transplantation and one-half of them were incubated with 1% collagenase in Eagle's culture media supplement with fetal calf serum and the other half of them were incubated without collagenase for 1 hr at 37°C. After incubation, these recovered mammary graft tissues were isografted into

←FIG. 23. (a) Photomicrograph of a 2-day isograft in the anterior chamber of the mouse eye

Note the amount of adipose and fibrous connective tissue and leukocytic reaction. Hematoxylin and eosin. ×600.

(b) Photomicrograph of a 2-day isograft in the anterior chamber of the mouse eye showing epithelial cell relationship to the edge of the isograft, as indicated by arrow

H indicates the presence of the peculiar mass resembling the so-called hyalin body. Hematoxylin and eosin. ×1,400.

(c) Photomicrograph of a 5-day isograft in the anterior chamber of the mouse eye

Note single layer cell lining of ducts. Arrow indicates melanin pigments derived from the affixed iris. Gomori and Grocott's methenamine silver. ×1,400.

(d) Photomicrograph of a 14-day isograft in the anterior chamber of the mouse eye

L indicates a ductal lumen filled with mammary epithelial cells. Arrow indicates melanin pigments derived from the affixed iris. Hematoxylin and eosin. ×1,400.

From Ref. *45*.

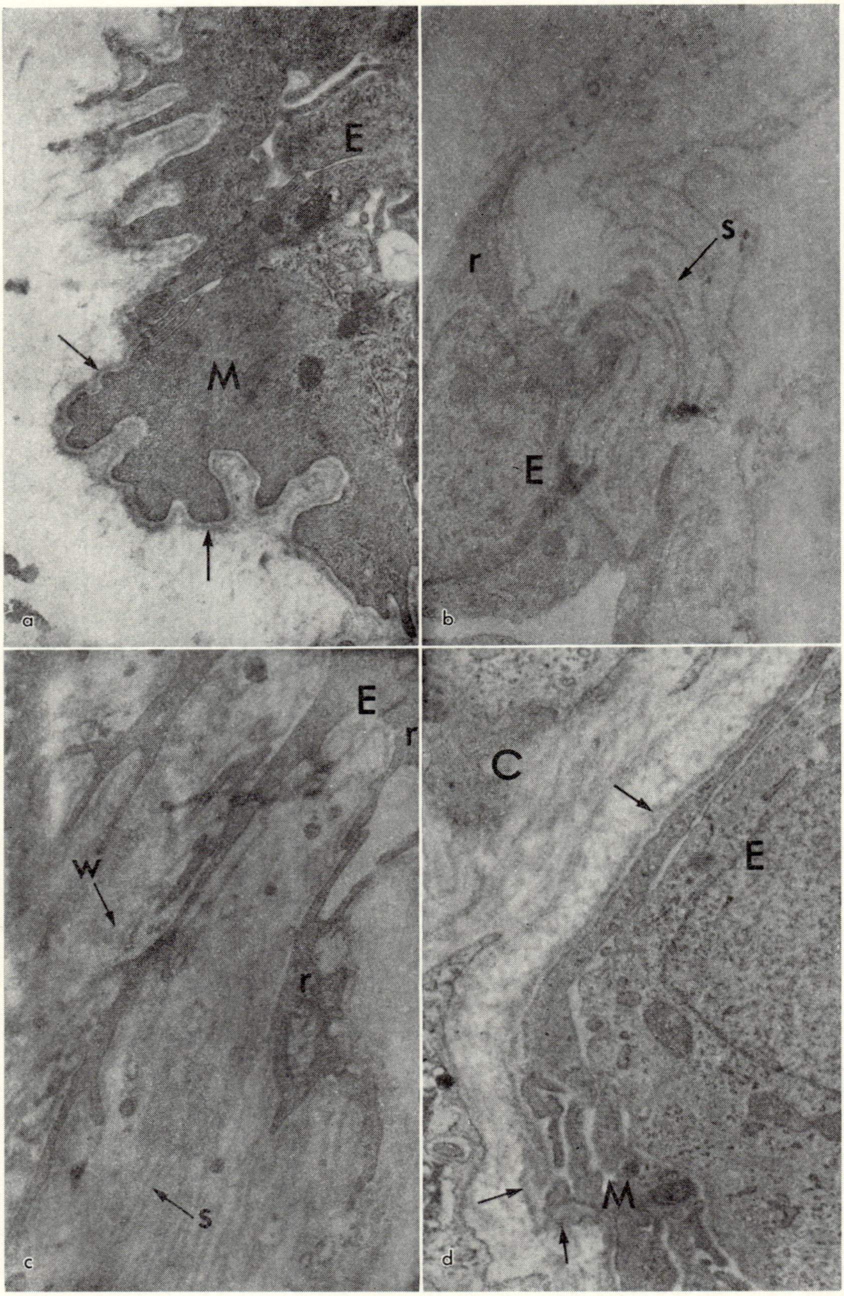
E
M
a
r
s
E
b
E
r
w
r
s
c
C
E
M
d

the gland-free 4th mammary fat pads of 6 new Balb/c female host mice which simultaneously received single pituitary isografts subcutaneously. Twelve days after retransplantation, the mammary grafts were examined as whole mounts. The 12-day isografts pretreated with collagenase grew into the host adipose tissue. This was evidenced by budding into the host's stroma, a diminished amount of surrounding fibrous connective tissue, and a retained tubular structure (Fig. 25c). Those isografts not pretreated with collagenase did not show any tubular structure or growth into the stromal tissue. Dense surrounding fibrous stromal tissue appeared to restrict growth of the mammary isograft (Fig. 25d).

The most contrasting observation obtained during early stages of isografting was the persistence of fairly well preserved mammary duct configurations in the anterior chamber of the eye 24 hr after transplantation, whereas in the gland-free 4th mammary fat pads all of the grafted duct-segments were completely disorganized and the basement membrane of the mammary grafts disappeared within 24 hr after transplantation. However, in the anterior chamber of the eye, the basement membrane never completely disappeared and the mammary epithelial cells were found to lie in the stroma immediately adjacent to the mammary duct-segments after escaping through a partially disrupted basement membrane.

Kratochwil (*48*) reported that trypsin-isolated epithelial rudiments of mammary anlagen from 12- to 16-day-old mouse embryos did not develop in the absence of mesenchyme, but were successfully recombined with 12-day-old mammary mesenchyme in organ culture. Only 16-day-old em-

←FIG. 24. (a) Electron micrograph of a control mammary duct-segment excised prior to transplantation

Myoepithelial cell (M) and duct epithelial cell (E) form an irregular basal surface with the cytoplasmic processes, which is surrounded by the basal lamina (lamina densa), as indicated by the arrows, consisting of even thickness and high electron densities. ×15,000.

(b and c) Electron micrograph of 2-day isografts in the anterior chamber of the mouse eye

Epithelial cells and their processes reveal the cytoplasm rich with free ribosomes (r). The basal lamina demonstrated unusual appearance such sa scalloped (s) or whirl-like (w) shapes. ×15,000.

(d) Electron micrograph of a 5-day isograft in the anterior chamber of the mouse eye

The intracytoplasmic organelles of the epithelial cell are well preserved. The basal lamina was usually single-layered with occasional infolding or irregularity. Myoepithelial cell is shown by (M). ×15,000.

From Ref. *45*.

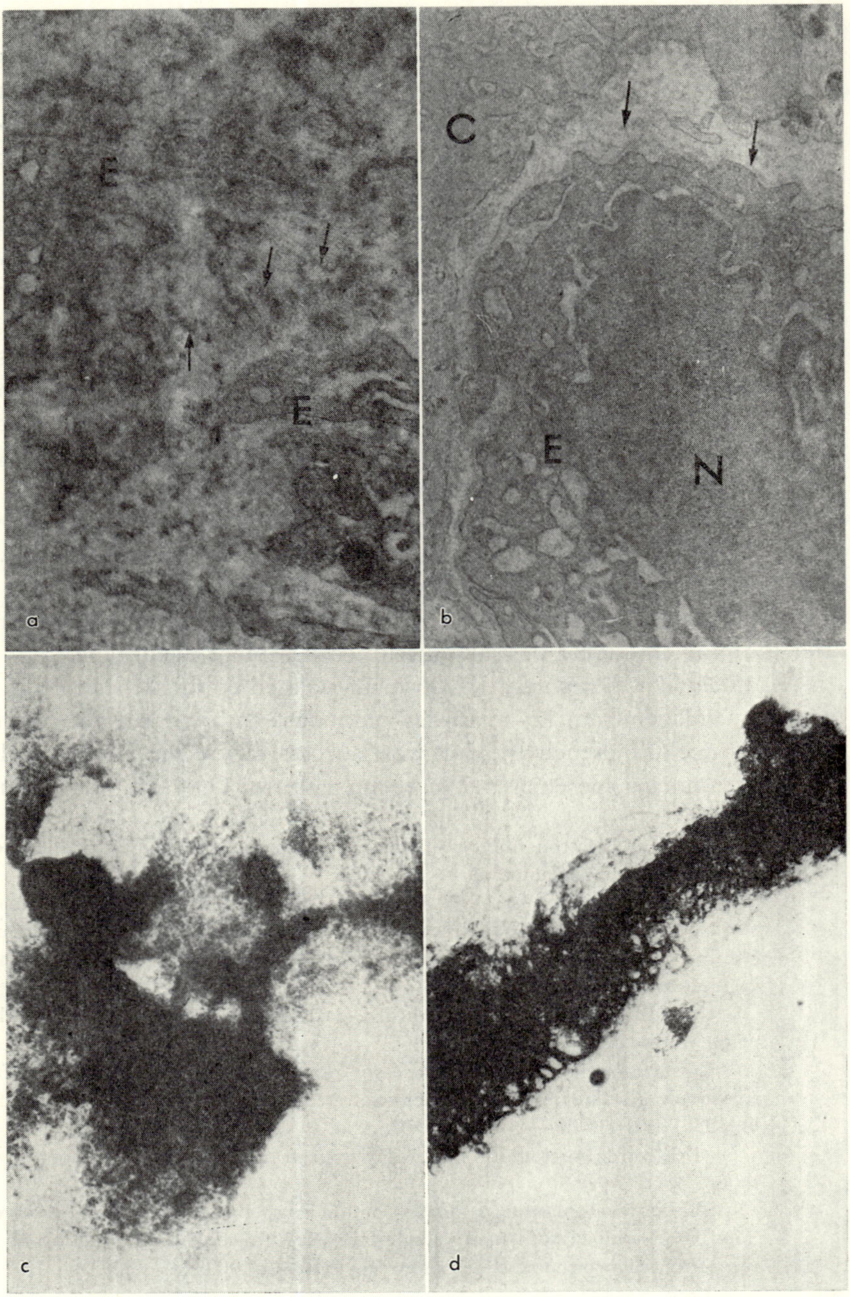
E
E
a
C
E
N
b
c
d

bryonic mammary epithelial cells were able to recombine with salivary mesenchyme and continued to develop *in vitro*. The morphogenetic pattern of the resulting glandular structure was similar to the salivary gland. When mammary or salivary gland epithelia were exposed to the simultaneous presence of both types of mesenchyme, their morphogenesis was strongly inhibited and typical of neither organ (*48*).

Recently, this line of work was advanced by the combination of *in vitro* and *in vivo* experimental procedures (*64*). In this work, embryonic mammary epithelial and mesenchymal components and the salivary mesenchyme were isolated by trypsinization *in vitro*. Isolated mammary epithelium and isolated mesenchyme were placed together in a dish and incubated overnight prior to isografting, allowing recombination through direct contact. Recombinants were isografted under the kidney capsule of 4-week-old female hosts. The results are summarized in Table XII. When the hosts were lactating, lactose synthetase B protein activity was compared between grafts and the host's lactating mammary glands. As shown in Table XIII, the recombinant graft tissue responded to endogenous hormonal stimulation and synthesized a milk protein, α-lactalbumin. Isografts of heterotypic recombinants of embryonic mammary epithelium with salivary mesenchyne underwent development morphogenetically resembling that of the salivary gland. However, cytodifferentiation of the

←FIG. 25. (a) Electron micrograph of a 14-day isograft in the anterior chamber of the mouse eye

Arrow indicates irregular density in the basal lamina. Note degenerative changes in the epithelial cell (E). ×15,000.

(b) Electron micrograph of a 21-day isograft in the anterior chamber of the mouse eye

Arrow indicates interruption of the basal lamina. Note also multilaminations of the basal lamina. Epithelial cells (E) were undergoing necrosis, as indicated by dilated endoplasmic reticular sacs (er) and a severely shrunken nucleus (N), whereas the connective tissue cells (C) were well developed. ×15,000.

(c) Photomicrograph of a 12-day retransplanted isograft pretreated with collagenase

Note the presence of a ductal structure and end budding in the recipient's adipose stromal tissue. Whole mount preparation stained with alum carmine. ×100.

(d) Photomicrograph of a 12-day retransplanted isograft not pretreated with collagenase

Note the dense connective tissue surrounding the isograft which did not proliferate. Whole mount preparation stained with alum carmine. ×100.

From Ref. *45*.

TABLE XII. Development of 16-Day Mammary Gland Epithelia Combined with Mammary and Salivary Mesenchyme, 3 Weeks after Transplantation under the Kidney Capsule in 4-Week-old Syngeneic Female Mice

Source of mesenchyme	No. of explants	No. of grafts recovered (%)	Developmental response of mammary epithelium
Renal stroma	20	4 (20)	Degeneration
Mammary (16 day)	18	11 (61)	Mammary gland-like
Salivary (14 day)	24	18 (75)	Salivary gland-like

From Ref. *64*.

TABLE XIII. Lactose Synthetase B Protein Activity in Glands Developing from 16-Day Mammary Epithelium Combined with 14-Day Salivary Mesenchyme under the Kidney Capsule and in Mammary Glands in Lactating Host Mice

Case No.	B protein activity (pmol/mg wet tissue/30 min)	
	Mammary *in situ*	Mammary epithelium plus salivary mesenchyme grafts
1	1,918	290
2	2,370	213
3	1,716	2,024
4	1,176	752

From Ref. *64*.

epithelium was like that of the mammary gland (*64*). Ceriani *et al.* (*8*) reported fetal mammary anlagen which started to proliferate soon after adipose cells appeared in the surrounding mesenchymal tissue. He further stated that the failure of mammary anlagen explants to assume characteristic ductal configurations was related to the breakdown of epithelial-mesenchymal interactions, as indicated by the lack of the basal lamina. The basal lamina has a role in orderly growth and reconstruction following injuries in several types of tissues (*26*, *74*). In invasive carcinoma, the basal lamina is absent.

Epithelial-mesenchymal interactions required for epithelial cell organization and differentiation in early organogenesis has been demonstrated (*10*, *11*, *29*, *50*, *60*). In a recent work (*45*) using the anterior chamber of the eye, the adipose tissue originally surrounding the transplanted duct-segments was chiefly replaced by rather dense fibrous connective tissue in the 14- and 21-day grafts. Within this fibrous coat, parenchymal tissue survived with only a limited ductal system. In contrast to the gland-free

4th mammary fat pad, in the anterior chamber of the eye, there was no further supply of adipose stroma by the recipients for the transplants. In order to elicit further growth the surviving mammary grafts were retransplanted from the anterior chamber of the eye to the gland-free 4th mammary fat pads. Only grafts which were incubated with collagenase prior to retransplantation survived on retransplantation and grew into the adipose stroma adjacent to the retransplanted mammary grafts. It appeared that an overgrowth of collagenous connective tissue in the stroma was a definite limiting factor in the growth of mammary parenchymal tissue (*45*). Greene (*28*) stated that the growth rate of tumors in the anterior chamber of the rabbit eye was inversely proportional to its stromal requirements. That some factor or factors may influence the mechanism of epithelial-stromal (or mesehchymal) interactions or the growth regulatory mechanism has been documented (*3*, *6*, *15*, *22*, *25*, *56*).

During embryogenesis of mouse mammary glands, epithelioid aggregates were observed to develop into mammary anlagen (*61*, *73*). Moscona (*53*, *54*) proposed, from his *in vitro* experiments with cell culture of various combinations of embryonic cell types, that morphogenetic cell contacts are mediated by specific products elaborated by the cells. Such extracellular materials may be involved in the processes of sorting out preferential convergence and type-specific grouping of cells into aggregates. Steinberg (*71*) reviewed the literature and discussed the problems concerning the reconstruction of tissues by dissociated cells and concluded that although early workers envisioned the tissue movements as resulting from pressures or other inhomogenities in the immediate environment, a considerable body of evidence has meanwhile been accumulated to show that the movements are due to intrinsic properties of the individual tissues themselves, but beyond this statement, we find ourselves in an area of uncertainty.

CONCLUSION

The literature on histogenesis of normal mammary glands isografted from normal adult mice was reviewed. However, the experiments which were directly concerned with carcinogenesis and precancerous changes were not included.

The following may be concluded: mammary transplants excised from any portion of the duct system of both male and female donor mice, even quiescent glands of a two-year-old mouse, or of a masculinized female donor, seem to have equal capability for regeneration and for milk secretion at parturition of the host mice. The ultimate size of the regenerating graft may depend on (1) the amount of adipose stromal tissue available for the mammary parenchyma to grow into at the site of transplantation, (2) the duration of transplantation, (3) the hormonal stimulation, (4) the environmental conditions at the site of transplantation, other than the amount of adipose tissue, and (5) the conditions of the host animals, including their ages. Adipose tissue is an essential substance for the growth of mammary glands which seem to prefer white fat to interscapular brown fat. As long as adipose tissue is available, the actual site of the mammary graft does not interfere with its growth whether it is placed intraperitoneally, retroperitoneally, or subcutaneously, even though the mammary gland is one of the subcutaneous appendages of the skin. Proliferation of mammary ducts may occur from any part of the duct system and in any direction in reference to their nipples, or even from partially necrotic mammary explants which had been organ cultures prior to isografting into the gland-free fat pads. These findings are supported by other studies as follows: single mammary glands at each site of transplantation can be reproduced following implantation of monolayer-cultured mammary cells, and also from small mammary duct-segments which were dissociated and scattered into the adjacent stromal tissue 24 hr following transplantation into the gland-free mammary fat pads. Contrary to adipose stromal tissue being beneficial to mammary growth, fibrous stromal tissue is a definite limiting factor of mammary growth. Another limiting factor is the environment of the host animal which includes the endogenous hormonal state and the aging of the animal, but probably most important the aging of the connective stroma. Mammary parenchyma may be successfully transplanted serially from an original donor's mammary gland to succeeding generations of host animals in the gland-free fat pads for far longer than the life span of any mouse as long as the environmental conditions in the host animal are continuously favorable. It is not known at present how the once-scattered mammary cells from each duct-segment transplant could aggregate in an orderly fashion and regenerate to a single mammary duct system at each site of transplantation and functionally differentiate in a manner indistinguishable from that of the host's mammary gland. This problem involves a number of important biological phenomena such as parenchyma-stromal interactions, dissociation and aggregation, cellular identification and sorting systems, reconstruction to a whole normal organ and cytodifferentiation. Using embryonic parenchymal and mesenchymal components of the mammary gland and other structures, and many attempts at exploring these biological and developmental problems have been undertaken. However, research utilizing mammary glands as an excellent experimental model, deserves more intense experimentation by investigators with diverse expertise in the field.

Acknowledgments

The present review work commenced during the author's tenure as Visiting Research Professor at Ludwig-Aschoff Haus, Pathologisches Institut der Universität Freiburg im Breisgau, Bundesrepublik Deutschland while on sabbatical leave from the University of Manitoba, Winnipeg, Manitoba, Canada. Thus, he wishes to thank Prof. Dr. med. Walter Sandritter, Director of the Institute, for permitting him to use the facilities, and also the staff of the University of Manitoba for granting him sabbatical leave. Thanks are also due to Ms. Linda Nahnybida for her assistance in collecting literature and reading the manuscript. Ms. Roberta Van Aertselaer typed the manuscript. This work was partially supported by the Medical Research Council of Canada.

REFERENCES

1. Barrnett, R. J. (1962). The morphology of adipose tissue, with particular reference to its histochemistry and ultrastructure. In *Adipose Tissue as an Organ*, ed. Kinsell, L. W., pp. 3–78. Springfield, Ill.: Charles C. Thomas.
2. Bern, H. A., Brown, D., and Ingraham, R. L. (1968). A note on the transplantability of organ-cultured mouse mammary tissues. *J. Natl. Cancer Inst.* **40**, 1267–1271.
3. Bern, H. A., Jones, L. A., Mills, K. T., Kohrman, A., and Mori, T. (1976). Use of the neonatal mouse in studying long-term effects of early exposure to hormones and other agents. *J. Toxicol. Environ. Health* Suppl. **1**, 103–116.
4. Blair, P. B. and Moretti, R. L. (1967). The mammary fat pad as a privileged transplantation site. *Transplantation* **5**, 542–544.
5. Blair, P. B. and Moretti, R. L. (1970). Transplantation of isologous male mammary gland tissue into the mammary fat-pads of female mice. *Transplantation* **10**, 44–52.
6. Browning, H. (1952). The action of tumors on normal tissue synchronously transplanted into the anterior chamber of the mouse eye. *Cancer Res.* **12**, 13–18.
7. Ceriani, R. L. (1970). Fetal mammary gland differentiation *in vitro* in response to hormones. I. Morphological findings. *Dev. Biol.* **21**, 506–529.
8. Ceriani, R. L., Pitelka, D. R., Bern, H. A., and Colley, V. B. (1970). Ultrastructure of rat mammary-gland anlagen *in vivo* and after culture with hormones. *J. Exp. Zool.* **174**, 79–100.

9. Chew, E. C. and Hoshino, K. (1970). Early histogenesis of transplanted mouse mammary glands. II. Within 96 hours following isografting. *Z. Anat. Entwicklungsgesch.* **132**, 318–324.
10. Cunha, G. R. (1972). Epithelia-mesenchymal interactions in primordial gland structures which become responsive to androgenic stimulation. *Anat. Rec.* **172**, 179–195.
11. Cunha, G. R. (1972). Tissue interactions between epithelium and mesenchyme of urogenital and integumental origin. *Anat. Rec.* **172**, 529–541.
12. Currie, R. W., Hoshino, K., and Kim, Y. T. (1977). Functional responses of neonatal mouse mammary glands to gestational hormonal stimuli. *Anat. Rec.* **187**, 563.
13. Daniel, C. W. and DeOme, K. B. (1965). Growth of mouse mammary glands *in vivo* after monolayer culture. *Science* **149**, 634–636.
14. Daniel, C. W., DeOme, K. B., Young, J. T., Blair, P. B., and Faulkin, L. J., Jr. (1968). The *in vivo* life span of normal and preneoplastic mouse mammary glands: A serial transplantation study. *Proc. Natl. Acad. Sci. U.S.* **61**, 53–60.
15. DeCosse, J. J., Gossens, C. L., Kuzma, J. F., and Unsworth, B. R. (1973). Breast cancer: Induction of differentiation by embryonic tissue. *Science* **181**, 1057–1058.
16. DeOme, K. B. and Faulkin, L. J., Jr. (1959). Mammary tumor development from hyperplastic alveolar nodules and normal lobules transplanted into mammary gland-free fat pads and in the dorsal subcutis of female C3H/He Crgl mice. *Proc. Am. Assoc. Cancer Res.* **3**, 16–17.
17. DeOme, K. B., Faulkin, L. J., Bern, H. A., and Blair, P. B. (1959). Development of mammary tumors from hyperplastic alveolar nodules transplanted into gland-free mammary fat pads of female C3H mice. *Cancer Res.* **19**, 515–520.
18. Eichwald, E. J. and Silmser, C. R. (1955). Skin. *Transplant. Bull.* **2**, 148–149.
19. Eichwald, E. J., Silmser, C. R., and Weissman, I. (1958). Sex-linked rejection of normal and neoplastic tissue. I. Distribution and specificity. *J. Natl. Cancer Inst.* **20**, 563–575.
20. Erwin, A. G. (1967). Male mammary gland tissue in female mice. *Proc. Can. Fed. Biol. Soc.* **10**, 97.
21. Faulkin, L. J. and DeOme, K. B. (1958). The effect of estradiol and cortisol on the transplantability and subsequent fate of normal, hyperplastic, and tumourous mammary tissue of C3H mice. *Cancer Res.* **18**, 51–56.
22. Faulkin, L. J., Jr. and DeOme, K. B. (1960). Regulation of growth and spacing of gland elements in the mammary fat pad of the C3H mouse. *J. Natl. Cancer Inst.* **24**, 953–969.
23. Feldman, M. (1958). The antigen determined by a Y-linked histocompatibility gene. *Transplant. Bull.* **5**, 15–16.

24. Fischer, A. (1937). The theory of the developmental physiology of malignant tumors. *Am. J. Cancer* **31**, 1–20.
25. Gersh, I. and Catchpole, H. R. (1949). The organization of ground substance and basement membrane and its significance in tissue injury, disease, and growth. *Am. J. Anat.* **85**, 457-507.
26. Giacometti, L. and Parakkal, P. F. (1969). Skin transplantation: Orientation of epithelial cells by the basement membrane. *Nature* **223**, 514–515.
27. Gladwin, R. C. (1971). Demonstration of basement membranes in renal biopsies by silver-methenamine on thin epony resin sections. *J. Clin. Pathol.* **24**, 669–670.
28. Greene, H.S.N. (1942). The use of the mouse eye on transplantation experiments. *Cancer Res.* **7**, 491–500.
29. Grobstein, C. (1967). Mechanisms of organogenic interaction. *Natl. Cancer Inst. Monogr.* **26**, 279–299.
30. Hauschka, T. S. (1955). Probable Y-linkage of a histocompatibility gene. *Transplant. Bull.* **2**, 154–155.
31. Hirsch, B. B. (1957). The influence of sex on transplantability of isologous thymic tissue in normal C57BL mice. *Transplant. Bull.* **4**, 58.
32. Hoshino, K. (1962). Morphogenesis and growth, potentiality of mammary glands in mice. I. Transplantability and growth potentiality of mammary tissue of virgin mice. *J. Natl. Cancer Inst.* **29**, 835–851.
33. Hoshino, K. (1963). Morphogenesis and growth potentiality of mammary glands in mice. II. Quantitative transplantation of mammary glands of normal male mice. *J. Natl. Cancer Inst.* **30**, 585–591.
34. Hoshino, K. (1964). Regeneration and growth of quantitatively transplanted mammary glands of normal female mice. *Anat. Rec.* **150**, 221–236.
35. Hoshino, K. (1965). Brown fat as a stroma for mammary growth. *Anat. Rec.* **151**, 363.
36. Hoshino, K. (1965). Development and function of mammary glands of mice prenatally exposed to testosterone propionate. *Endocrinology* **76**, 789–794.
37. Hoshino, K. (1967). Transplantibility of mammary gland in brown fat pads of mice. *Nature* **213**, 194–195.
38. Hoshino, K. (1970). Induction of cancer in mammary isografts from male donors to CBA female host mice. *J. Natl. Cancer Inst.* **44**, 819–825.
39. Hoshino, K. (1970). Indefinite *in vivo* life span of serially isografted mouse mammary gland. *Experientia* **26**, 1393–1395.
40. Hoshino, K. (1975). Quantitative transplantation of mammary duct-segments in mice and rabbits for morphological, endocrinological studies as well as mammary carcinogenesis. *Proc. Can. Assoc. Lab. Anim. Sci.* 237–240.
41. Hoshino, K. and Bernet, M. A. (1964). 3-Methylcholanthrene concentration and clearance in some adipose tissues in mice. *Cancer Res.* **24**, 648–651.

42. Hoshino, K. and Gardner, W. U. (1961). Growth potentialities of the normal mammary tissue in mice. *Anat. Rec.* **139**, 240.
43. Hoshino, K. and Gardner, W. U. (1967). Transplantability and life span of mammary gland during serial transplantation in mice. *Nature* **213**, 193–194.
44. Hoshino, K., Gardner, W. U., and Pawlikowsky, R. A. (1965). The incidence of cancer in quantitatively transplanted mammary glands and its relation to age and milk agent of the donor and host mice. *Cancer Res.* **25**, 1792–1803.
45. Hoshino, K., Martin, F., and Machino, M. (1976). Early histogenesis of transplanted mouse mammary glands. III. Parenchymal-stromal interaction. *Dev. Growth Differ.* **18**, 79–94.
46. Hoshino, K. and Moore, J. E. (1968). Sex-linked histoincompatibility of pituitary isografts in the C57BL strain of mice. *Int. J. Cancer* **3**, 374–381.
47. Johansson, B. (1959). Brown fat: Review. *Metabolism* **8**, 221–240.
48. Kratochwil, K. (1969). Organ specificity in mesenchymal induction demonstrated in the embryonic development of the mammary gland of the mouse. *Dev. Biol.* **20**, 46–71.
49. Krohn, P. L. (1962). Review lectures on senescence. II. Heterochronic transplantation in the study of ageing. *Proc. Roy. Soc. London, Ser. B.* **157**, 128–147.
50. Lasfargues, E. Y. (1957). Cultivation and behaviour *in vitro* of the normal mammary epithelium of the adult mouse. *Anat. Rec.* **127**, 117–129.
51. Meissier, B. and Leblond, C. P. (1957). Preparation of coated radio-autographs by dipping section in fluid emulsion. *Proc. Soc. Exp. Biol. Med.* **96**, 7–10.
52. Moretti, R. L. and Blair, P. B. (1966). The male histocompatibility antigen in mouse mammary tissue. I. Growth of the male mammary gland in female mice. *Transplantation* **4**, 596–604.
53. Moscona, A. A. (1961). Tissue reconstruction from dissociated cells in growth in living systems. Proc. Int. Symp. on Growth, Pardue Univ., ed. Zarrow, M. X., pp. 197–220.
54. Moscona, A. A. (1967). The development *in vitro* of chimeric aggregations of dissociated embryonic chick and mouse cells. In *Molecular and Cellular Aspects of Development*, Rev. ed., ed. Bell, E., pp. 19–27. New York, Evanston, London: Harper & Row.
55. Nandi, S. (1958). Endocrine control of mammary-gland development and function in the C3H/He Crgl mouse. *J. Natl. Cancer Inst.* **21**, 1039–1063.
56. Nicoll, C. S. (1965). Growth autoregulation and the mammary gland. *J. Natl. Cancer Inst.* **34**, 131–140.
57. Peer, L. A. (1959). Transplantation of fat. In *Transplantation of Tissues*, vol. II, ed. Peer, L. A., pp. 178–189. Baltimore: Williams & Wilkins.

58. Prehn, R. T. (1953). Tumors and hyperplastic nodules in transplanted mammary glands. *J. Natl. Cancer Inst.* **13**, 859–871.
59. Prehn, R. T. and Main, J. M. (1956). The influence of sex on isologous skin grafting in the mouse. *J. Natl. Cancer Inst.* **17**, 35–36.
60. Propper, A. and Gomot, L. (1967). Interactions tissulaires au cours de l'organogenese de la glande mammaire de l'embryon de Lapin. *C. R. Acad. Sci. (Paris)* **264**, 2573–2575.
61. Raynaud, A. (1961). *Milk: The Mammary Gland and Its Secretion*, vol. 1, ed. Kon, S. K. and Cowie, A. T., pp. 3–162. New York: Academic Press.
62. Russell, P. S. and Monaco, A. P. (1965). Introduction and terminology. In *The Biology of Tissue Transplantation*, pp. 1–5. Boston: Little, Brown and Co.
63. Sachs, L. and Heller, E. (1958). The sex-linked histocompatibility antigens. *J. Natl. Cancer Inst.* **20**, 555–561.
64. Sakakura, T., Nishizuka, Y., and Dawe, C. J. (1976). Mesenchyme-dependent morphogenesis and epithelium-specific cytodifferentiation in mouse mammary gland. *Science* **194**, 1439–1441.
65. Shimkin, M. B., Wyman, R. S., and Andervont, H. B. (1946). Mammary tumors in mice following transplantation on mammary tissue. *J. Natl. Cancer Inst.* **7**, 77–78.
66. Sidman, R. L. (1956). Histogenesis of brown adipose tissue *in vivo* and in organ culture. *Anat. Rec.* **124**, 581–601.
67. Sidman, R. L. and Fawcett, D. W. (1954). The effect of peripheral nerve section on some metabolic responses of brown adipose tissue in mice. *Anat. Rec.* **118**, 487–507.
68. Snell, G. D. (1956). A comment on Eichwald and Silmser's communication. *Transplant. Bull.* **3**, 29–31.
69. Snell, G. D. and Stimpfling, J. H. (1966). Genetics of tissue transplantation In *Biology of the Laboratory Mouse*, 2nd ed., ed. Green, E. L., pp. 457–462. Toronto: McGraw-Hill.
70. Staff of Cancer Research Genetics Laboratory, University of California, Berkeley, California (1963). Current applications of a method of transplantation of tissues into gland-free mammary fat pads of mice. In *Methodology in Mammalian Genetics*, ed. Burdette, W. J., Appendix VII, pp. 565–569. San Francisco: Holden Day.
71. Steinberg, M. S. (1967). Reconstruction of tissues by dissociated cells. In *Molecular and Cellular Aspects of Development*, Rev. ed., ed. Bell, E., pp. 28–42. New York: Harper & Row.
72. Thompson, J. S. (1963). Transplantation of whole mammary glands in mice. *Transplantation* **1**, 526–534.
73. Turner, C. W. and Gomez, E. T. (1933). The normal development of the

mamary gland of the male and female albino mouse. *Univ. Missouri Res. Bull.* **182**, 3–42.

74. Vrachko, R. and Benditt, E. P. (1972). Basal lamina: The scaffold for orderly cell replacement: Observations on regeneration of injured skeletal muscle fibers and capillaries. *J. Cell Biol.* **55**, 406–419.
75. Williams, M. F. and Hoshino, K. (1970). Early histogenesis of transplanted mouse mammary glands. I. Within 21 days following isografting. *Z. Anat. Entwicklungsgesch.* **132**, 305–317.
76. Young, L.J.T., Medina, D., and DeOme, K. B. (1971). The influence of host and tissue age on life span and growth rate of serially transplanted mouse mammary gland. *Exp. Gerontol.* **6**, 49–56.

II – 3

PROLACTIN RECEPTORS IN THE MAMMARY GLAND

Kaoru KOHMOTO and Senkiti SAKAI

Department of Animal Breeding, University of Tokyo, Tokyo, Japan

The mammary gland has long been known to be a target organ of prolactin (*6*). However, the interaction between prolactin and mammary cells had not been studied until the existence of a specific receptor site for prolactin was recently demonstrated in rabbits (*28*), rats (*8*), and mice (*8*, *23*). Studies on the mode of action of glucagon clarified that this hormone acts on the surface membrane of its target cells, where it activates membrane-bound adenylate cyclase and converts ATP to cyclic AMP as a second messenger, suggesting that this may be the general method of action of polypeptide hormones (*21*). Further, research on the estrogen receptor in the uterine cytosol demonstrated the existence of hormone-receptor interaction for the first time and suggested that each hormone may have a specific receptor site in target cells (*10*). These ideas were extended to the mode of action of other polypeptide hormones, and lead to the idea that each polypeptide hormone has a specific site of action on the cell surface. When we turn our attention to the role of hormones as mediators of communication between organs, it is important to clarify the whole process of the sequence of transmission of information, *i.e.*, hormone-receptor interaction, subsequent activation of membrane-bound enzyme systems such as adenylate cyclase, transport of the second messenger to the nucleus, transcription of gene information and translation of messenger RNA at the ribosomes. However, nothing is known thus far about the second messenger for prolactin in the mammary gland, except for some negative results on cyclic AMP (*34*). Therefore, of the whole process of the information transmission system, we only have some limited knowledge about the interaction between prolactin and its receptors in the mammary gland of rabbits, rats and mice. However it is valuable to describe here the nature of the interaction and the behavior of the receptor site in view of the importance of the knowledge about the receptor site for prolactin in the elucidation of mammary development and lactogenesis.

1. Iodination of Prolactin

For the development of studies on prolactin receptors, techniques of radioiodination of prolactin were really essential. It is known that ovine prolactin radioiodinated by the chloramine-T method completely lost its biological activity as judged by pigeon crop assays. Chloramine-T is a still popular oxidant for iodinating peptide hormones for radioimmunoassays. Although the chloramine-T method does a great deal of damage to the biological activity of prolactin, this method maintains the antigenicity of the hormone unimpaired. To avoid destruction of the biological activity of prolactin, we used the lactoperoxidase method which was established by Marchalonis (*17*) to iodinate immunoglobulin, later modified by Thorell and Johansson (*32*) to iodinate insulin, growth hormone and luteinizing hormone (LH), and by Frantz and Turkington (*9*) for the iodination of prolactin. We modified the method to give prolactin the smallest chance of damage. Our method is as follows:

Reagents

1) 0.5 mCi $Na^{125}I$ (carrier-free, New England Nuclear Corp.) in 10 μl 0.1N NaOH;

2) 25 μl 0.5M phosphate buffer, pH 6.9;

3) 5 μg ovine prolactin in 10 μl 0.05M phosphate buffer, pH 7.3, freshly prepared;

4) 5 μg lactoperoxidase in 5 μl 0.05M phosphate buffer, pH 7.3, stored frozen;

5) Four portions of 25 μg H_2O_2 in 10 μl, totaling 100 μg H_2O_2 in 40 μl phosphate buffer, 0.05M, pH 7.3, freshly prepared.

The above-listed reagents were added to a polystyrene tube (10× 75 mm) with microsyringes in this order. The reaction was started by addition of the first 10 μl hydrogen peroxide solution. One, 3, and 6 min after the initiation of the reaction, hydrogen peroxide (10 μl each) was added. Ten minites after the first addition of hydrogen peroxide, the reaction was terminated by dilution of the reaction mixture with 0.5 ml 0.05M phosphate buffer (pH 7.3), and the whole mixture was layered on a Sephadex G-75 column (1×17 cm in size) pretreated with 1 ml of 4% bovine serum albumin (BSA) and equilibrated with the phosphate buffer (pH 7.3, 0.05 M). Free iodine was separated by elution with the phosphate buffer. Each 1-ml fraction was collected in polystyrene tubes containing 0.2 ml of 4% BSA. The specific radioactivity of the prolactin iodinated in this way was 70–90 mCi/mg as calculated by the method of Greenwood *et al.* (*11*).

Ovine prolactin iodinated by this method was shown to be unimpaired, in terms of electrophoretic mobility on polyacrylamide gel electrophoresis, antigenicity in radioimmunoassay and biological activity as judged by the pigeon crop-sac assay (*23*). The biological activity was estimated to be 1.1 times that of the native prolactin (NIH-P-S9) according to the method of Tanabe *et al.* (*31*). We used only 100 μg of hydrogen peroxide divided into 4 additions instead of adding the whole amount at the beginning to avoid oxidation of the prolactin. Therefore, the loss of biological activity by the chloramine-T method may not result from iodination itself but from oxidation of prolactin. Frantz and Turkington, who used 300 μg of H_2O_2, observed a more-rapidly moving radioactivity peak on disc electrophoresis than the normal peak of prolactin. Sakai also observed a radioactivity with faster mobility when he used 300 μg of H_2O_2 in his preliminary experiments. The development of the technique to iodinate prolactin with high specific radioactivity and unimpaired biological activity lead to the study on the interaction between prolactin and its receptor site in the mammary gland.

2. *The Existence and Characterization of a Prolactin Receptor in the Mouse Mammary Gland*

The existence of prolactin receptors and their kinetic properties were demonstrated and studied by different methods in different laboratories. Shiu *et al.* (*29*) and Frantz *et al.* (*8*) used particulate fractions of the mammary gland of rabbits, rats and mice, whereas Birkinshaw and Falconer (*2*) used autoradiography. We used mammary slices from lactating mice. Our method is as follows.

The thoracic third mammary glands from mice on days 2 to 10 of lactation (mostly day 7), killed after 5 hr of litter removal followed by 1 hr of suckling, were cut into 0.5-mm-thick slices by a tissue slicer (Hotta

Rika Co., Tokyo). Later we found that suckling was unnecessary. However, the removal of litters gave better results. Ten to 25 mg slices were incubated in a glass test tube (18×110 mm) containing 1 or 1.5 ml Medium 199 with 6 ng of ^{125}I-prolactin (approximately 200,000–300,000 cpm) and 0.5% BSA at pH 7.4 in an atmosphere of 95% O_2 and 5% CO_2 for up to 3 hr. The amount of tissue should be less than 20 mg/ml of medium because a linear relation between radioactivity uptake and tissue weight was observed in this range. When the incubation was terminated, slices were washed in saline, blotted on filter paper and weighed on a torsion balance. Radioactivity was counted in a gamma spectrometer with a counting efficiency of 27–30%. The total uptake of ^{125}I-prolactin was expressed as cpm/mg wet weight of tissues. Slices were also incubated in a medium containing 5 μg of native prolactin in addition to 6 ng/ml of ^{125}I-prolactin at the same time to assess nonspecific uptake of radioactivity (diffusion into the intracellular space and nonspecific binding) in the same way. Specific binding was calculated by subtraction of the nonspecific uptake from the total uptake.

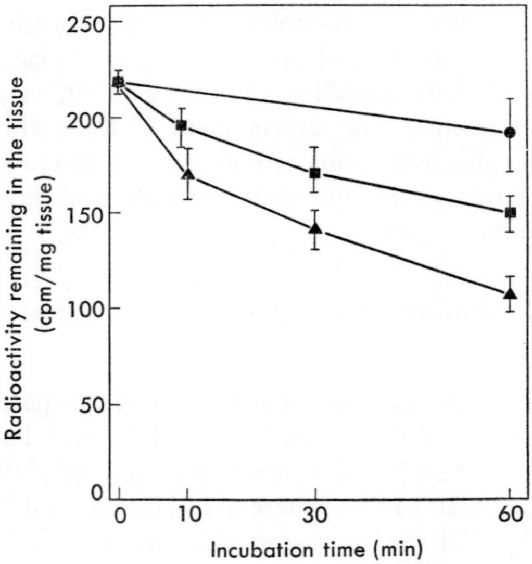

FIG. 1. Release of radioactivity from mammary tissues preincubated with 6 ng/ml of ^{125}I-prolactin for 60 min at 37°C, then incubated in Medium 199 at 0 (●), 25 (■), and 37 (▲) °C

The bars indicate standard errors for six experiments.

1) Time- and temperature-dependent nature of uptake and release of ^{125}I-*prolactin*

Both the uptake of prolactin by mammary slices and the release from the tissue are highly dependent on the temperature and time length of incubation (Fig. 1). Mammary slices incubated at 37°C contained the largest amount of prolactin, and those incubated at 0°C took up the least amount of prolactin. The use of tissue slices rather than dispersed single cells or particulate fractions always brings about a problem of diffusion. Therefore, it seems important to investigate the general pattern of diffusion of protein molecules. For this purpose, ^{131}I-labeled human serum albumin was incubated with mammary slices substituting for ^{125}I-prolactin. The results showed that the pattern of radioactivity uptake by the slices is completely different from that observed with ^{125}I-prolactin, increasing rapidly and reaching a plateau within 15–30 min after the initiation of incubation, and that diffusion does not depend on the incubation

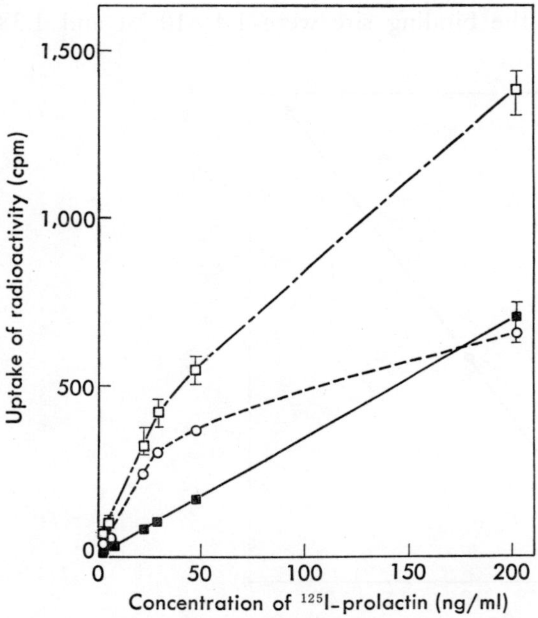

FIG. 2. Binding as a function of concentration of ^{125}I-prolactin

The broken line shows specific binding (○). The correction was made by subtracting nonspecific uptake (■) from total uptake (□). The bars show standard errors of six experiments.

temperature so much as the total uptake of ^{125}I-prolactin. There seemed to exist a process which gradually accumulated ^{125}I-prolactin after its quick diffusion. When 5 μg/ml of native prolactin was added to the medium, the pattern of radioactivity uptake by the tissue slices resembles that observed with ^{131}I-labeled human serum albumin. Therefore, the behavior of ^{125}I-prolactin in the presence of a large amount of native prolactin was thought to represent nonspecific uptake mainly due to diffusion of prolactin. The difference between the total uptake and the nonspecific uptake was called the specific binding of prolactin.

To examine the features of specific binding, mammary slices were incubated in various concentrations of ^{125}I-prolactin with or without native prolactin at 37°C for 60 min. The results are shown in Fig. 2. Here again, the total uptake of radioactive prolactin showed a different pattern from that seen in the presence of a large amount (5 μg/ml) of native prolactin (nonspecific uptake). The nonspecific uptake was related linearly to the concentration of ^{125}I-prolactin. A Lineweaver-Burk plot (double reciprocal plot) was made from the data (Fig. 3). The dissociation constant and the number of the binding site were 1.4×10^{-9}M and 1.38×10^{-15}

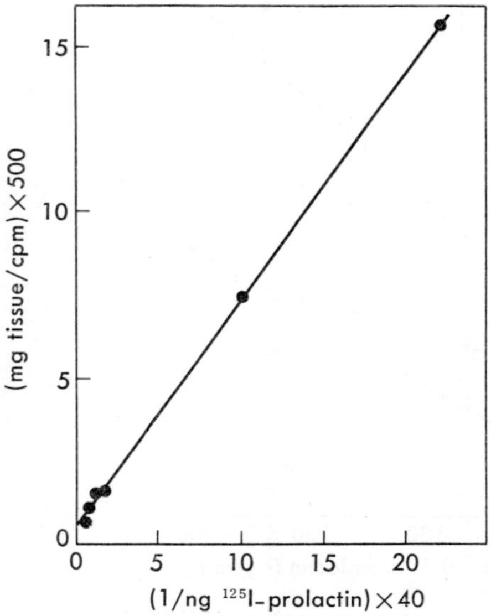

FIG. 3. Lineweaver-Burk plot of specific binding of ^{125}I-prolactin
The reciprocal of specific binding of prolactin in Fig. 2 is plotted on the ordinate, and that of concentration on the abscissa. $K_m=1.4\times10^{-9}$M.

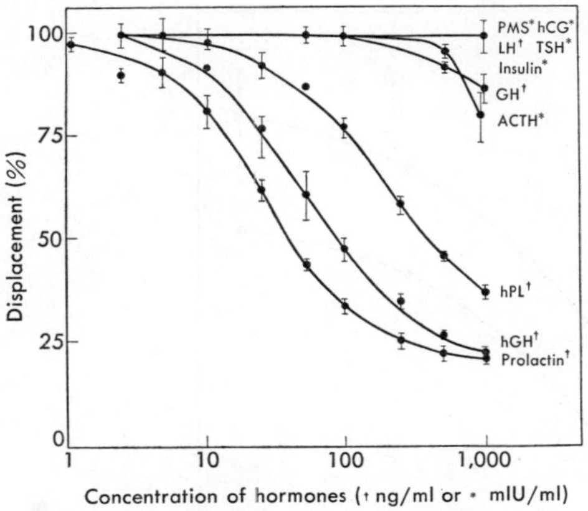

FIG. 4. Displacement of ^{125}I-prolactin with various hormones at various concentrations

mol/mg wet tissue, respectively. The figures indicate that a small number of saturable binding sites with a high affinity to prolactin exist in the lactating mouse mammary gland.

The specificity of the binding was tested by a displacement study (Fig. 4). Ovine prolactin, human growth hormone, and human choriomammotropin (placental lactogen), which are all known to be lactogenic, displaced ^{125}I-prolactin in a dose-response manner, whereas ovine LH, bovine thyroid stimulating hormone (TSH), human chorionic gonadotropin, pregnant mare serum gonadotropin and bovine insulin did not displace ^{125}I-prolactin. Large amounts of bovine growth hormone (GH) and bovine adrenocorticotropic hormone (ACTH) displaced iodinated prolactin to a small extent which was likely caused by contamination of prolactin. These results demonstrate the existence of a binding site which is saturable, specific for lactogenic hormones and has a high affinity to prolactin.

2) Kinetic figures of the interaction between prolactin and the receptor

The time course change of the specific binding was further investigated (Fig. 5). Figure 6 was plotted under an assumption that the specific binding between prolactin and the receptors is a reversible reaction of the second order:

$$H + R \underset{k_{-1}}{\overset{k_1}{\rightleftharpoons}} HR\,,$$

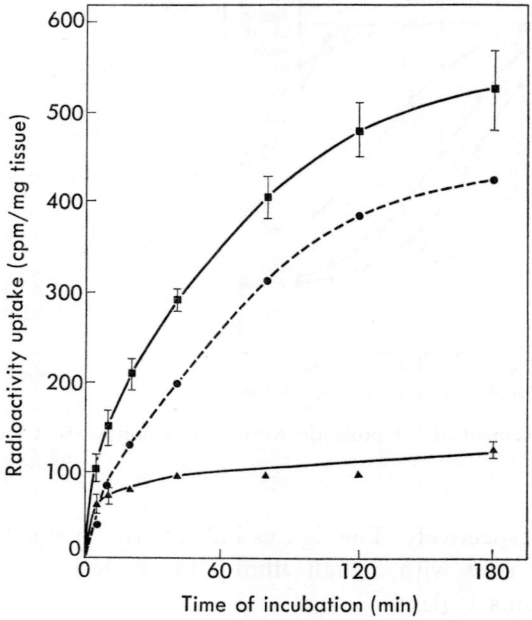

FIG. 5. Time dependence of specific binding of ^{125}I-prolactin to mammary tissues

Mammary tissues were incubated with 6 ng/ml of ^{125}I-prolactin. Total uptake of prolactin (■), nonspecific uptake (▲), and specific binding (●) are shown in this figure.

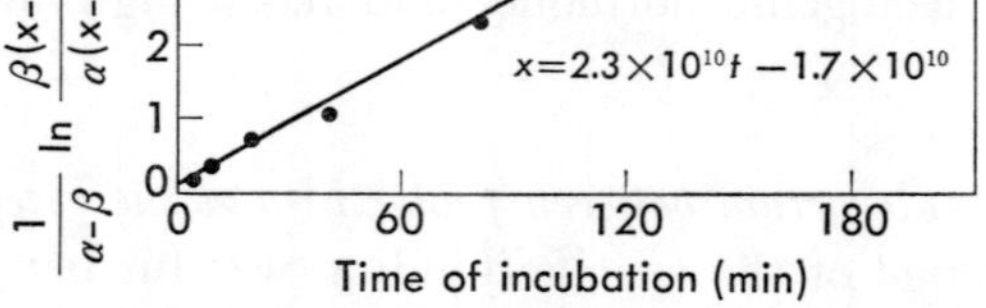

FIG. 6. Estimation of the rate constant of association based on the specific binding in Fig. 5

In the figure, x represents the concentration of prolactin-receptor complex; α and β represent the roots of the equation: $x^2-(a+b+K)x+4ab=0$, where a, b, and K are concentrations of prolactin (1.28×10^{-10}M), concentration of receptor (1.38×10^{-15} mol/mg of tissue), and dissociation constant (5.8×10^{-10}M), respectively.

where H, R, HR, k_1, and k_{-1} represent free hormone, unassociated receptor, hormone-receptor complex, and rate constants of association and dissociation, respectively. The linearity of the line supports this assumption of reversible reaction of the second order. Similar results were also obtained by Shiu and Friesen (*28*) in the rabbit mammary particulate fraction. They showed that the prolactin released from receptors had the same biological activity as the prolactin before binding to receptors. The intactness of the hormone after dissociation from receptors was demonstrated by Cuatrecasas (*7*) in the interaction between insulin and its receptors in fat cells.

The rate constant of association ($k_1 = 2.3 \times 10^7 \text{M}^{-1}\ \text{min}^{-1}$) was measured from Fig. 6, and the dissociation constant ($K_d = 5.8 \times 10^{-10}\text{M}$) from the equilibrium data. The rate constant of dissociation was calculated from these constants ($k_{-1} = 1.3 \times 10^{-2}\ \text{min}^{-1}$). The half time of dissociation $T_{1/2} = 52$ min) was calculated from the rate constant of dissociation. The value of the dissociation constant was smaller than that obtained from the Lineweaver-Burk plot, indicating a higher affinity. This was probably due to the shorter incubation time in the previous study (60 min) causing an underestimation of the specific binding. Other thermodynamic constants, such as entropy, heat capacity and free energies, of the prolactin-receptor interaction in the mammary gland of any species have not yet been determined.

3. *Development of the Binding Site for Prolactin during Pregnancy and in Lactogenesis*

1) *Simplified method for determination of the number of the binding site*

For the determination of the number of binding site, a Lineweaver-Burk plot, Scachard plot, or other methods are used. However, these methods require a considerably large amount of tissue. When we assess the number of binding sites of pregnant mice, we always have to deal with small amounts of tissues which contain only a small number of receptor sites. A simple method was used, therefore, for an approximate estimation of the specific binding site, on the basis of the following equation:

$$H + R \underset{k_{-1}}{\overset{k_1}{\rightleftharpoons}} HR$$

$$\frac{d[HR]}{dt} = k_1[H][R] - k_{-1}[HR] \tag{1}$$

$x=[HR]$, concentration of hormone-receptor complex;
$a-x=[H]$, where a is the initial concentration of ^{125}I-prolactin;
$b-x=[R]$, where b is the total number of the specific binding site; and
$K=k_1/k_{-1}$, where K represents the dissociation constant.

Equation (1) can be expressed as Eq. (2).

$$\frac{dx}{dt}=k_1(a-x)(b-x)-k_{-1}x=k_1\{x^2-(a+b+K)x+ab\} \tag{2}$$

Let the roots of $x^2-(a+b+K)x+ab=0$ be α and β ($\alpha \geq \beta$), then they are expressed as Eqs. (3) and (4).

$$\alpha=\frac{a+b+K+\sqrt{(a+b+K)^2-4ab}}{2} \tag{3}$$

and

$$\beta=\frac{a+b+K-\sqrt{(a+b+K)^2-4ab}}{2} \tag{4}$$

The differential equation (2) can be integrated as Eq. (5).

$$\frac{1}{\alpha+\beta}\ln\frac{\beta(x-\alpha)}{\alpha(x-\beta)}=k_1t \tag{5}$$

Therefore, the solution of the differential equation (2) is expressed as (6).

$$x=\frac{\alpha\{1-e^{-(\alpha-\beta)k_1t}\}}{\dfrac{\alpha}{\beta}-e^{-(\alpha-\beta)k_1t}} \tag{6}$$

If a and K are much greater than b, as in our experimental conditions, then α and β will be expressed as Eqs. (7) and (8).

$$\alpha \simeq a+K \tag{7}$$

$$\beta \simeq \frac{ab}{a+K} \tag{8}$$

Let the value of x at equilibrium ($t \to \infty$) be x_e, then x_e is equal to β.

$$x_e=\beta \tag{9}$$

From Eqs. (3), (4), (7), and (8), α is much greater than β, and the following formulas will be given.

$$\alpha \gg \beta = x_e \geq x \tag{10}$$

$$\alpha - x \simeq \alpha \tag{11}$$

$$\alpha - \beta \simeq \alpha \tag{12}$$

From Eqs. (5), (11), and (12), the following formulas (13) and (14) will be given.

$$\frac{1}{a+K} \ln \frac{x_e}{x_e - x} = k_1 t \tag{13}$$

$$x = x_e \{1 - e^{-(a+K)k_1 t}\} \tag{14}$$

Finally from Eqs. (7), (8), and (14), the next formula is given.

$$b = \frac{1 + \dfrac{K}{a}}{1 - e^{-(a+K)k_1 t}} x \tag{15}$$

If the temperature is constant, k_1 and K are constant. If the time is long enough, Eq. (15) is expressed as Eq. (16).

$$b = \left(1 + \frac{K}{a}\right) x \tag{16}$$

Actually, we compare the radioactivity of the bound ^{125}I-prolactin in the same experiment, instead of always calculating the number of binding site if temperature and incubation time are fixed. It should be noticed that the nature of binding, such as dissociation constant and rate constants, is assumed to be unchanged through pregnancy and lactation, and that this presumption is not yet proven experimentally. However, a change of these constants is not conceivable in the interaction of any kind of hormone. The data reported thus far show that the dissociation constant is unchanged in different physiological conditions (*4*, *26*).

2) Changes of the number of the binding site for prolactin during pregnancy and lactogenesis

Change in the number of the binding site for prolactin during pregnancy is described by Holcomb *et al.* (*13*) in rats and Sakai and Kohmoto (*25*) in mice. The general pattern of the change is similar in these two reports. It remains low during pregnancy, starts increasing with late pregnancy, and continues to increase until it reaches a plateau soon after parturition. The number of the binding site at late pregnancy and lactogenesis is about 2–3 times as much as that of midpregnancy, and the level

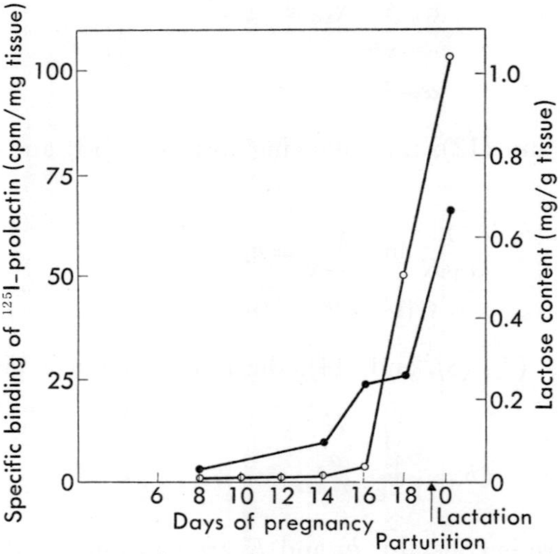

FIG. 7. Specific binding sites of ^{125}I-prolactin (●) and lactose content (○) in the mammary gland during pregnancy and lactogenesis

of the plateau during lactation is about 5 times as much as that of parturition. Figure 7 shows the changes of the binding site for prolactin during pregnancy along with the lactose content of the mouse mammary gland.

From these results, we suppose that binding sites are not abundant during pregnancy and are induced before parturition and that this is the reason why lactation is not initiated during pregnancy regardless of the presence of a large amount of choriomammotropin (placental lactogen), which is also lactogenic (*14*). Holcomb *et al.* (*13*) suggested the possible masking of the binding site by a large amount of choriomammotropin present in the blood of pregnant rats, which is associated with the binding site of prolactin so that the binding site cannot be detected by ^{125}I-prolactin. Since the half time of dissociation in our kinetic data is about 1 hr, as shown above, half the amount of the bound prolactin dissociates in 1 hr when all the receptors are associated with choriomammotropin. Therefore about three quarters of the binding site become free from choriomammotropin and available for the ^{125}I-prolactin binding in 2 hr of incubation. We conclude, therefore, that prolactin receptors may be underestimated to a small extent in the presence of a large amount of placental lactogen but that induced prolactin receptors are more than the underestimated number of the receptors. It can be assumed, however, that there is no difference in the kinetic characters between prolactin and choriomammotropin, although we only know that choriomammotropin shares the same receptor site as prolactin (*24*). Our further study shows that hysterectomy during pregnancy did not largely increase the specific binding of ^{125}I-prolactin, and that the increase of specific binding after hysterectomy is less than the amount of increase after ovariectomy (*12*).

The next question is what induces prolactin receptors? Posner *et al.* (*20*), Aragona *et al.* (*1*), and Ranke *et al.* (*22*) reported that prolactin itself induced its own receptors in the rat liver, whereas Sherman *et al.* (*26*) reported that testosterone, medroxyprogesterone, and cortisol had an effect on the decrease of prolactin binding in the rat liver. Prolactin may induce its own receptors also in the mammary gland. We suspected the possibility that glucocorticoid is an inducer of prolactin receptors in the mammary gland. To examine this hypothesis, the following experiments were conducted. Mammary tissues from 8-day-pregnant D strain mice were organ-cultured in Medium 199 containing 5 μg/ml bovine insulin with or without 1 μg/ml cortisol. The specific binding of prolactin was determined after 3 days in culture. The results are summarized in Fig. 8. Mammary tissues cultured in the medium containing cortisol had a sig-

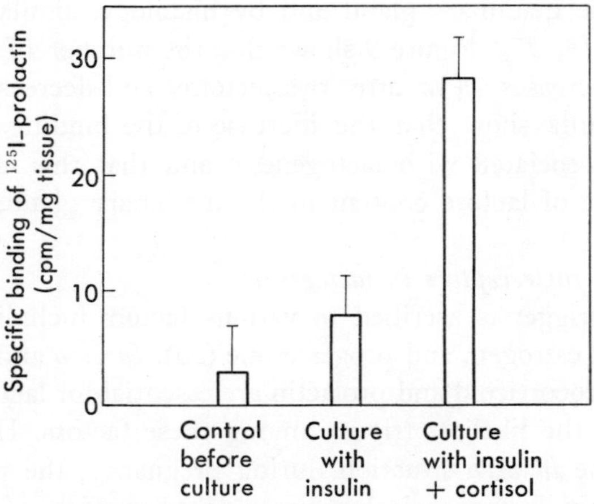

FIG. 8. Induction of specific binding sites for prolactin *in vitro*

Mammary explants from 8-day-pregnant mice were organ-cultured for 3 days in Medium 199 with insulin or insulin+cortisol. Explants cultured with insulin+cortisol had more binding sites than the controls before culture or those cultured with insulin alone ($p<0.05$).

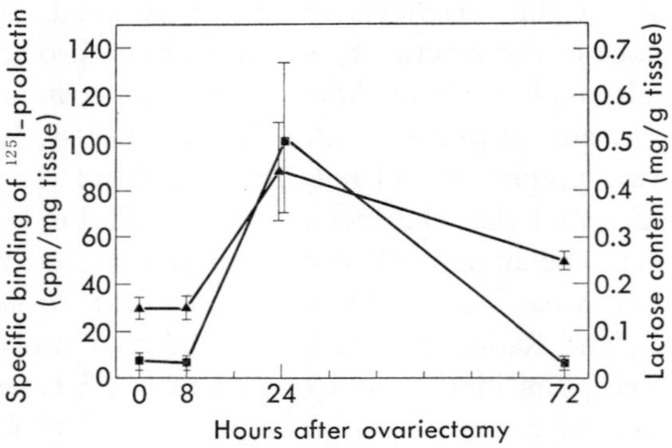

FIG. 9. Specific binding sites (▲) for prolactin and lactose content (■) in the mammary gland after ovariectomy on day 13 of pregnancy (mean±SE of 5 mice)

Mice aborted between 8 and 24 hr after ovariectomy.

nificantly larger amount of specific binding than those cultured without cortisol ($p<0.05$).

The change in the number of prolactin receptors was investigated further in ovariectomized pregnant KA mice (*12*). Pregnant mice aborted within 24 hr after ovariectomy and initiated milk secretion as judged by lactose content in the mammary gland and by histology, similar to the observation in rats (*15*, *27*). Figure 9 shows that the number of binding sites for prolactin increases 24 hr after ovariectomy and decreases again in 72 hr. These results show that the increase of the binding sites for prolactin is always associated with lactogenesis and that this change is parallel to the change of lactose content in the mammary gland.

3) *The role of prolactin receptors in lactogenesis*

The lactogenic trigger is ascribed to various factors including prolactin, glucocorticoid, estrogen, and progesterone (*33*). *In vivo* and *in vitro* studies show that glucocorticoid and prolactin are essential for lactogenesis and that prolactin is the likeliest trigger among these factors. However, when looking into the *in vivo* situation during pregnancy, the prolactin surge does not explain lactogenesis because a large amount of choriomammaotropin is present in the blood of pregnant animals, which is also highly lactogenic, but does not initiate milk secretion.

Glucocorticoid is one of the important factors (*18*, *19*, *30*). Harigaya *et al.* (*12*) observed mammary secretion and a higher specific binding of

^{125}I-prolactin in the mammary gland of pregnant mice injected with glucocorticoid than in the saline controls. On the other hand, Kuhn (*15*, *16*), based on his findings that ovariectomy in pregnant rats resulted in lactose synthesis and that only progesterone can inhibit lactogenesis, suggested that the withdrawal of progesterone was the lactogenic trigger. Our study showed high lactose content and significantly increased specific binding in pregnant mouse mammary glands after the injection of glucocorticoids. Furthermore, an injection of progesterone prevented abortion and receptor induction, accompanied by low lactose content in the mammary gland (*12*). A small dose of progesterone (0.2 mg/mouse), prevented abortion associated with an increased amount of prolactin binding when compared with high doses of progesterone (1 and 5 mg). Considering these results and the induction of prolactin receptors by glucocorticoid *in vitro*, we conclude that progesterone acts to inhibit glucocorticoid action on receptor induction.

The transport of the hormonal signal of prolactin to the nucleus of mammary epithelial cells to initiate the synthesis of milk is a sequence of reactions probably mediated by the prolactin-receptor interaction and the second messenger for prolactin. Processes after the interaction between prolactin and its receptor site, and transport of hormonal signal to the nucleus, are not yet clarified. Our investigation revealed that prolactin receptors are not abundant in the mammary gland of pregnant mice. Therefore, it is probable that the hormonal signal of prolactin is not properly transmitted to the nucleus to initiate milk secretion and that the induction of the receptors may make this process possible.

The receptor site for prolactin is one of the useful concepts to elucidate lactogenesis. However, our knowledge about prolactin-receptor interaction in the mammary gland is scanty. Research should be extended to all the stages of mammary development including carcinogenesis (*3*–*5*), and other aspects of transmission of information following the hormone-receptor interaction. These kinds of studies may contribute greatly to the clarification of all the events in mammary development.

SUMMARY

The technique of radioiodination of prolactin by the lactoperoxydase method (which is a prerequisite for study of the prolactin-receptor interaction) was introduced. Prolactin labeled by this method retained most of its biological activity as measured by the pigeon crop assay with a high specific radioactivity. Using ^{125}I-prolactin, the existence of a binding site for prolactin, which is saturable and specific to lactogenic hormones with high affinity ($K_d=1.4\times10^{-9}$M), was demonstrated in the lactating mouse mammary gland. The number of the binding site (1.38×10^{-15} mol/mg tissue) was also estimated. The kinetic data for association fit a reversible second-order reaction. A simplified method for estimating the approximate number of binding sites was worked out, based on the second-order reversible reaction model. The number of prolactin receptors estimated in this way increase during late pregnancy and continue to increase after parturition to a plateau on days 2–10 of lactation. It is suggested that prolactin receptors are induced before lactogenesis. Glucocorticoid is one of the factors responsible for the induction of prolactin receptors. Mammary explants from 8-day-pregnant mice organ-cultured with insulin and cortisol for 3 days showed a larger number of specific binding sites for prolactin than those cultured with insulin alone. Pregnant mice aborted, initiated lactose synthesis and increased specific binding of ^{125}I-prolactin to the mammary tissues after ovariectomy. This increase was prevented by progesterone. From these results, it is suggested that glucocorticoid induces prolactin receptors in lactogenesis, and that the induction of the receptor is inhibited by progesterone during pregnancy.

REFERENCES

1. Aragona, C., Bohnet, H. G., and Friesen, H. G. (1976). Prolactin binding sites in the male rat liver following castration. *Endocrinology* **99**, 1017–1022.
2. Birkinshaw, M. and Falconer, I. R. (1972). The localization of proalctin labelled with radioactive iodine in rabbit mammary tissue. *J. Endocrinol.* **55**, 323–334.
3. Costlow, M. E., Buschow, R. A., and McGuire, W. L. (1974). Prolactin receptors in an estrogen receptor-deficient mammary carcinoma. *Science* **184**, 85–86.
4. Costlow, M. E., Buschow, R. A., and McGuire, W. L. (1976). Prolactin receptors and androgen-induced regression of 7,12-dimethylbenz(a)anthracene-induced mammary carcinoma. *Cancer Res.* **36**, 3324–3329.
5. Costlow, M. E., Buschow, R. A., and McGuire, W. L. (1976). Prolactin receptors in 7,12-dimethylbenz (a) anthracene-induced mammary tumors following endocrine ablation. *Cancer Res.* **36**, 3941–3943.
6. Cowie, A. T. and Tindal, J. S. (1971). *The Physiology of Lactation*. London: Edward Arnold.

7. Cuatrecasas, P. (1971). Properties of the insulin receptor of isolated fat cell membranes. *J. Biol. Chem.* **246**, 7265–7274.
8. Frantz, W. L., MacIndoe, J. H., and Turkington, R. W. (1974). Prolactin receptors: Characteristics of the particulate fraction binding activity. *J. Endocrinol.* **60**, 485–497.
9. Frantz, W. L. and Turkington, R. W. (1972). Formation of biologically active ^{125}I-prolactin by enzymic radioiodination. *Endocrinology* **91**, 1545–1548.
10. Gorski, J., Toft, D., Shyamala, G., Smith, D., and Notides, A. (1968). Hormone receptors: Studies on the interaction of estrogen with the uterus. *Recent Prog. Horm. Res.* **24**, 45–72.
11. Greenwood, F. C., Hunter, W. M., and Glover, J. S. (1963). The preparation of ^{131}I-labelled human growth hormone of high specific radioactivity. *Biochem. J.* **89**, 114–123.
12. Harigaya, T., Sakai, S., and Kohmoto, K. (1978). Induction of mammary prolactin receptors and lactose synthesis after ovariectomy in the pregnant mouse. *Endocrinol. Japon.* **25**, 157–161.
13. Holcomb, H. H., Costlow, M. E., Buschow, R. A., and McGuire, W. L. (1976). Prolactin binding in rat mammary gland during pregnancy and lactation. *Biochim. Biophys. Acta* **428**, 104–112.
14. Kohmoto, K. and Bern, H. A. (1970). Demonstration of mammotrophic activity of the mouse placenta in organ culture and by transplantation. *J. Endocrinol.* **48**, 99–107.
15. Kuhn, N. J. (1969). Progesterone withdrawal as the lactogenic trigger in the rat. *J. Endocrinol.* **44**, 39–54.
16. Kuhn, N. J. (1969). Specificity of progesterone inhibition of lactogenesis. *J. Endocrinol.* **45**, 615–616.
17. Marchalonis, J. J. (1969). An enzymic method for the trace iodination of immunoglobulins and other proteins. *Biochem. J.* **113**, 299–305.
18. Nandi, S. and Bern, H. A. (1961). The hormones responsible for lactogenesis in BALB/cCrgl mice. *Gen. Comp. Endocrinol.* **1**, 195–210.
19. Oka, T. and Topper, Y. J. (1971). Hormone-dependent accumulation of rough endoplasmic reticulum in mouse mammary epithelial cells *in vitro*. *J. Biol. Chem.* **246**, 7701–7707.
20. Posner, B. I., Kelly, P. A., and Friesen, H. G. (1974). Induction of a lactogenic receptor in rat liver: Influence of estrogen and the pituitary. *Proc. Natl. Acad. Sci. U. S.* **71**, 2407–2410.
21. Rall, T. W. and Sutherland, E. W. (1958). Formation of a cyclic adenine ribonucleotide by tissue particles. *J. Biol. Chem.* **232**, 1065–1076.
22. Ranke, M. B., Stanley, C. A., Tenore, A., Rodbard, D., Bongiovanni, A. M., and Parks, J. S. (1976). Characterization of somatogenic and lactogenic binding sites in isolated rat hepatocytes. *Endocrinology* **99**, 1033–1045.

23. Sakai, S., Kohmoto, K., and Johke, T. (1975). A receptor site for prolactin in lactating mouse mammary tissues. *Endocrinol. Japon.* **22**, 379–387.
24. Sakai, S. and Kohmoto, K. (1976). Binding of mouse choriomammotropin to prolactin receptors in the mouse mammary gland. *Endocrinol. Japon.* **23**, 499–503.
25. Sakai, S. and Kohmoto, K. (1978). Development of prolactin receptors in the mouse mammary gland during pregnancy and lactogenesis. Unpublished.
26. Sherman, B. M., Stagner, J. I., and Zamudio, R. (1977). Regulation of lactogenic hormone binding in rat liver by steroid hormone. *Endocrinology* **100**, 101–107.
27. Shinde, Y., Ôta, K., and Yokoyama, A. (1965). Lactose content of mammary glands of pregnant rats near term: Effect of removal of ovary, placenta and foetus. *J. Endocrinol.* **31**, 106–114.
28. Shiu, R.P.C. and Friesen, H. G. (1974). Properties of a prolactin receptor from the rabbit mammary gland. *Biochem. J.* **140**, 301–311.
29. Shiu, R.P.C., Kelly, P. A., and Friesen, H. G. (1973). Radioreceptor assay for prolactin and other lactogenic hormones. *Science* **180**, 968–971.
30. Talwalker, P. K., Nicoll, C. S., and Meites, J. (1961). Induction of mammary secretion in pregnant rats and rabbits by hydrocortisone acetate. *Endocrinology* **69**, 802–808.
31. Tanabe, Y., Shoda, Y., and Saeki, Y. (1954). A local method of prolactin assay using a comparison of the responses in the two crop-sacs of the same pigeon. *Bull. Natl. Inst. Agric.* **9**, 57–65 (in Japanese with English summary).
32. Thorell, J. I. and Johansson, B. G. (1971). Enzymic iodination of polypeptides with ^{125}I to high specific activity. *Biochim. Biophys. Acta* **251**, 363–369.
33. Tucker, H. A. (1974). General endocrinological control of lactation. In *Lactation*, ed. Larson, B. L. and Smith, V. R., pp. 277–326. New York, London: Academic Press.
34. Turkington, R. W., Majumder, G. C., Kadohama, N., MacIndoe, J. H., and Frantz, W. L. (1972). Hormonal regulation of gene expression in mammary cell. *Recent Prog. Horm. Res.* **28**, 417–449.

II – 4

4 — II

SOME ASPECTS OF CASEIN BIOSYNTHESIS IN THE MAMMARY GLAND

Senichi Komine

Department of Biochemistry, School of Medicine, Kyorin University, Tokyo, Japan

Milk contains specific materials such as lactose, short carbon chain fatty acids (C_6–C_{10}), casein, α-lactablumin, *etc.* They do not exist in any other organs, so the mammary gland is a very interesting organ which produces the specific materials mentioned above only during the lactating period. The process of synthesis of these materials in the mammary gland has been investigated by many researchers, but only the chemical process by which glucose becomes lactose has been proven, and the mechanism of casein biosynthesis and its secretion has almost been clarified.

Generally, most biochemical research on the mammary gland have been done from the viewpoint of biochemical metabolism, such as protein, lactose metabolism, *etc.* So the general reviews dealing with the biochemical mechanisms in the mammary gland are very scanty. Presently, only "Lactation" (*17*) can be referred to.

The biosynthetic mechanism of the special milk fatty acids, the control mechanism of lactose metabolism and other biochemical problems of the mammary gland are very interesting subjects for review; herein the author describes some biochemical aspects of casein biosynthesis for the reason of its specifity and its relatively large quantity in milk composition.

Before viewing the biochemical aspects, we must understand the general histology of the mammary secretory cells and the morphological aspect of casein secretion. These problems were reviewed in "Lactation" (*17*), and also by Werner *et al.* (*46*) with many electron microscopic pictures. Casein and other milk proteins made in the rough endoplasmic reticulum are concentrated in the Golgi body where they are included in the small vesicle called the secretory vesicle which reaches the plasma membrane. After binding to the plasma membrane, milk proteins are secreted from the vesicle to the outside of the cell. This type of secretion is called the reverse pinocytosis type.

The above-mentioned process is recognized as the main pathway of casein biosynthesis in the cell, but the possibility of the existence of other pathways of casein biosynthesis can be postulated by the results of our experiments.

The description of casein biosynthesis problems should be divided into different items, such as (1) the effects of hormones, (2) locality of synthesis in the cell, (3) the change of ribosomes, (4) casein phosphorylation, (5) secretory mechanism, (6) messenger RNA for casein, (7) the synthetic material of casein, and (8) the energy source for casein biosynthesis.

1. Effects of Hormones

Insulin, prolactin, and hydrocortisone are indispensable in the biosynthesis of milk proteins, of which insulin is especially essential *in vitro*. Since the original work of Lockwood *et al.* (*21*), this fact has been confirmed by many investigators. Recently Rillema (*28*, *29*) reported that the initial effect for the enhancement of milk protein biosynthesis was the increase of RNA synthesis speed. But the process of the chemical changes in the mammary cell by hormones is still unknown. Recently, cyclic AMP (cAMP) as the second messenger in the cell for hormones has been discussed. We investigated whether or not casein biosynthesis could be explained by the cAMP theory. At first, we estimated the activities of adenyl cyclase in immature, pregnant and lactating mice mammary glands and the activities were compared with the abilities of casein biosynthesis. It stood to reason that the ability for casein synthesis increased rapidly during the late pregnancy to lactating period; but in any stage, the activities of adenyl cyclase did not show marked variation. After the addition of insulin, prolactin, and hydrocortisone into the organ culture medium, the development of the organ and the ability for casein biosynthesis and the activity of adenyl cyclase were studied by using mice mammary glands. The addition of hormones was effective for the development of the organ and the ability for casein biosynthesis but was not effective for increasing the activity of adenyl cyclase. With the addition of cAMP into the organ

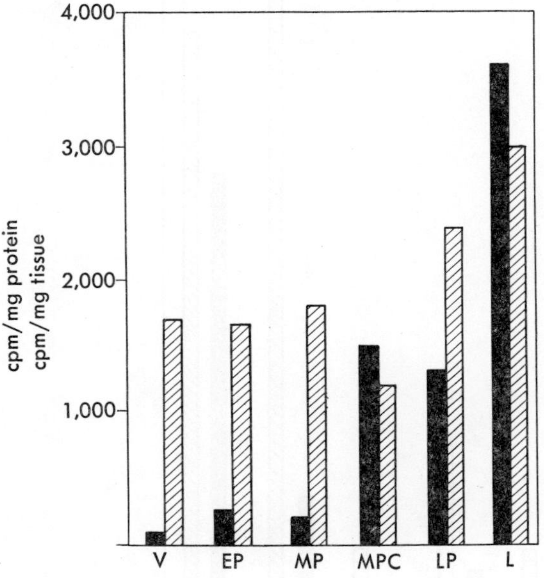

FIG. 1. Changes in the activities of casein biosynthesis and adenyl cyclase at different stages

▨ ^{14}C-cAMP; ■ ^{32}P-casein. V, virgin; EP, early-preg. (6–7 days); MP, mid-preg. (8–10 days); MPC, [MP+(insulin+prolactin+hydrocortisone)]; LP, late-preg. (18 days); L, lactating (2 days).

culture medium, the ability for casein biosynthesis did not increase as shown in Fig. 1. So we consider that the hormonal effect on casein biosynthesis could not be explained by the cAMP theory. Sapag-Hagar and Greenbaum (*33*) reported that the activity of adenyl cyclase in the rat mammary gland increased with the progress of pregnancy to reach maximum activity at the end of pregnancy. It should be noted that insulin acts to decrease the amount of cAMP in tissues (*24*, *26*), and hydrocortisone is not effective in increasing cAMP (*7*). As far as is known, there have been no reports showing that prolactin is effective in increasing cAMP. There are no reports on whether casein biosynthesis is enhanced by cyclic GMP or not.

As shown in Fig. 2, we found through experiments with mice mammary glands in organ culture that the effects of insulin, prolactin and hydrocortisone appeared more markedly in the incorporation of ^{14}C-labeled amino acid with the casein molecule than in the case of ^{32}P-labeled

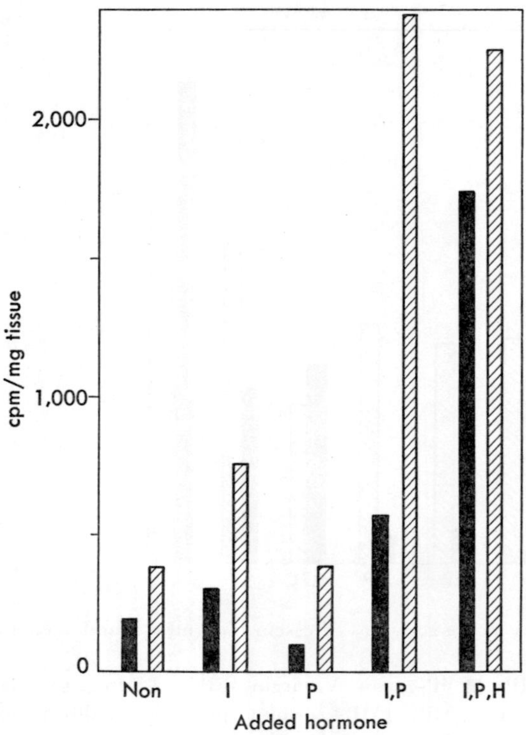

FIG. 2. The additional effect of hormones for casein biosynthesis
▨ ^{14}C-amino acids; ■ ^{32}P-orthophosphoric acid. I, insulin; P, prolactin; H, hydrocortisone.

phosphoric acid. These results indicate that these hormones have stronger actions on the peptide synthesis of casein than on the phosphrylation of casein. The concentration of prolactin in the blood increased rapidly a few days before and after parturition (*14*, *37*) and the concentration of adrenal steroids increased during the late pregnancy (*25*, *35*, *40*, *45*). According to these results, development of the mammary gland and the synthetic ability of the milk proteins seem to depend upon the concentration of hormones in the blood. But Shiu and Friesen (*35*) reported that the number of the prolactin receptors per cell membrane protein weight was most abundant in the adrenal cortex, about twice as much as in the mammary gland, and also that prolactin receptors were found even in the liver and kidney, with about one-third the number of receptors found in the mammary gland. Therefore hormonal effects on the mammary gland may depend on both the amount of hormone receptors and hormone concentration in the blood. A further discussion of the prolactin receptor appears below.

2. Locality of Casein Biosynthesis, Change of Ribosomes, Casein Phosphorylation, and Secretory Mechanism

Milk proteins are synthesized on the rough endoplasmic reticulum, and these casein peptides are concentrated and phosphorylated in the Golgi bodies (*27*, *46*). The rough endoplasmic reticulum develops and engorged protein granules appear in the Golgi bodies during pregnancy. Milk proteins have been synthesized using membrane-bound ribosomes *in vitro* (*9*, *10*, *43*). However, the possibility that casein may synthesize on free ribosomes and that phosphorylation could be performed outside the Golgi bodies cannot be neglected. We have observed in mice mammary glands that the quantity of ribosomes increased from onset of pregnancy until lactation, but the ratio of free to bound ribosomes remained constant throughout the period (*ca.* 1 : 4). The amount of polysomes also increased and the ratio of free to bound polysomes was the same as that of ribosome.

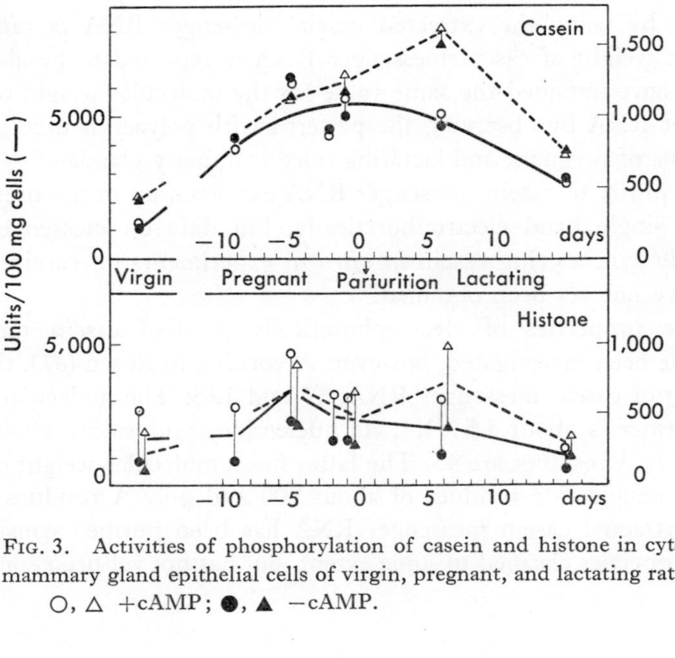

FIG. 3. Activities of phosphorylation of casein and histone in cytosol of the mammary gland epithelial cells of virgin, pregnant, and lactating rats ○, △ +cAMP; ●, ▲ −cAMP.

Bingham and Farrell (*4*) suggested that casein was phosphorylated in the Golgi body and indicated the existence of casein kinase there. Contrary to these findings, Asaga, our collaborator, found that casein kinase in the cytosol of the rat mammary gland cells increased remarkably from pregnancy to lactation, as shown in Fig. 3. Moreover, the same enzyme was found in mitochondria by Clari (*6*). So there is a possibility that casein is synthesized and phosphorylated in locations other than the rough endoplasmic reticulum and the Golgi bodies.

3. Messenger RNA for Casein

Recently, the messenger RNA for particular proteins, such as casein, has been identified (*11*, *13*, *31–33*, *36*). The following methods have been used for this classification: (1) ultracentrifugation, (2) column chromatography using a Sepharose 4B, with RNA separated by the quality of the molecular weight, (3) oligo (dT) cellulose or poly U-Sepharose column chromatography, with messenger RNA identified by polyacrylamide (*11*, *30*) or agarose gel electrophoresis (*32*), and (4) ribosomes containing casein messenger RNA are precipitated by the addition of casein antibody (*13*). Usually, the casein messenger RNA is extracted by a combination of the methods described above and then the ability for casein biosynthesis is evaluated by using the extracted casein messenger RNA *in vitro*. The molecular weight of casein messenger RNA is reported to be about 10–*15*S. We have obtained the same value for the molecular weight of casein messenger RNA by observing the patterns with polyacrylamide gel electrophoresis of pregnant and lactating mice mammary glands.

The purity of casein messenger RNA extracted up to the present has shown a single band electrophoretically, but data on messenger RNA specifically synthesizing casein *in vitro* in experiments on casein biosynthesis have not yet been obtained.

Some properties of electrophoretically purified casein messenger RNA have been investigated, however. According to Rosen (*31*), there are two kinds of casein messenger RNA, 15 and 12S. The molecular weight of the former is about 4.5×10^5, its nucleotide residues are about 1,300 and its poly A residues are 45. The latter has a molecular weight of about 3.2×10^5, neucleotide residues of about 900 and poly A residues are 41. So the extracted casein messenger RNA has been purified considerably and its properties clarified to some extent, but has not yet been completely purified.

4. *Precursors of Casein*

The problem of the synthetic materials for casein has already been solved so recent studies on this aspect are very scarce. When radio isotope labeled amino acids are infused into the vein, they were rapidly incorporated into casein (*1–3*, *5*). It was also observed that glycine converted to serine in the mammary gland (*5*). According to these results, it is reasonable to conclude that the synthetic materials for casein were the free amino acids in the blood. But Barry (*3*) observed that when rabbit serum proteins labeled with ^{14}C-glycine was infused into another rabbit's vein, the ^{14}C-glycine appeared in the casein. Moreover, the activity of the total cathepsin in the mammary gland increased from late pregnancy to lactation, during which the activity reached levels more than 10 times that of the virgin period (*12*). The author has also compared proteolitic activity in the lactating rat mammary gland by using bovine albumin as the substrate with other organs. The activity in the mammary gland showed about five-sevenths of the liver's activity and this value was the same for the kidney. It was recognized that the removal percentage of amino acids from the blood into the mammary gland was about 35% by the method of the arterio-venous circulation in the mammary gland (*34*), so if the source of milk proteins depended upon the free amino acids in the blood, 400 liters of blood must flow into the mammary gland for the production of only 1 liter of milk, even if the removal was 100% (*8*). Thus, the synthetic material of casein may be the amino acids pooled in the secretory cell of the mammary gland, and these pooled amino acids may be constructed by free amino acids coming from the blood and the proteoclastic amino acids mainly derived from serum albumin.

5. *Energy Source for Casein Biosynthesis*

Milk contains many of the special materials which are produced only in the mammary gland. These materials are synthesized very actively in the mammary cells during lactation. Thus, vast energy is needed for their biosynthesis. Glucose, acetate, lactate, *etc.*, are probably used as the energy source of biosynthesis. The concentrations of these in mammary cells may increase respectably during the lactation period. Therefore, the blood vessels in the mammary gland also develop enormously, together with the development of the mammary gland during late pregnancy to lactation (*23*, *41*). This theory is also supported by data observed by the differential

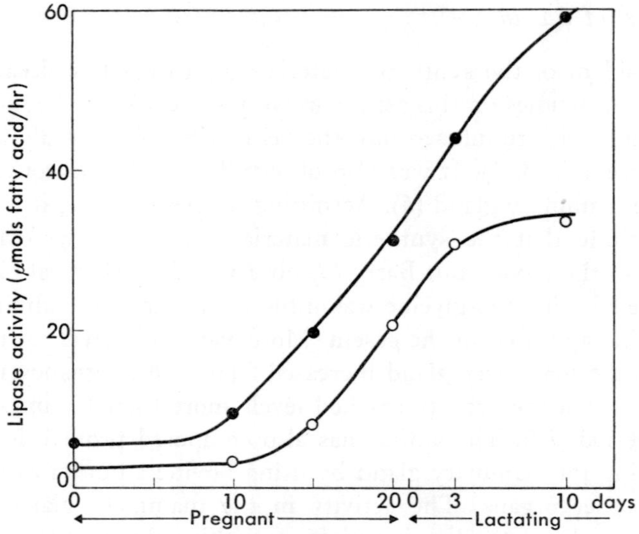

FIG. 4. Activities of lipase in mice mammary glands from pregnancy to lactation

● estimated at pH 6.6 using phosphate buffer; ○ estimated at pH 7.6 using Hepes-Tris buffer.

concentrations of glucose, lactate, *etc.*, between the mammary artery and the vein (*16*, *18–20*, *42*, *44*).

Otherwise, the normal virginal mouse mammary gland consists mostly of fat cells and during lactation a small amount of capillary plexuses surrounding the fat cells, but during lactation, the fat cells are displaced by secretory cells (*23*). This fact was observed in our laboratory too, so Anzai, our collaborator, became interested in the lost fat. He investigated the variation of lipase activities in mice mammary glands during pregnancy and lactation. As shown in Fig. 4, the lipase activity increased linearly from about the 10th day of pregnancy, and reached maximum activity 3 days after parturition. The total fatty acids in the mammary gland also increased from the 10th day of pregnancy, and reached a maximum at the 15–20th day of pregnancy and decreased rapidly after parturition. It can be assumed from these results that the fat stored in the mammary gland during the normal cyclic stage and early pregnancy, and can be used as the energy required for synthesis during the late pregnancy and lactating period. The following observations of Anzai also support this report that the variation of acetyl-CoA-carboxylase in the mammary gland showed almost the same pattern of the lipase. According to McBride and Edward (*22*), the activity of lipoprotein lipase in the guinea pig's mammary gland increased rapidly immediately before parturition, and reached a maximum on the 7th day after parturition. So, during lactating period, the fat which not only derived from the mammary gland but also from other organs (*38*, *39*) may mobilize to the mammary secretory cells, and in these cells the activities of lipase and lipoprotein lipase may increase markedly, so that this fat may be used as a biosynthetic energy source for the composition of milk, including casein. So far it has been observed that fat cells are replaced with secretory cells in the rabbit or mouse mammary gland during the lactating period, However, according to the electron microscopic observation reported by Kraehenbuhl (*15*), the big fat globule in the mammary epitherial cell was decomposed and consumed rapidly during late pregnancy, then the organelles in the cell reverted to its original place, and this resulted in lactation.

SUMMARY

The author commented about some problems of casein biosynthesis and its secretion, based on our experiments, with the following summary.

1) Hormonal effects on casein biosyntheses could not be explained by cAMP theory. Insulin, prolactin, and hydrocortisone were effective in increasing the ability of casein biosynthesis, but the activity of adenyl cyclase was not influenced by their addition to the organ culture medium. Also the activities did not show remarkable changes between immature, pregnant, and lactating mice. Even with the addition of cAMP in the culture medium an elevation of ability for casein biosynthesis did not occur.

Hormonal effects on casein biosynthesis appeared more effectively in peptide synthesis than in phosphorylation.

2) Casein mainly synthesizes on the rough endoplasmic reticulum, and phosphorylation may be done in the Golgi body. But other synthesizing and phosphorylating routes for casein must not be neglected.

3) The size of messenger RNA for casein was between 10–15S, but it has not yet been extracted in a completely pure form.

4) Synthetic material of casein is not limited to the free amino acids in the blood. Serum albumin may also be used as a material. In this case, serum albumin may be hydrolyzed by the protease contained in the mammary gland, and then incorporated into the amino acids pooled in the cell together with the free amino acids coming from the blood.

5) For the energy of biosynthesis of milk components including casein, fat stored in the mammary gland may be used together with glucose, lactate, acetate *etc.*, because the activity of lipase in the mammary gland increases rapidly during late pregnancy to the lactating period.

REFERENCES

1. Askonas, A. B., Campbell, N. P., and Work, S. T. (1954). The biosynthesis of proteins. 2. Synthesis of milk proteins by the goat. *Biochem. J.* **58**, 326–331.
2. Barry, M. J. (1952). The source of lysine, tyrosine and phosphorus for casein synthesis. *J. Biol. Chem.* **195**, 795–803.
3. Barry, M. J. (1961). *Milk: The Mammary Gland and Its Secretion*, vol. 1, ed. Kon, S. K. and Cowie, A. T. pp. 389–419. New York, London: Academic Press.
4. Bingham, W. E. and Farrell, M. H., Jr. (1974). Casein kinase from the Golgi apparatus of lactating mammary gland. *J. Biol. Chem.* **249**, 3647–3651.
5. Campbell, N. P. and Work, S. T. (1952). The biosynthesis of proteins. 1. Uptake of glycine, serine, valine and lysine by the mammary gland of the rabbits. *Biochem. J.* **52**, 217–228.
6. Clari, G. (1976). Phosphorylation of casein by mitochondrial protein kinase. *Mol. Biochem.* **13**, 67–71.
7. Friedmann, N., Exton, J. H., and Park, O. R. (1967). Interaction of adrenal steroids and glucagon on gluconeogenesis in perfused rat liver. *Biochem. Biophys. Res. Commun.* **29**, 113–119.
8. Folley, S. J. (1949). Biochemical aspcets of mammary gland function. *Biol. Rev.* **24**, 316–352.
9. Gaye, P. and Denamur, R. (1970). Preferential synthesis of β-lactoglobulin by the bound ribosomes of the mammary gland. *Biochem. Biophys. Res. Commun.* **41**, 266–272.
10. Gaye, P., Viennot, N., and Denamur, R. (1972). *In vitro* synthesis of α-lactalbumin and β-lactoglobulin by microsomes and bound polysomes from the mammary gland of lactating sheep. *Biochim. Biophys. Acta* **262**, 371–380.
11. Gaye, P., Houdebine, L., and Denamur, R. (1973). Isolation of active messenger RNA for α_s casein from bound polysomes of mammary gland. *Biochem. Biophys. Res. Commun.* **51**, 637–644.
12. Greenbaum, L. A. and Greenwood, C. F. (1954). Some enzymic changes in mammary gland of rats during pregnancy, lactation and mammary involution. *Biochem. J.* **56**, 625–631.
13. Houdebine, L. and Gaye, P. (1976). Purification of the mRNAs for ewe α_s-casein and β-casein. *Eur. J. Biochem.* **63**, 9–14.
14. Ingalls, G. W., Convery, M. E., and Hafs, D. H. (1973). Bovine serum LH,

GH and prolactin during late pregnancy, parturition and early lactation. *Proc. Soc. Exp. Biol. Med.* **143**, 161–167.
15. Kraehenbuhl, P. J. (1977). Dispersed mammary gland epitherial cells. 1. Isolation and separation procedures. *J. Cell. Biol.* **72**, 390–405.
16. Kronfeld, S. D., Raggi, F., and Ramberg, F. C. (1968). Mammary blood flow and ketone body metabolism in normal, fasted and ketotic cows. *Am. J. Physiol.* **215**, 218–227.
17. Larson, L. B. and Smith, R. V. (eds.) (1976). *Lactation*, vols. 1–3. London, New York: Academic Press.
18. Linzell, L. J. (1960). Valvular incompentence in the venous drainage of the udder. *J. Physiol.* **153**, 481–491.
19. Linzell, L. J. (1966). Measurement of venous flow by continuous thermodilution and its application to measurement of mammary blood flow in the goat. *Circ. Res.* **18**, 745–765.
20. Linzell, L. J. (1960). Mammary-gland blood flow and oxygen, glucose and volatile fatty acid uptake in conscious goat. *J. Physiol.* **153**, 492–509.
21. Lockwood, D. H., Turkington, R. W., and Topper, Y. J. (1966). Hormone dependent development of milk protein synthesis in mammary gland *in vitro*. *Biochim. Biophys. Acta* **130**, 493–501.
22. McBride, W. O. and Edward, D. K. (1963). The lipoprotein lipase of mammary gland and the correlation of its activity to lactation. *J. Lipid Res.* **4**, 17–20.
23. Nishinakazawa, H. (1970). Anatomical studies on the vascular system of the mammary gland of the mammals. *Bull. Fac. Agric. Kagoshima Univ.* **20**, 1–56.
24. Oye, I. and Sutherland, E. W. (1966). The effect of epinephirine and other agents on adenyl cyclase in the cell membrane of avian erythrocytes. *Biochim. Biophys. Acta* **127**, 347–454.
25. Paape, J. M. and Desjardins, C. (1971). Nursing duration and suckling intensity: Effects on plasma corticosterone, circulating leukocytes and mammary nucleic acids. *Proc. Soc. Exp. Biol. Med.* **138**, 12–20.
26. Rall, T. W. and Sutherland, E. W. (1958). Formation of a cyclic adenosine ribouncleotide by tissue particles. *J. Biol. Chem.* **232**, 1065–1076.
27. Reynolds, M. and Folley, J. S. (eds.) (1969). *Lactogenesis*. Philadelphia, Pa.: Univ. Pennsilvania Press.
28. Rillema, A. J. (1975). Characteristics of prolactin stimulation of uridine metabolism in mammary gland explants. *Endocrinology* **96**, 1307–1311.
29. Rillema, A. J. (1975). Rapid effects of insulin on uridine metabolism in mammary gland explant. *Am. J. Physiol.* **228**, 1531–1534.
30. Rosen, M. J. (1975). Regulation of casein messenger RNA during the development of the rat mammary gland. *Biochemistry* **14**, 2895–2903.
31. Rosen, M. J. (1976). Isolation and characterization of purified rat casein messenger ribonucleic acids. *Biochemistry* **15**, 5263–5270.

32. Rosen, M. J. (1976). Quantitation of casein messenger ribonucleic acid sequences using a specific complementary DNA hybridization probe. *Biochemistry* **15**, 5272–5280.
33. Sapag-Hagar, M. and Greenbaum, A. L. (1973). c-AMP-phosphodiesterase and of the level of 3′, 5′ cyclic adenosine monophosphate in rat mammary gland during pregnancy and lactation. *Biochem. Biophys. Res. Commun.* **53**, 982–987.
34. Seldon-Peters, M.C.J. and Barry, M. J. (1956). The uptake of glutamine and other amino acids from the blood stream by the lactating mammary gland. *Biochem. J.* **63**, 673–680.
35. Shiu, P.C.R. and Friesen, G. H. (1974). Properties of a prolactin receptor from the rabbit mammary gland. *Biochem. J.* **140**, 301–311.
36. Shuster, C. R., Houdebine, L., and Gaye, P. (1976). Studies on the synthesis of casein messenger RNA during pregnancy in the rabbit. *Eur. J. Biochem.* **71**, 193–199.
37. Smith, L. K. and Schanbacher, L. F. (1973). Hormone induced lactation in the bovine. 1. Lactational performance following injection of 17β-estradiol and progesterone. *J. Dairy Sci.* **56**, 738–743.
38. Smith, W. R. and Walsh, A. (1975). Composition of liver lipids of the rat pregnancy and lactation. *Lipid* **10**, 643–645.
39. Smith, W. R. and Walsh, A. (1976). Effect of lactation on lipolysis in rat adipose tissue. *Lipid* **11**, 418–420.
40. Smith, G. V. and Convey, M. E. (1971). Influence of acute and chronic suckling on plasma corticosterone and mammary nucleic acids. *Proc. Soc. Exp. Biol. Med.* **136**, 588–591.
41. Soemarwoto, N. I. and Bern, H. A. (1958). The effect of hormones on the vascular pattern of the mouse mammary gland. *Am. J. Anat.* **103**, 403–422.
42. Spincer, J., Rook, F.A.J., and Tower, G. K. (1969). The uptake of plasma constituents by the mammary gland of the sow. *Biochem. J.* **111**, 727–732.
43. Stein, O. and Stein, Y. (1967). Lipid synthesis, intracellular transport and secretion. II. Electron microscopic radioautographic study of mouse lactating mammary gland. *J. Cell Biol.* **34**, 251–263.
44. Verbeke, R. and Peeters, G. (1965). Uptake of free plasma amino acids by the lactating cow's udder and amino acid composition of udder lymph. *Biochem. J.* **94**, 183–189.
45. Voogt, L. J., Star, M., and Meites, J. (1969). Influence of cycling, pregnancy, labor and suckling on corticosterone-ACTH levels. *Am. J. Physiol.* **216**, 655–658.
46. Werner, W. F., Marion, R. L., Jürgen, K., Heide, Z., and Thomas, W. K. (1976). Involvement of vesicle material in casein secretion and surface regeneration. *J. Cell Biol.* **69**, 173–195.

II – 5

HORMONAL CONTROL OF THE INDUCTION OF LACTOSE SYNTHESIS IN THE RAT

Akira Yokoyama and Katuaki Ôta
Faculty of Agriculture, Nagoya University, Nagoya, Japan

Since the classical work of Halban (*21*) and Hammond (*22*), much information concerning the role of the pituitary gland, ovary, placenta and fetuse, and other endocrine organs in the hormonal control of the initiation of lactation has been accumulated (see *9*, *50* for review). However, the interaction among several hormones and/or endocrine glands relating to lactogenesis has not been clarified.

In order to determine the time of onset of copious milk secretion (lactogenesis) and to elucidate the hormonal control of lactogenesis, a quantitative evaluation of milk is required. In small experimental animals quantitative assessment of milk secretion is very difficult. Therefore, specific milk components such as lactose and casein which can be measured quantitatively are used as indicators of lactogenesis. In the strictest sense, therefore, we should use the term "the initiation of the synthesis of lactose, casein, *etc.*" instead of lactogenesis.

Shinde *et al.* (*46*), studying the appearance of lactose in the mammary gland, reported that the appearance could be advanced by ovariectomy and/or feto-placentectomy performed on days 18 or 19 of pregnancy in the rat, and suggested that the loss of placenta might contribute to the initiation of lactation. Since the administration of progesterone could suppress the appearance of lactose following ovariectomy and feto-placentectomy (*31*, *46*) and since a decrease in the plasma concentration of progesterone preceded normal parturition in the pregnant rat (*36*, *54*), withdrawal of the suppressing effect of progesterone is suggested as a trigger of initiation of milk synthesis in the mammary glands of the rat (*31*, *52*). Holcomb *et al.* (*23*) reported that progesterone might be responsible for reducing the binding activity of prolactin in the mammary gland during pregnancy. Kohmoto (*29*) also found that ovariectomy increased the prolactin receptor in the mammary gland in pregnant mice. The findings that progesterone appeared to repress the formation of α-lactalbumin, which is a subunit of the lactose synthetase, in the mammary gland of the mouse *in vitro* could support the suggestion concerning the suppressing role of progesterone in the initiation of milk synthesis (*51*).

It has been well established that prolactin and glucocorticoids play indispensable roles in the initiation of lactation in the rat (see *9*, *11*, *50* for review). An increase in the rate of secretion of prolactin and glucocorticoids would then occur with the onset of milk synthesis. An abrupt increase in the plasma concentration of prolactin occurs at the end of pregnancy (*1*, *6*, *32*, *36*, *38*). However, consistent results concerning the circulating concentration of glucocorticoids have not been obtained. Therefore, the first part of this paper deals with the changes in the concentration of plasma corticosterone and of pituitary prolactin of the rat in late pregnancy and at parturition, with special reference to the 24-hr variation in steroid secretion.

Considering the mechanism of lactogenesis, we have to pay attention to the responsiveness of the mammary gland as well as the mechanism of release of the lactogenic hormone complex. In this connection, it is very interesting to determine the stage of pregnancy at which the mammary gland is able to initiate lactose synthesis in response to lactogenic stimuli and to compare the responsiveness to stimuli in the pregnant mammary gland with that in the pseudopregnant mammary gland. The comparison of the responsiveness of the mammary gland between the pregnant and the pseudopregnant rat is expected to throw light on the involvement of the placenta in the endocrine mechanism of lactogenesis.

The important role of placental hormones not only in the development of the mammary gland during pregnancy but also in the initiation of synthesis of milk has been reported (*37*, *39*). The second part of this paper is mostly concerned with this aspect.

Primigravid Wistar-Imamichi rats, weighing 200–280 g at mating, were used. They were housed singly in wooden cages and kept in a temperature-(24 ± 2°C) and light-(14L: 10D lights on 05.00 hr) controlled animal room. Commercial diet (CA-1, Nihon CLEA Co., Ltd., Japan) and water were given *ad libitum*. Animals were mated on the day of proestrous. Pseudopregnancy was induced by mating with vasectomized rats. The day on which plugs in the vaginal smear or sperms and plugs were found was designated day 0 of pseudopregnancy and pregnancy, respectively. Operations were carried out under ether anesthesia.

Lactose contents of the six posterior mammary glands were measured by a method using β-galactosidase and glucose oxidase. DNA and RNA contents of the glands were measured by the diphenylamine (*12*) and orcinol reactions (*7*), respectively, after extraction according to the Schmidt-Thanhauser-Schneider technique (*44*). Plasma concentration of corticosterone was determined by the fluorometric method of Guillemin *et al.* (*20*).

Duncan's multiple range test as modified by Kramer (*30*) and Student's *t*-test were used for statistical analysis.

1. Plasma Concentration of Corticosterone during Pregnancy and Daily Fluctuation of the Concentration in the Rat

Kamoun and his coworkers (*24*, *25*, *28*) reported a marked increase in the plasma concentration of corticosterone taking place in the last 3 or 4 days of pregnancy. Kuhn (*31*), on the other hand, could not find any appreciable changes in the concentration of the hormone throughout the period before and after parturition. Absence of detectable changes in the concentration of plasma corticoid throughout pregnancy was also reported by Voogt *et al.* (*53*), although they obtained a very high level of plasma corticosterone on the day of parturition. These inconsistencies, together with the finding that the administration of corticoid failed to initiate milk secretion in pregnant rats (*10*), puzzle us and make it desirable to elucidate the role of adrenal steroids in the mechanism of lactogenesis.

Recently a considerable body of evidence on the circadian rhythmicity in pituitary-adrenal function has been accumulated (see *13* for review). Therefore, the discrepancies between the results decribed above on the plasma level of corticosterone may be due to the 24-hr fluctuations in concentrations.

Chronological changes in the concentration of plasma corticosterone throughout pregnancy and at parturition were re-examined with special reference to the 24-hr variation in steroid secretion. The content of prolactin in the anterior pituitary of animals killed on days 15, 19, 20, 21, and 22 of pregnancy was also determined using a microdensitometer after disc electrophoresis on polyacrylamide gels (*55*).

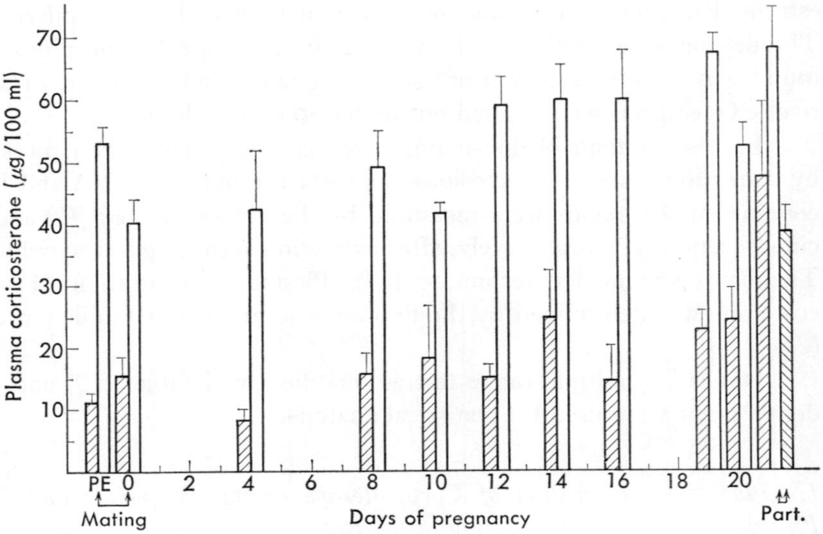

FIG. 1. Changes in plasma concentration of corticosterone in rats in proestrus and in pregnancy

▨ a.m. (10.00–10.30); □ p.m. (18.30–19.00), prepartum; ▧ p.m. (18.30–19.00), postpartum. Each bar represents the mean values obtained from 5 rats. Vertical line indicates ±SEM. PE, proestrus; Part., parturition. Ôta, Hosoe, Shimizu, and Yokoyama, unpublished data.

Blood samples were obtained by decapitation in the morning (10.00–10.30 hr) and evening (18.30–19.00 hr) of days 0, 4, 8, 10, 12, 14, 15, 16, 19, 20, 21, and 22 of pregnancy. Rats killed on day 0 of pregnancy had been housed with males on the morning of proestrous and separated at about 19.00 hr after checking the completion of mating. More than 80% of the mothers in our colony were found with newborn young on the morning of day 22 of pregnancy.

In order to minimize the disturbance to the animals before collection of blood samples, routine feeding, watering, and weighing were all omitted on the day of autopsy.

The plasma corticosterone levels (Fig. 1) in the morning remained low from the day of proestrus to day 20 of pregnancy. However, the level tended to increase slightly but progressively toward the end of pregnancy. A marked elevation of the plasma concentration was found on the morning of day 21 and the value was about two times higher than the morning levels of days 19 and 20. Evening levels of plasma corticosterone were significantly higher than morning levels except on day 21 of pregnancy and, contrary to the morning level, were maintained fairly consistently from day 0 to day 10 of pregnancy. A significant rise in the evening concentration was obtained on day 12 and the level was maintained throughout the remaining pregnancy period. The mean value of the corticoid concentration from day 12 to day 21 was significantly higher than that from day 0 to day 10. The present results on the morning levels of plasma corticosterone agree well with those of Kamoun *et al.* (*25*) and Koch (*28*), who reported a marked rise in the levels in the last 3 or 4 days of pregnancy. The findings on the evening levels of plasma corticosterone are well consistent with the report of Kuhn (*31*) who reported no appreciable change in the level near term. He also noted low corticosterone levels in two isolated morning samples. Therefore, discrepancies in the results of previous workers on the change in levels of plasma corticosterone in the rat during late pregnancy can be attributed to difference in the time of blood collection. Grota and Ader (*19*) reported the presence of a 24-hr periodicity of function of the adrenal gland in the pregnant rat which was essentially the same as that in non-pregnant cyclic animals (*14*, *57*). The present results demonstrate that the secretory activity of the adrenal cortex increases progressively during pregnancy, yet keeps its intrinsic circadian periodicity, until day 21 of pregnancy.

The mechanism by which evening levels of plasma corticosterone are maintained at high levels during the last half of pregnancy remains unclear. It is unlikely that fetal adrenal cortex contributes the increase, because the hypothalamo-pituitary-adrenal system in the fetal rat has been reported to begin functioning between the 17th and 18th day of intrauterine development (*8*, *15*, *34*; day 1 of pregnancy in these works corresponds to day 0 in our dating system). Barlow *et al.* (*5*), based on their observation of evening levels of plasma corticosterone in pregnant mice, suggested the possibility that the feto-placental unit provides the main secretory stimulus to the adrenal gland.

Both the content and concentration of prolactin in the pituitary gland of rats killed in the morning decreased significantly after day 19 of pregnancy (Fig. 2). The finding that the blood levels of pituitary prolactin in the rat in late pregnancy rises abruptly 2 or 3 days before parturition seems to coincide with the morning fall in pituitary prolactin content described above. On the other hand, no change in the evening level of pituitary prolactin, like plasma corticosterone levels, was observed. Circadian rhythmicity of plasma prolactin levels was reported in the pseudopregnant

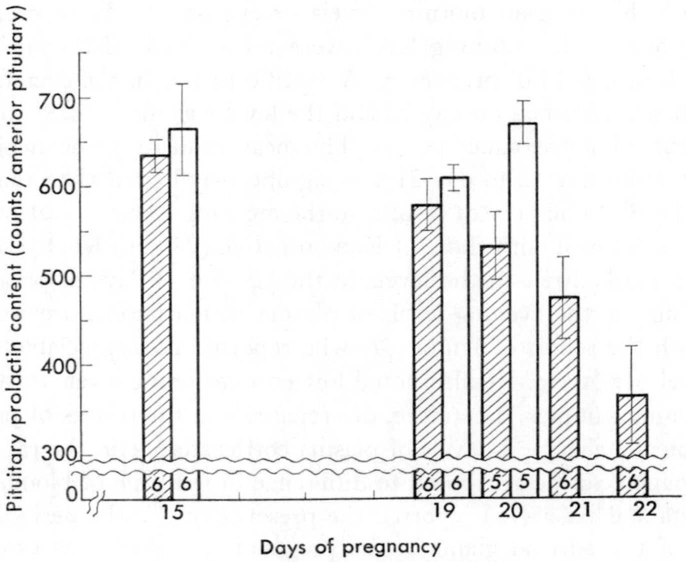

FIG. 2. Changes in the pituitary content of prolactin in rats in late pregnancy Hatched and open bars represent the mean values for rats killed in the morning or evening of a given day of pregnancy, respectively. Vertical lines indicate ± SEM. The number of rats in each group is shown at the bottom of the bar. From Ref. *41*.

rat (*17*, *18*, *33*). Smith and Neill (*48*) revealed that the rhythm in the hormone secretion in the first half of pregnancy disappeared in the mid-pregnancy. Our data on the pituitary content of prolactin seem to be consistent with this finding except for those on day 20.

Animals killed on the morning of day 22 of pregnancy were divided in 5 groups according to the stage of parturition, determined visually at the time of autopsy (Table I). The concentration of plasma corticosterone was depleted to its lowest value during delivery. The depletion began with the relaxation of symphysis pubis and the value reached a nadir in a group of rats in which parturition was still in progress (Table I, Group 3). The depletion in the plasma corticosterone level during the course of delivery is very difficult to explain, since the labor pains are thought to be a stress to the mother. Voogt *et al.* (*53*), and Arishima *et al.* (*4*) reported an increase in plasma corticosterone during delivery. At present no explanation is available for the difference in the corticoid level between ours and other workers. More detailed studies are required.

Both the content and concentration of prolactin in the pituitary gland

TABLE I. Concentrations of Plasma Corticosterone and Prolactin Content of the Anterior Pituitary of Rats on the Day of Parturition (Ôta, Ôta, and Yokoyama, 1974)

Group	Stage of parturition	Rat No.	Plasma corticosterone (μg/100 ml plasma)		Pituitary prolactin: Content (counts/AP[a])		Pituitary prolactin: Concentration (counts/mg AP[a])	
1	Relaxation of pubic symphysis, without bleeding	48	52.2	(42.6)[b]	549	(489.0)	93.0	(71.4)
		5-H	32.9		429		49.8	
2	Relaxation of pubic symphysis, with bleeding	1-T	47.6	(25.4)	711	(682.0)	84.6	(79.6)
		4-T	14.1		603		75.5	
		6-H	14.5		732		78.6	
3	During delivery of young	5	8.3	(11.8)	537	(514.5)	68.7	(65.4)
		30	15.3		492		62.1	
4	Post partum, not suckled	31	33.6	(22.6)	405	(361.5)	57.0	(47.9)
		44	11.5		318		38.7	
5	Post partum, suckled	32	24.2	(31.8)	408	(372.8)	45.3	(42.4)
		36	26.9		198		22.2	
		45	53.0		579		70.5	
		49	23.0		306		31.5	
	Day 21 of pregnancy	(6)[c]	39.9±4.1[d]		477.9±44.4		58.2±3.9	

Collection of blood and pituitary samples was performed at 10.00–10.30 hr on day 22 of pregnancy. The results of pituitary prolactin were expressed as the number of count of microdensitometer.

[a] Anterior pituitary.

[b] Mean.

[c] No. of rats used.

[d] Mean±SEM.

were as high as on day 19 of pregnancy in rats in which the delivery of young had not begun or was in progress (Groups 1–3 in Table I). In the post parturient rats (Groups 4 and 5) pituitary prolactin content and concentration were very low, except for one rat in Group 5, and the values were lower than at any other stages of pregnancy examined. These findings suggest the occurrence of a surge in prolactin secretion around the time of parturition and seem to agree with the findings of Nagasawa and Yanai (*38*) who reported an abrupt rise of circulating levels of prolactin just before parturition.

The observed increase in both prolactin and corticosterone secretion might be provoked by the change in the secretory pattern of gonadal steroids occurring around day 19 of pregnancy (*35*, *54*, *56* for progesterone).

However, it must be noted that no appreciable changes were found in the evening levels of either pituitary prolactin or plasma corticosterone.

The results on plasma levels of corticosterone seem to indicate that corticosterone is unlikely to be a lactogenic trigger in the rat.

2. Induction of Lactose Synthesis in the Mammary Glands of Pregnant and Pseudopregnant Rats by Ovariectomy

Shinde *et al.* (*46*) reported that the removal of the ovaries at the end of pregnancy could result in a marked increase in the lactose content about 40 hr after the operation. It has been reported that alveoli appear at about the middle of the pregnancy period in the rat and that explants from the mammary gland of mid-pregnanty mice cultured with suitable hormonal combinations can synthesize milk proteins (see *16* for review). Therefore, it is reasonable to consider that the mammary glands of mid-pregnancy are competent to synthesize milk in response to ovariectomy. The following experiments were designed to determine the stage of pregnancy at which mammary glands were able to initiate lactose synthesis in response to ovariectomy.

Ovariectomy was carried out between 17.30 and 18.00 hr on days 8, 10, 12, 14, 16, 18, 19, and 20 of pregnancy and the animal were killed by decapitation about 40 hr after ovariectomy. A sham operation was performed at some stages of pregnancy. Intact pregnant rats were killed at appropriate intervals after day 8 of pregnancy. Trunk blood was collected into a heparinized glass tube for corticosterone determination.

A small amount of lactose appeared first on day 10 of pregnancy in all rats ovariectomized on day 8. Lactose contents in the mammary gland of ovariectomized pregnant rats increased almost linearly thereafter to day 16 of pregnancy, then the level was maintained until the end of pregnancy (Fig. 3c). In the intact pregnant rats, lactose could be detected first on day 21 of pregnancy, as was reported by Shinde *et al.* (*46*).

The total DNA content of the 6 posterior mammary glands of the intact and ovariectomized rats increased linearly from days 8 to 20 of pregnancy, and the DNA content of the mammary glands in the rats killed 40 hr after ovariectomy was always higher than that in the normal pregnant rat killed on the equivalent day of pregnancy. The increase during the 40 hr after ovariectomy was very similar in the various stages of pregnancy (Fig. 3a). Therefore, lactose content/mg DNA increased from days 10 to 16 of pregnancy and declined slightly towards the end of pregnancy (Fig. 3c).

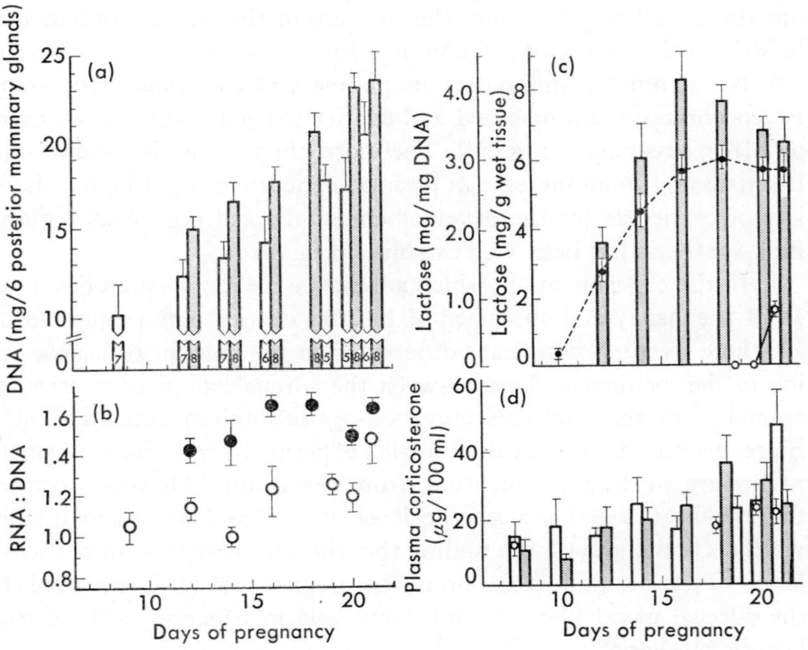

FIG. 3. Changes in nucleic acid and lactose contents of mammary glands and plasma corticosterone concentration during the course of pregnancy in normal and ovariectomized (ovx) (40 hr) rats

(a) and (d), open bars, normal; hatched bars, ovx; ○, sham-ovx in (d) only. (b), ○, normal; ●, ovx (c), ○, normal and ●, ovx (mg lactose/g wet tissue); hatched bars, ovx and open bar, normal (mg lactose/mg DNA). Vertical lines indicate ± SEM. Figures at the bottom of the bars in (a) show the number of rats used for mammary gland analysis; in (d) 8 sham-ovx, 8 ovx, and 5 normal rats were used in each group. From Ref. *46*.

The ratio of RNA to DNA in ovariectomized rats was fairly constant throughout the experimental period and it was comparable to that observed on day 21 of normal pregnancy when lactose was first detected (Fig. 3b).

It is likely, therefore, that the lactose was formed not only by the cells newly formed after ovariectomy but also by cells existing before. These findings are interesting in relation to the *in vitro* experiments using the mammary glands of the pregnant mouse, which have demonstrated that only the newly formed daughter cells are able to synthesize milk (see *49* for review). Since the RNA: DNA ratio was fairy consistent throughout the experimental period, the increase in the lactose content may not be due to the increased activity of a single cell.

No significant differences in plasma corticosterone were found between normal, sham-operated and ovariectomized pregnant rats except on day 18 of pregnancy (Fig. 3d). Therefore, the increase in lactose could not be attributed to an increase in plasma corticosteroids, although the necessity of corticoids for the development of the cell organelles required for milk synthesis has been well established *in vitro* (*35*).

In the experiments in which adrenals were removed on day 10 or day 14 of pregnancy and autopsied 40 hr after ovariectomy performed on day 14, there were no significant differences in the amount of lactose appearing in the mammary gland between the adrenalectomized-ovariectomized animals and sham adrenelectomized-ovariectomized animals (Table II). Since the number of rats used in this experiment was still very small, it is premature to draw a conclusion from the results. However, considering these results, together with the level of corticoid described in the previous section and with the finding that the administration of corticosteroid failed to initiate milk secretion in the pregnant rat (*10*), it is unlikely that the adrenal gland plays an important role in triggering the initiation of lactose synthesis.

It has been well known that the rat placenta secretes lactogenic hormone and that the secretion of placental lactogen begins around day 10 of pregnancy (*26*). Pregnancy is maintained if the pituitary is removed after day 12 of pregnancy but not before day 12. Therefore, it is very in-

TABLE II. Effect of Adrenalectomy on Lactose Contents of the Mammary Glands in the Pregnant Rat Killed 40 hr after Ovariectomy (Yokoyama and Ôta, unpublished data)

Operation[a] (day of pregnancy)	Lactose mg/g wet tissue[b]	Mean±SEM	
Sham 10+ovx 14	4.19		
	2.98		
Sham 14+ovx 14	5.43	4.47±0.56	
	5.26		
adx 10+ovx 14	2.95		N.S.
	4.53	3.25±0.42	
	3.59		
adx 14+ovx 14	3.25		

[a] ovx: ovariectomy, adx: adrenalectomy; operation was performed on the evening (between 17.00–18.00 hr) and animals were killed about 40 hr after ovariectomy.
[b] Values obtained from the individual animal. N.S.: not significant.

TABLE III. Effect of Ovariectomy on Lactose Contents of the Mammary Gland in Pregnant and Pseudopregnant Rats (Ôta, Horiba, Shani, and Yokoyama, unpublished data)

Animals	No. of animals	Operation	Day of autopsy	Lactose: No. of rats with significan amount of lactose	Lactose: Mean±SEM (mg/mg DNA)
Pregnant	3	Sham	14	0	—
	3	ovx	14	3	2.12±0.38
	5	Sham	18	0	—
	5	ovx	18	5	5.36±0.45
Pseudo-pregnant	2	Sham	14	1	0.25
	3	ovx	14	2	0.20
	5	Sham	18	2	0.035
	6	ovx	18	4	0.15±0.02

Operation was performed about 40 hr before the time of autopsy (09.30–10.00 hr).

teresting to note that the appearance of an appreciable amount of lactose on day 12 of pregnancy coincides very well with beginning of the secretion of placental lactogen. In our colony of rats, pseudopregnancy usually lasts for about 13–14 days and if we remove the uterus on day 7 of pseudopregnancy it can be prolonged up to 17 days. Therefore, the hysterectomized pseudopregnant rat seems to be a good tool for assessing the biological role of placental lactogen in the initiation of lactose synthesis in response to ovariectomy in the pregnant rat.

Ovaries were removed on days 12 and 16 of pseudopregnancy. The animals were decapitated 40 hr after ovariectomy. Contrary to the pregnant rats, a small amount of lactose appeared in about half of the sham-operated pseudopregnant rats irrespective of the day of autopsy. Ovariectomy performed on days 12 and 16 could not stimulate lactose synthesis in the mammary gland in the pseudopregnant rats to the same extent seen in the pregnant rats. Lactose could be detected in the mammary gland in 2/3 of the animals in this group. The amount was much less in the pseudopregnant than in the pregnant rat, similar to that obtained in the sham-operated pseudopregnant (PSP) animals (Table III).

No increase in the DNA content of the mammary gland was induced by ovariectomy in the pseudopregnant animals (Fig. 4a). The content of DNA in the mammary glands of the sham-operated pseudopregnant rats slightly decreased on day 18, while the content in the ovariectomized

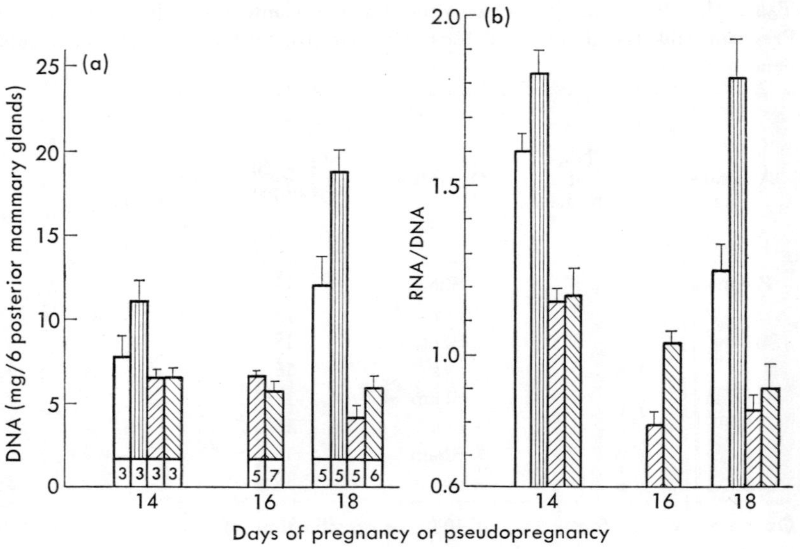

FIG. 4. Nucleic acid contents and RNA/DNA ratio of mammary glands of ovariectomized pregnant (ovx) or ovariectomized-hysterectomized pseudopregnant (ovx-hystx) rats

▧ sham-operated pregnancy; ▥ ovx. pregnancy; ▨ sham-operated pseudopregnancy; □ ovx-hystx pseudopregnancy. Values are means ± SEM. Figures at the bottom of bars indicate the number of rats used. Animals were operated on about 40 hr before autopsy. Ôta, Horiba, Shani, and Yokoyama, unpublished data.

group was similar to that obtained on days 14 and 16 in both the ovariectomized and the sham-operated rats. Therefore, on day 18 the DNA content seemed to increase after ovariectomy, although no significant difference was found between these two values. Since estrous smears appeared in some animals on day 18, the obtained decrease in the DNA reflects an involutionary change of the mammary gland which might be ascribed to a rise in circulatory estrogen.

The RNA: DNA ratio obtained in the ovariectomized pseudopregnant rats killed on days 14 and 18 was not different from that in the corresponding sham-operated animals (Fig. 4b). The discrepancy in the value of the RNA: DNA ratio between this series of experiments and the series described previously cannot be explained. However, the ratio in the ovariectomized pregnant rats, in this as well as in the previous series, was siginificantly higher than those in the sham-operated rats.

The DNA content in the sham-operated pregnant rats on day 14 was not different from that in rats killed on the equivalent day of pseudopregnancy, as shown in Fig. 4a. Although these findings are inconsistent with that obtained by Anderson and Turner (*3*, see *2* for review), who reported that the DNA content was higher in pregnant rats than in the pseudopregnant, the findings may indicate that the hormonal environment for the development of the mammary gland in the pregnant rat was similar to the hysterectomized pseudopregnant rat during at least the first 12–14 days. In fact, Pepe and Rothchild (*42*) reported that progesterone concentration in the peripheral blood of hysterectomized pseudopregnant rats was not significantly different from that obtained on a comparable day of pregnancy. Moreover, these findings on the DNA content are somewhat strange in view of the well-known mammogenic activity of the placenta in the rat; Kelly *et al.* (*26*) used the radioreceptor assay and reported that one of two peaks in mammaotrophin obtained during the pregnancy period was found between days 12 and 13.

The increase in the DNA content and the appearance of a large amount of lactose obtained from the mammary glands of pregnant animals after ovariectomy should be ascribed to the mammogenic and lactogenic activity of the placenta, respectively. These activities of the placenta at the end of pregnancy were reported by Nagasawa and Yanai (*37*, *39*). The present results also suggest that progesterone might hold in check not only the initiation of the synthetic activity of the mammary gland in response to the lactogenic activity of the placenta, but also the growth of the mammary gland in response to the placental mammogenic activity. This suggestion agrees well with that proposed by Kuhn (*31*) for explaining the sudden increase in lactose after ovariectomy in pregnant rats.

The difference in the response of the mammary gland to ovariectomy between the pregnant and pseudopregnant rats could be discussed from several view points: the presence or absence of lactogenic activity of the placenta, the difference in the responsiveness of the mammary gland, the difference in the secretory pattern of the lactogenic hormone complex after ovariectomy and the possible combinations of these possibilities.

Prolactin and adrenocorticotropic hormone (ACTH) or adrenal corticoids are essential components of the lactogenic hormone complex in the rat (see *9*, *50* for review). If prolactin and adrenal corticoids are administered in large amounts, they can be expected to nullify the possible difference in the hormone level between the pregnant and the pseudopregnant rats which may occur after ovariectomy. Therefore, the responsiveness of the mammary gland to the lactogenic hormone was compared between pseudopregnant and pregnant rats treated with a large amount of prolactin and corticoid. In order to make the endogenous hormone levels uniform, adrenals and uterus with fetuses or with decidual tissue were also removed at the time of ovariectomy. Ovaries were removed on the evening of day 12 of pregnancy or pseudopregnancy. The deciduoma was induced in both horns by scratching the antimesometrial site of the uterus on day 5 of pseudopregnancy. Animals subjected to ovariectomy, adrenalectomy, and hysterectomy (triply-operated animals) were injected subcutaneously with prolactin (0.5 mg NIH-P-S 11 in 0.1 ml saline) and cortisone acetate (1 mg Corton, Merck-Banyu, suspended in 0.1 ml distilled water). Ovariectomized rats and sham-operated rats were injected with saline. The injections were started immediately after the operation and repeated in the morning (around 09.00 hr) and afternoon (around 18.00 hr) on the day following the operation. Animals were decapitated about 40 hr after the operation. A preliminary experiment revealed that the content of lactose obtained in the triply-operated animals killed 40 hr after the operation was higher than that from animals killed 72 hr after the operation, notwithstanding the fact that the latter animals received twice as much hormones after the operation.

The results of the contents of lactose and DNA in the 6 posterior mammary glands in ovariectomized pregnant and pseudopregnant rats treated with saline agreed well with those obtained in animals without saline treatment described in the previous section (Fig. 4).

In all mammary glands of the triply-operated pseudopregnant rats a considerable amount of lactose was detected after the hormone teatment, although the amount was significantly lower than that obtained in similarly treated or sham operated-saline treated pregnant rats.

No increase in DNA content was obtained after the administration of hormones to the triply-operated pseudopregnant animals, and the amount was significantly less than that in similarly treated pregnant rats.

These results clearly indicate that the alveolar cells of the mammary gland in the pseudopregnant rat are competent to synthesize lactose if a sufficient amount of the lactogenic hormone complex is provided. Therefore, the findings that almost no synthetic response could be detected after ovariectomy in the pseudopregnant animals might be attributed either to an insufficient level of the lactogenic hormone complex in the circulation or to a low sensitivity of the alveolar cells to the horomone complex. An insufficiency of the hormone level is unlikely because a large amount of

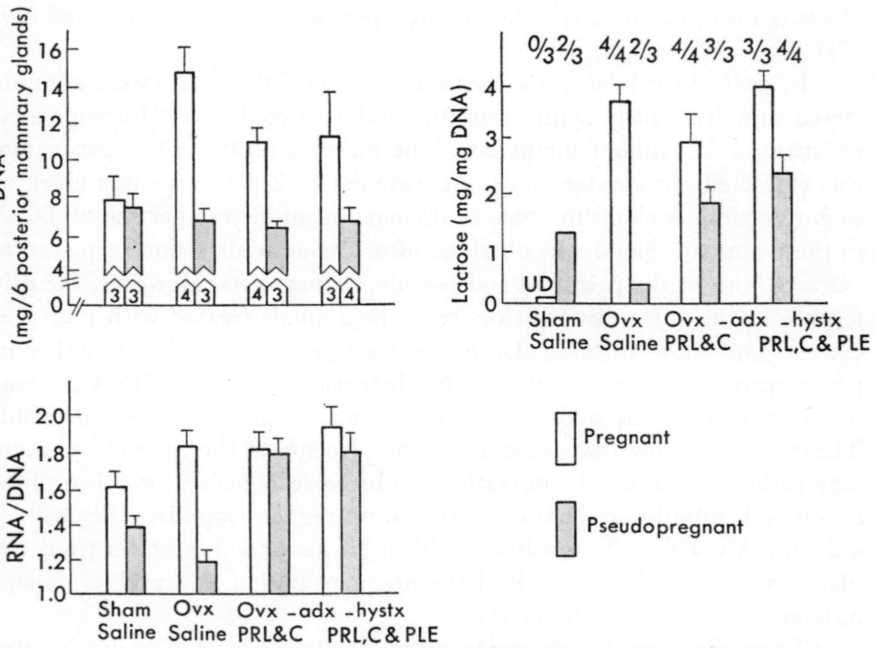

FIG. 5. Nucleic acid and lactose contents of mammary glands in ovariectomized (ovx) or ovariectomized, adrenalectomized and hysterectomized (ovx-adx-hystx) pregnant and pseudopregnant rats

Open bars, pregnant; hatched bars, pseudopregnant; PRL, prolactin; C, cortisone acetate; PLE, placental extracts; UD, undetectable. Figures at the bottom of bars and the top of the bars indicate the number of rats used and the number of rats showing positive lactose synthesis per number of rats used, respectively. Values are means ± SEM. Values of lactose for ovx-saline and sham-saline in pseudopregnant rats represent the average of two rats showing positive lactose synthesis. Ôta, Sakamoto, and Yokoyama, unpublished data.

hormones was administered exogenously. The only difference found between the pregnant and pseudopregnant rats in the present experimental conditions is the presence of placentae and fetuses at the time of operation in the pregnant rat. Therefore, it can be assumed that the placenta might play a role in rendering the alveolar cells sensitive to prolactin and other lactogenic hormones and thus the placenta might be indispensable for inducing proliferation of the alveolar cells and lactose synthesis. Oka and Topper (*40*) demonstrated, by using the mouse mammary gland, that prolactin treatment *in vivo* enabled the alveolar cells to respond to insulin and caused proliferation *in vitro*. Lactogenic-mammotrophic activity of the rat placenta measured by a specific radioreceptor assay has been reported (*26*, *27*).

In order to validate this assumption, placental extracts were administered simultaneously with prolactin and corticoids to triply-operated pregnant and pseudopregnant rats. The placenta on day 12 of pregnancy was extracted with water and the equivalent of 2 placentae was given at each injection. A slight increase in the amount of lactose per mg of DNA in the mammary gland was obtained after the administration of placental extracts both in the pregnant and pseudopregnant rats. However, the difference in the value obtained between the animals treated with placental extracts and those without placental extracts was not significant either in pregnant or pseudopregnant rats. No increase in the total DNA content was obtained by the addition of the extract to prolactin and corticoid. These results imply that presence of the placenta at the time of ovariectomy rather than after the operation might be responsible for cell proliferation and initiation of lactose synthesis in pregnant rats. In other words, only the alveolar cells sensitized with a hormone or hormones from the placenta, even in the first half of the pregnant period, can proliferate and differentiate to synthesize lactose.

There are some discrepancies in the circulating level of prolactin after ovariectomy in the pregnant rat. Vermouth and Deis (*52*) reported a rapid rise in serum prolactin levels after ovariectomy performed on day 19 of pregnancy. On the other hand, no increase of prolactin levels was reported by Bridges and Goldman (*6*) and Simpson *et al.* (*47*). Although no information concerning the blood level of prolactin was available in the present experiment, the finding presented here that the amount of lactose per cell did not increase after the administration of prolactin and corticoid may lead us to support the conception that changes in the plasma level of prolactin and corticoid do not constitute a lactogenic signal (*31*).

Since corticoid and prolactin may not be considered as triggers for initiation of lactose synthesis as described in this paper, the role of the placenta in providing receptors to the lactogenic hormone complex deserves much consideration. In this connection, it is very interesting to note that prolactin appeared to have an important effect in increasing prolactin binding sites in the rat liver (*43*). Withdrawal of progesterone seems to further enhance the formation of receptors in the alveolar cells of the mammary gland, as was suggested by Kohmoto (*29*).

Acknowledgments

Work reported in this paper was supported in part by research grants from the Ministry of Education, Science and Culture of Japan (Nos. 836021, 111509, 210709, and 156179). We are grateful to R. Ogawa for animal care and Yôko Niwa for secretarial assistance. We are indebted to the National Institute of Arthritis, Metabolism and Digestive Diseases, Bethesda, Maryland, USA, for gifts of bovine prolactin.

REFERENCES

1. Amenomori, Y., Chen, C. L., and Meites, J. (1970). Serum prolactin levels in rats during different reproductive states. *Endocrinology* **86**, 506–510.
2. Anderson, R. R. (1974). Development and structure of the mammary gland. Endocrinological control. In *Lactation: A Comprehensive Treatise*, vol. 1, ed. Larson, B. L. and Smith, V. R., pp. 97–140. New York: Academic Press.
3. Anderson, R. R. and Turner, C. W. (1968). Mammary gland growth during pseudopregnancy and pregnancy in the rat. *Proc. Soc. Exp. Biol. Med.* **131**, 167–171.
4. Arishima, K., Nakama, S., Morikawa, Y., Hashimoto, Y., and Eguchi, Y. (1977). Maternal-foetal interrelations of plasma corticosterone concentrations at the end of gestation in the rat. *J. Endocrinol.* **72**, 239–240.
5. Barlow, S. M., Morrison, P. J., and Sullivan, F. M. (1974). Plasma corticosterone levels during pregnancy in the mouse: The relative contributions of the adrenal glands and foeto-placental units. *J. Endocrinol.* **60**, 473–483.
6. Bridges, R. S. and Goldman, B. D. (1975). Ovarian control of prolactin secretion during late pregnancy in the rat. *Endocrinology* **97**, 496–498.
7. Ceriotti, G. (1955). Determination of nucleic acids in animal tissues. *J. Biol. Chem.* **214**, 59–70.
8. Cohen, A. (1963). Corrélations entre l'hypophyse et le cortex surrénal du nouveau-né. *Arch. Anat. Micr. Morph. Exp.* (*Paris*) **52**, 277–407.
9. Cowie, A. T. and Tindal, J. S. (1971). *The Physiology of Lactation*, Monogr. Physiol. Soc. No. 22. London: Edward Arnold.
10. Davis, J. W. and Liu, T.M.Y. (1969). The adrenal gland and lactogenesis. *Endocrinology* **85**, 155–160.
11. Denamur, R. (1971). Reviews of the progress of dairy science. Section A. Physiology: Hormonal control of lactogenesis. *J. Dairy Res.* **38**, 237–264.
12. Dische, Z. and Schwarz, K. (1937). Microchemical methods for determining various pentoses in the presence of one another and of hexoses. *Microchim. Acta* **2**, 13–19: Cited from Watanabe, K. and Miura, K. (1957). In *Zikken Kagaku Koza*, vol. 23, Biochemistry I, ed. Japan. Soc. Chem. Chap. 2, pp. 243–331. Tokyo: Maruzen (in Japanese).
13. Dunn, J. D. (1974). Circadian variation in aderenocortical and anterior pi-

tuitary hormones. In *Biological Rhythms in Neuroendocrine Activity*, ed. M. Kawakami, pp. 119–139. Tokyo: Igaku Shoin.

14. Dunn, J., Scheving, L., and Millet, P. (1972). Circadian variation in stress-evoked increases in plasma corticosterone. *Am. J. Physiol.* **222**, 402–406.
15. Eguchi, Y., Harai, O., Morikawa, Y., and Hashimoto, Y. (1973). Critical time in the hypothalamic control of the pituitary-adrenal system in fetal rats: Observations in fetuses subjected to hypervitaminosis A and hypothalamic destruction. *Endocrinology* **93**, 1–11.
16. Forsyth, I. A. (1971). Reviews of the progress of dairy science. Section A. Physiology: Organ culture techniques and the study of hormone effects on the mammary gland. *J. Dairy Res.* **38**, 419–445.
17. Freeman, M. E. and Neill, J. D. (1972). The pattern of prolactin secretion during pseudopregnancy in the rat: A daily nocturnal surge. *Endocrinology* **90**, 1292–1294.
18. Greef, W., Dullaart, J., and Zeilmaker, G. H. (1975). Serum luteinizing hormone, follicle-stimulating hormone, prolactin and progesterone concentrations and follicular development in the pseudopregnant rat after unilateral ovariectomy. *J. Endocrinol.* **66**, 249–256.
19. Grota, L. J. and Ader, R. (1970). Adrenocortical function in pregnant rats: Handling and the 24-hour rhythm. *Physiol. Behav.* **5**, 739–741.
20. Guillemin, R., Clayton, G. W., Lipscomb, H. S., and Smith, J. D. (1959). Fluorometric measurement of rat plasma and adrenal corticosterone concentration. *J. Lab. Clin. Med.* **53**, 830–832.
21. Halban, J. C. (1905). Die innere Sekretion von Ovarium und Placenta und ihre Bedeutung für die Funktion der Milchdrüse. *Arch. Gynäkol.* **75**, 353–441.
22. Hammond, J. (1917). On the causes responsible for the developmental progress of the mammary glands in the rabbit during the latter part of pregnancy. *Proc. Roy. Soc., Ser. B* **89**, 534–545.
23. Holcomb, H. H., Costlow, M. E., Buschow, R. A., and McGuire, W. L. (1975). Alterations in prolactin binding to rat mammary gland during pregnancy and lactation. *Clin. Res.* **23**, 552A.
24. Kamoun, A. (1970). Activité cortico-surrénale au cours de la gestation, de la lactation et du développement pré et post-natal chez le rat. I. Concentration et cinétique de disparition de la corticostérone. *J. Physiol. (Paris)* **62**, 5–32.
25. Kamoun, A., Mialhe-Voloss, C., and Stutinsky, F. (1965). Etude de l'activité surrénalienne au cours de la gestation chez la ratte. *C. R. Séancs. Soc. Biol.* **159**, 469–472.
26. Kelly, P. A., Shiu, R.P.C., Robertson, M. C., and Friesen, H. G. (1975). Characterization of rat chorionic mammotropin. *Endocrinology* **96**, 1187–1195.
27. Kelly, P. A., Tsushima, T., Shiu, R.P.C., and Friesen, H. G. (1976). Lacto-

genic and growth hormone-like activities in pregnancy determined by radioreceptor assays. *Endocrinology* **99**, 765–774.

28. Koch, B. (1969). Liaisons de la corticostérone au protéines plasmatiques et régulation du niveau du stéroide libre au cours de la gestation et la lactation chez la ratte. *Horm. Metab. Res.* **1**, 129–135.
29. Kohmoto, K. and Sakai, S. (1978). Prolactin receptors in the mammary gland. This volume, pp. 231-248.
30. Kramer, C. Y. (1956). Extension of multiple range tests to group means with unequal numbers of replications. *Biometrics* **12**, 307–310.
31. Kuhn, N. J. (1969). Progesterone withdrawal as the lactogenic trigger in the rat. *J. Endocrinol.* **44**, 39–54.
32. Linkie, D. M. and Niswender, G. D. (1972). Serum levels of prolactin, luteinizing hormone, and follicle stimulating hormone during pregnancy in the rat. *Endocrinology* **90**, 632–637.
33. McLean, B. K. and Nikitovitch-Winer, M. B. (1975). Cholinergic control of the nocturnal prolactin surge in the pseudopregnant rat. *Endocrinology* **97** 763–770.
34. Milkovic, S., Milkovic, K., and Paunovic, J. (1973). The initiation of fetal adrenocorticotropic activity in the rat. *Endocrinology* **92**, 380–384.
35. Mills, E. S. and Topper, Y. J. (1970). Some ultrastructural effects of insulin, hydrocortisone, and prolactin on mammary gland explants. *J. Cell Biol.* **44**, 310–328.
36. Morishige, W. K., Pepe, G. J., and Rothchild, I. (1973). Serum luteinizing hormone, prolactin and progesterone levels during pregnancy in the rat. *Endocrinology* **92**, 1527–1530.
37. Nagasawa, H. and Yanai, R. (1971). Quantitative participation of placental mammotropic hormones in mammary development during pregnancy in mice. *Endocrinol. Japon.* **18**, 507–510.
38. Nagasawa, H. and Yanai, R. (1972). Changes in serum prolactin levels shortly before and after parturition in rats. *Endocrinol. Japon.* **19**, 139–143.
39. Nagasawa, H. and Yanai, R. (1973). Effects of adrenalectomy and/or deficiency of pituitary prolactin secretion on initiation and maintenance of lactation in mice. *J. Endocrinol.* **58**, 67–73.
40. Oka, T. and Topper, Y. J. (1972). Is prolactin mitogenic for mammary epithelium? *Proc. Natl. Acad. Sci. U.S.* **69**, 1693–1696.
41. Ôta, K., Ôta, T., and Yokoyama, A. (1974). Plasma corticosterone concentrations and pituitary prolactin content in late pregnancy and their withinday fluctuations in the rat. *J. Endocrinol.* **61**, 21–28.
42. Pepe, G. J. and Rothchild, I. (1974). A comparative study of serum progesterone levels in pregnancy and in various types of pseudopregnancy in the rat. *Endocrinology* **95**, 275.
43. Posner, B. I., Kelly, P. A., and Friesen, H. G. (1975). Prolactin recep-

tors in rat liver: Possible induction by prolactin. *Science* **188**, 57–59.

44. Schneider, W. C. (1946). Phosphorus compounds in animal tissue. III. A comparison of methods for the estimation of nucleic acids. *J. Biol. Chem.* **164**, 747–751.
45. Shani, J., Ôta, K., Tomogane, H., and Yokoyama, A. (1977). Induction of lactose synthesis in the mammary glands of pregnant rats by ovariectomy. *J. Endocrinol.* **72**, 103–104.
46. Shinde, Y., Ôta, K., and Yokoyama, A. (1965). Lactose content of mammary glands of pregnant rats near term: Effect of removal of ovary, placenta and foetus. *J. Endocrinol.* **31**, 105–114.
47. Simpson, A. A., Simpson, M.H.W., and Kulkarni, P. N. (1973). Prolactin production and lactogenesis in rats after ovariectomy in late pregnancy. *J. Endocrinol.* **57**, 426–429.
48. Smith, M. S. and Neill, J. D. (1976). Termination of the two daily surges of plasma prolactin initiated by mating in the rat. *Endocrinology* **98**, 696–701.
49. Topper, Y. J. (1970). Multiple hormone interactions in the development of mammary gland *in vitro*. *Rec. Prog. Horm. Res.* **26**, 287–308.
50. Tucker, H. A. (1974). Development and maintenance of lactogenesis. General endocrinological control of lactation. In *Lactation, A Comprehensive Treatise*, vol. 1, ed. Larson, B. L. and Smith, V. R., pp. 277–326. New York: Academic Press.
51. Turkington, R. W. and Hill, R. L. (1969). Lactose synthetase: Progesterone inhibition of the induction of α-lactalbumin. *Science* **163**, 1458–1460.
52. Vermouth, N. T. and Deis, R. P. (1974). Prolactin release and lactogenesis after ovariectomy in pregnant rats: Effect of ovarian hormones. *J. Endocrinol.* **63**, 13–20.
53. Voogt, J. L., Sar, M., and Meites, J. (1969). Influence of cycling, pregnancy, labor and suckling on corticosterone-ACTH levels. *Am. J. Physiol.* **216**, 655–659.
54. Wiest, W. G. (1970). Progesterone and 20α-hydroxypregn-4-en-3-one in plasma, ovaries and uteri during pregnancy in the rat. *Endocrinology* **87**, 43–48.
55. Yokoyama, A., Tomogane, H., and Ôta, K. (1971). Effect of ovariectomy and of oestrogen administration on the decrease in pituitary prolactin content which occurs on the afternoon of pro-oestrus in the rat. *Experientia* **27**, 1221–1222.
56. Yoshinaga, K., Hawkins, R. A., and Stocker, J. F. (1969). Estrogen secretion by the rat ovary *in vivo* during the estrous cycle and pregnancy. *Endocrinology* **85**, 103–112.
57. Zimmermann, E. and Critchlow, V. (1967). Effects of diurnal variation in plasma corticosterone levels on adrenocortical response to stress. *Proc. Soc. Exp. Biol. Med.* **125**, 658–663.

II – 6

EFFECTS OF CONCURRENT PREGNANCY AND CONTINUOUS SUCKLING ON TWO CONSECUTIVE LACTATIONS

Hideo MIZUNO and Naoto SENSUI*

*Faculty of Agriculture, Shizuoka University, Shizuoka, Japan and College of Agriculture and Veterinary Medicine, Nihon University, Tokyo, Japan**

Various changes in the mammary gland occur in regular sequence throughout pregnancy, parturition, lactation, and postweaning periods in many species of mammals and the sequential hormone control on them has been extensively studied. In dairy cows, however, the lactation period usually advances simultaneously with the next pregnancy. Although concurrent pregnancy does not appear have an effect on lactation during earlier months of gestation, there is a marked inhibitory effect on the milk yield during the latter part of gestation. The mechanism by which pregnancy counteracts milk production has not been completely determined. Furthermore, it has been widely recognized that a non-milking period of appropriate length (dry period) is normally essential for attainment of optimum lactation after the next parturition. The physiological reason why such a dry period is necessary remains to be determined. In this connection, it is interesting that prepartum milking on subsequent lactation has been advocated for its favorable effects (see Chapter II-9).

Concurrent pregnant-lactation can also be established by mating at postpartum estrus in rats and mice. Many studies have been carried out on the effects of lactation on reproduction (*2*, *6*, *13*, *22*, *36–40*, *42*). On the other hand, there seems to be relatively small number of studies on the effects of concurrent pregnancy on the physiology of the mammary glands and also on the effects of suckling on subsequent lactation in these animals (*4*, *14–16*, *20*, *21*, *30*).

This paper describes the effects of concurrent pregnancy and suckling on the changes in mammary function in mice at the transitional stages from the regression of the preceeding lactation to the initiation of the subsequent lactation.

1. Concurrent Pregnancy and Lactation

Mice of the dd strain which had been bred in our laboratory were used. Primiparous pregnant mice were kept in individual cages. To establish concurrent lactating pregnancy, males cohabited with females from a few days before the expected date of parturition. Births were checked at 9.00 a.m. every morning and the day when a litter was found was designated as day 1 of lactation, *i.e.*, the day following delivery. Males were removed and the litter size was adjusted to 6 pups on day 1 of lactation. Each lactating non-pregnant group and lactating pregnant group was divided into 2 groups; the naturally-weaning group and the continuously suckled group. In the former group, original litters were not weaned forcedly to avoid abrupt mammary involution and cohabited with the mothers throughout the lactation period. In the latter group, original litters were replaced on day 14 of lactation with foster litters consisting of six 5-day-old pups. In some groups in the first experiment, foster litters of six 10-day-old pups were used. They became almost independent of mother's milk after day 22 of lactation and the weight gains of litters consisting of pups more than 18 days old could not be used as a reliable index of lactational performance.

1) Experiment 1

The delay in implantation of embryos has been well studied in concurrently lactating pregnant mice and rats (*6*, *22*, *40*, *42*). The length of concurrent pregnancy was examined in other groups of mothers, being 28.5 ± 0.7 days in the lactating pregnant period in the original litter group and 28.6 ± 1.1 days in those with replaced litter groups, ranging from 22 to 31 days, respectively. However, the mothers were killed on days 18, 22, and 26 of lactation irrespective of day of concurrent pregnancy; the mothers which had given birth were excluded from this experiment.

The concurrently lactating pregnant mother tended to be superior in lactational performance to the lactating non-pregnant mother until day 22 of lactation. However, between day 22 and day 26 the average litter gain in the lactating pregnant group was almost completely inhibited

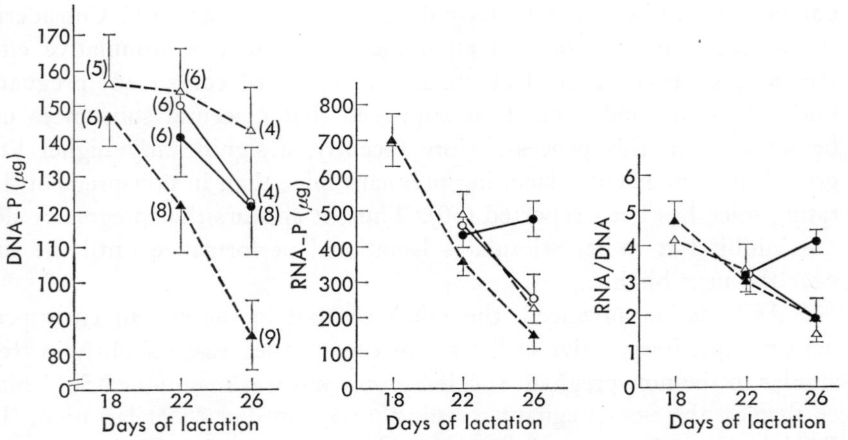

FIG. 1. Changes in the DNA (left) and RNA (middle) contents and the RNA/DNA ratio (right) in the inguinal mammary glands of lactating mice that are concurrently pregnant with original litter (△), non-pregnant with original litter (▲), concurrently pregnant with replaced litter (○), and non-pregnant with replaced litter (●)

Figure in parenthesis shows the number of mice. Mean ± SE.

whereas it increased, though at a lower rate than in earlier stage, in the lactating non-pregnant group.

The data on the mammary nucleic acids determined at corresponding stages are summarized in Fig. 1. The DNA and RNA contents and the RNA/DNA ratio decreased steadily from day 18 towards day 26 of lactation in the non-pregnant naturally-weaning group while the DNA content declined to a lesser extent and RNA and RNA/DNA were rather higher on day 26 than on day 22 in the non-pregnant suckled group. These results are in good agreement with a number of previous reports (*3*, *4*, *29*, *31*) that continuous suckling can retard the regressing process in the mammary gland and maintain its secretory activity after natural weaning. The DNA content tended to be higher in the concurrent pregnant group than in the non-pregnant group but the RNA/DNA ratio was not different between these groups on day 18 and day 22. Similar results had been obtained in a previous study in mice (*16*) and also in rats during the early stage of concurrent pregnancy (*20*, *35*). These data on nucleic acids suggest that the increased milk production reflected in litter growth in the pregnant lactating group may be due to the larger amount of mammary parenchyma rather than to its enhanced secretory activity. Considering the average duration of delayed implantation, such a stimulative effect seems to be exerted until about day 14 or 15 of concurrent pregnancy under present conditions. It is supposed that placental substances may be involved in this process. More recently, a significantly higher litter growth in concurrently lactating pregnant mice than in non-pregnant lactating mice has been reported (*30*). Thus, it appears that pregnancy does not inhibit but rather stimulates lactational performance until the time near the next birth.

As lactation advanced, the DNA content in the concurrently pregnant groups, irrespective of litter replacement, decreased slightly in trend similar to the non-pregnant suckled group and was maintained 50% higher than in the non-pregnant weaning group on day 26 of lactation. The RNA content, however, decreased rapidly and was about half that in the non-pregnant suckled group, though still significantly higher than in the non-pregnant weaning group, and the RNA/DNA ratio was reduced to about the same level of that in the non-pregnant weaning group on day 26.

The lactose content in the mammary glands decreased in all groups towards day 26 of lactation. On day 26 of lactation a somewhat higher lactose content was observed in concurrently pregnant groups in which litters could obtain substantially no milk than in non-pregnant suckled group in which litters continued to gain weight. The lactose content in the mammary gland is not always an indicator of the secretory function of the gland but only shows the milk retained if the litter has been allowed to suckle until the time the mother is killed.

These results indicate that concurrent pregnancy can effectively retard mammary regression in the sense of cell number but cannot maintain the secretory function sufficient to support litter growth towards the end of advancing pregnancy, even if suckling stimulus is continuously given.

2) Experiment 2

Our attempt to control the time of implantation by subcutaneous injection of estradiol, which had been reported to be effective (*42*), did not succeed. Therefore, this series of experiments was carried out to obtain more precise information on changes occurring at the stage of transition to the second lactation. The mothers were killed randomly and grouped in days of pregnancy by checking the external features of the fetuses. A group of primiparous pregnant mice was used as a reference, in which the day the vaginal plug was found was designated as day 1 of pregnancy.

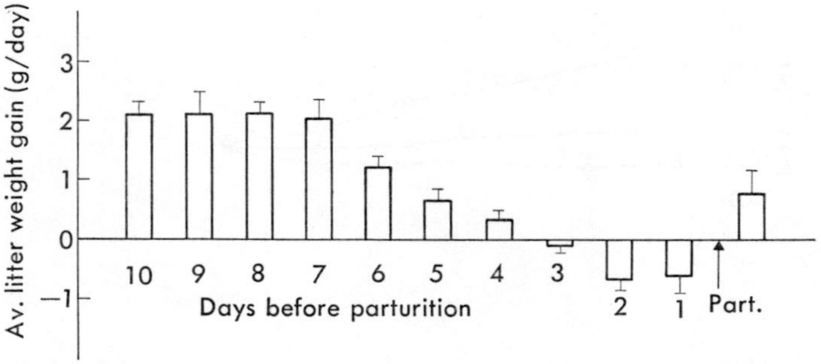

FIG. 2. The average daily gain in litter weight of concurrently lactating pregnant mice during a 10-day period before the next birth
Mean ± SE (n = 12).

Groups of day 14–15 to day 19 of pregnancy were obtained and these corresponded to day 23–24 to day 28 of concurrent lactation on the average, showing that the delay of implantation was about 8 days on the average. The average number and weight of fetuses were not significantly different between groups at any stage of pregnancy, indicating that fetal development was not influenced by concurrent pregnancy under the present conditions. This result was in accordance with that of Bruce and East (*2*) but contrary to that of McCarthy (*13*).

The average daily gain of litter weight in the concurrently pregnant suckled group was calculated during a period of 10 days counted back from the birth of the second litter (Fig. 2). It shows that milk secretion continued at a nearly constant rate but began to decline from 7 days before and stopped substantially from 2 days before the second birth. A sudden rise was observed from parturition to day 1 of lactation. Bruce (*4*) has described quite similar results on litter growth in concurrently pregnant lactating rats.

The data on nucleic acids are plotted in Fig. 3. In both concurrently pregnant groups, irrespective of litter replacement, the level of DNA was maintained almost constant while the RNA content decreased gradually and therefore the RNA/DNA ratio decreased from day 14–15 to day 19 of concurrent pregnancy. This confirms the results in Experiment 1 and suggests that lower lactational performance at a later stage in concurrent pregnancy might result not from the reduced mammary cell number but from the depressed secretory activity of cells. This contradicts the result obtained by Paape and Tucker (*20*) that mammary DNA content

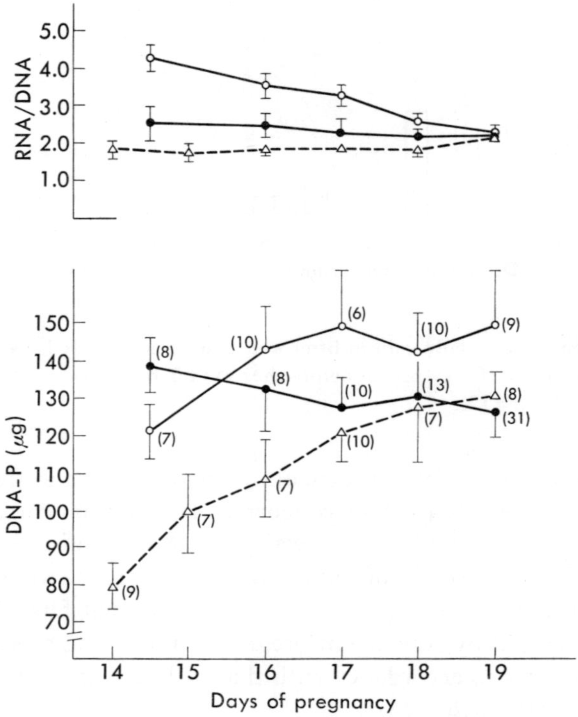

FIG. 3. Changes in the DNA content (bottom) and the RNA/DNA ratio (upper) in the inguinal mammary glands of mice that are concurrently pregnant with original litter (●) and concurrently pregnant with replaced litter (○) and of primiparous pregnant mice (△)

Figure in parenthesis shows the number of mice. Mean±SE.

decreased markedly with advancing concurrent pregnancy in rats. In their experiment, rats in which the time of blastocyst implantation was adjusted by estradiol injection gave birth until day 24±1 of lactation. Such hastened concurrent pregnancy may exert adverse effects more potently on established lactating glands when pregnancy is maintained without harmful effects on fetal development. There is some evidence that pregnancy was disturbed in rats which had mated at postpartum estrus if extensive suckling stimulus was given before day 10 of pregnancy (*36*, *37*). In fact, in their experiment a significant reduction in DNA content of the mammary gland was not observed in concurrently pregnant rats carrying 6 or fewer fetuses at day 19 to 20 of lactation (*35*). Furthermore, in their experiment the mammary DNA content was maintained almost constantly at higher levels over a period from day 12 to day 24 if intensive suckling was given in non-pregnancy. On the other hand, in our experiment the mammary DNA content decreased slightly but definitely towards the later stage of lactation even if suckling was continued in non-pregnant mothers (Fig. 1). To investigate the effect of concurrent pregnancy on lactation, it seems more suitable to establish pregnancy at recurring estrus during prolonged lactation rather than to control the time of blastocyst implantation after mating at postpartum estrus. Delayed implantation did not occur in concurrent pregnancy during prolonged lactation in rats (*4*).

In the primiparous pregnant group, the DNA and RNA increased steadily as pregnancy progressed but RNA/DNA ratios remained nearly constant from day 16 onwards and tended to increase slightly on day 19 of pregnancy. Whether maintenance of the total DNA at a constant level during the last 4 to 5 days of concurrent pregnancy is due to compensation by newly-proliferated secretory cells or to the maintenance of existing old cells or to a combination of these two processes was not answered in the present experiment. However, the mammary DNA content in concurrently lactating pregnant mice appeared to be less than the sum of the DNA content in the regressing mammary glands of naturally-weaning mice (see Experiment 1) and the DNA content in developing mammary glands of primiparous pregnant mice, when comparison was made by adjusting day of lactation with day of pregnancy. Therefore, it is possible that mammary cell proliferation might occur to a lesser extent in concurrent pregnancy than in normal pregnancy, supposing that pregnancy does not accelerate the regression of existing older cells. This may recall histological studies in which the rate of cell division in the mammary glands is lower in simultaneously pregnant lactating rats and cows than in pregnant rats and cows (*1*, *23*).

The reason why continuous suckling maintained mammary gland cell numbers and secretory activity in the lactating non-pregnant mother while it maintained mammary cell numbers to a similar extent but could not maintain secretory activity in the concurrently pregnant mother has yet to be clarified. Does the hormonal milieu responsible for maintaining gestation and for proliferating the mammary cells adversely affect mammary secretory function? If so, why does the inhibitory effect become marked towards the end of pregnancy? Is the responsiveness to the galactopoietic hormones of existing older cells maintained by suckling stimulus different from the responsiveness in newly-proliferating cells during advancing pregnancy? If so, is the maintenance of total DNA content during concurrent pregnancy due to compensation by newly-differentiated cells? These problems are complicated by their concern with the mechanism by which initiation of milk secretion is triggered off at parturition in the primiparous animal.

The precise process of lactogenesis varies from species to species and many problems have to be studied further (see Chapter II-5). However, it may be safe to say in general that the stimulatory factors become dominant, the inhibitory factors are withdrawn and the balance between these factors shifts to favor the onset of milk secretion at parturition. On the other hand, continuous suckling can extend the normal lactation period but a definite decline in lactational performance occurs (*28*, *29*, *31*). Hormones required for the maintenance of lactation are reported to become insufficient during prolonged lactation (*28*, *29*). For the mechanism causing these hormonal changes, the idea that a reduction in the sensitivity of the hypothalamus to suckling stimulus has been postulated, since prolactin and corticoids liberated in response to milking stimulus decreased during later stages of lactation (*11*, *12*, *19*). Similarly, a decrease in the suppressing effect of suckling stimulus on gonadotropic hormones with advancing lactation (*7*, *32*) supports this concept. Thus, a limited amount of milk secretion can be continued by the relatively low levels of hormones liberated in response to suckling insofar as no inhibitory factors appear. Then it is possible that the changes in hormone levels associated with the advance of concurrent pregnancy will hold in check secretory

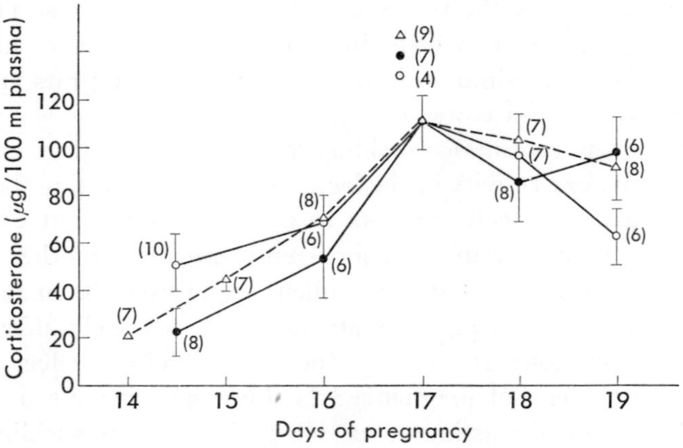

FIG. 4. Changes in the plasma level of corticosterone of mice Remarks are the same as Fig. 3.

activity at later stages of lactation despite continuous suckling stimulus.

On the other hand, it has been shown that corticoids can induce milk secretion in pregnant mice (*17*), rats (*27*), and heifers (*34*) but prolactin could not. Corticoids may be a rate-limiting factor for prolonged lactation in rats (*28*, *29*). The blood levels of corticosterone were determined by essentially the same method of Guillemin *et al.* (*8*). Mice were killed at 9.00–10.00 a.m. No significant difference was detectable in corticosterone levels between concurrently pregnant groups, irrespective of suckling stimulus, and the primiparous pregnant group (Fig. 4). A more extensive analysis of various hormone levels in the blood of concurrently pregnant animals is necessary.

Morphometric study of mice has shown that mammary gland cells at the time of parturition and at the onset of lactation are not yet fully differentiated (*9*, *10*). Thus, it may be possible that the mammary cells newly-differentiated by concurrent pregnancy occupied the glands, replacing older cells, and therefore the total cell numbers could apparently be maintained at a certain level while secretory activity decreased towards the end of concurrent lactating pregnancy.

2. Continuous Suckling and Subsequent Lactation

All mothers in the concurrently pregnant group with original litters or with replaced litters cohabited with the litters until day 1 of the second lactation, *i.e.*, the day on which a newborn litter was found at 9.00 a.m. On day 1 of the second lactation, the old litter was removed from the cage and the number of the newly-born litter was adjusted to 6 pups. The litter weight was measured daily at 9.00 a.m. When any pups were found to be dead, only surviving pups were weighed and then foster pups of the same age were added to make the litter size 6. As a control, a group of primiparous normal lactating mice was used.

The continuously suckled group showed a higher rate of mortality among newly-born pups on day 1 of lactation. From our observations on the day of birth, they did not seem to be stillborn. The average weight of surviving pups was very slightly lower than in other groups. Nevertheless, the litter size (surviving plus dead pups) was not significantly different compared with the first birth or with the births in other groups. No deteriorative influence of continuous suckling throughout pregnancy on the number and the development of the fetuses has been detected under present conditions (see Experiment 2). Crushing by the old litter may be

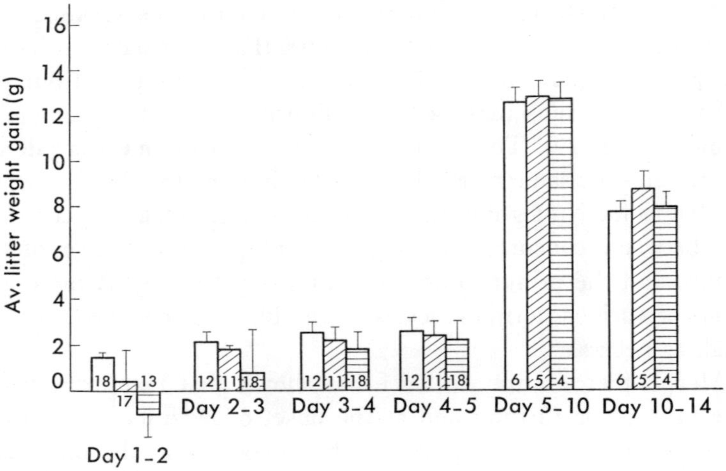

FIG. 5. The average litter weight gains during the second lactation of mice that have been concurrently pregnant with original litter (▨) and concurrently pregnant with replaced litter (⊟)

That of primiparous normal lactating mice is shown as control (□). Figure in bottom of each column shows the number of mice. Mean±SE.

ruled out since the presence of males at the first birth or the presence of an original litter that was larger than the replaced litter did not cause such high mortality among newborn pups. Therefore, the higher mortality of newborn pups at day 1 of lactation may be due to a lesser amount of available milk after birth and not due to the weakness of pups. It seemed unlikely in this experiment that the mother's nipple had been damaged by pre- and early postpartum suckling by the older pups (*24*). But the competition for available milk between old litters and newborn litters might be partially responsible, since an abrupt increase in the weight of old litters just at parturition was observed (Fig. 2).

The gains in litter weight during the second lactation are presented in Fig. 5. Between day 1 and day 2, the loss of pups and the average litter gain were 9% and 0 g in the naturally-weaning group, and 17% and −1.0 g in the continuously suckled group, respectively. Further, an 8% loss of pups occurred between day 2 and day 3 in the latter group. However, the litter growth in these groups recovered as lactation progressed and no significant difference existed in litter gain during a period of 10 days from day 5 to day 14, compared with the primiparous normal lactating control group.

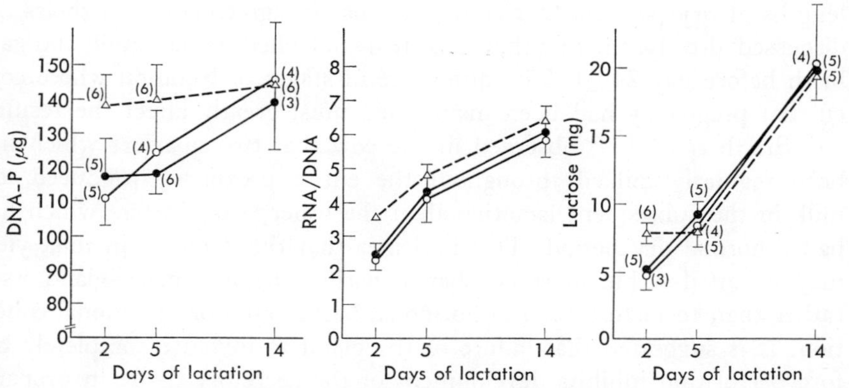

FIG. 6. Changes in the DNA content (left) and the RNA/DNA ratio (middle) and the lactose content (right) in the inguinal mammary glands of mice during the second lactation subsequent to concurrently pregnant lactation with original litter (●) and to concurrently pregnant lactation with replaced litter (○) Those from primiparous normal lactating mice are shown as controls (△). Figure in parenthesis shows the number of mice. Mean±SE.

The mothers were killed after 4 hr separation from litters on days 2, 5, and 14 of lactation and mammary nucleic acids and lactose contents were determined (Fig. 6). There were shifts towards lower mammary DNA, RNA, and RNA/DNA ratio and lactose content in concurrently pregnant groups compared with primiparous lactating controls on day 2 of lactation. The levels of these parameters in each group increasingly agreed towards day 14 of lactation. Thus the unfavorable effect on litter growth at the early stage of subsequent lactation observed in concurrently pregnant groups seemed to be attributable to reduced cell numbers and insufficient secretory activity of the mammary glands.

The original litter appeared to become independent of mother's milk almost from day 22 and completely from the later stage of lactation. Accordingly, the non-suckling period before the next parturition, *i.e.*, dry period, was considered to be about 4 to 5 days on the average in the concurrently pregnant group with original litters. Therefore, the present results show that a non-existent or very short dry period may exert an inhibitory effect on the onset of the next lactation. Paape and Tucker (*21*) studied the effect of various lengths of dry periods on subsequent lactation in rats. The mammary glands in rats given 0-day dry period had higher cell numbers at early lactation (day 1) but contained reduced numbers of cells in later stages compared with those rats given other lengths of dry periods. Our results are not in agreement with theirs. As discussed already, the rats they used had controlled implantation and gave birth before day 24±1. The difference in stages of lactation where concurrent pregnancy had been maintained must greatly affect the results.

Smith *et al.* (*25*) observed in the cow that two quarters which had been regularly milked throughout the entire pregnancy produced less milk in the subsequent lactation than the other two quarters which had had a normal dry period. This indicates that the decrease in milk yield may be attributable to some change within the mammary gland itself rather than to factors such as hormonal background or nutritional condition. It is suggested that failure of the gland to involute completely before parturition inhibits development of the secretory tissue in preparation for the next lactation (*5*, *25*, *41*). On the other hand, Swanson *et al.* (*26*) observed that in prepartum half udders, 6 weeks' difference in the dry period did not significantly affect dry weight, DNA or alveolar concentration at the end of pregnancy. Thus, they concluded that subsequent subnormal lactation after a short dry period might be due to subnormal function rather than structure. In our experiment, the mammary DNA contents in concurrently lactating pregnant groups with replaced litters (0-day dry period) or with original litters (short dry period) were maintained approximately at the same level as that at the end of primiparous pregnancy (see Experiments 1 and 2). However, not only mammary cell numbers but also secretory activity of individual cells were subnormal early in the second lactation. It is speculated that cell division occurring around parturition (*33*) may be suppressed by reasons yet to be elucidated. It must be emphasized here that the amount of DNA reflects the total number of cells, irrespective of their nature, and thereby does not always indicate the number of actual secretory epithelial cells, but also reflects myoepithelial cells, adipocytes, fibroblasts, and others. Thus, attempts have been made to estimate the extraparenchymal DNA and the mammary stromal tissues (*18*, *20*). At present, no specific parameters are known for the mammary epithelial cells. Moreover, it is not known whether the mammary secretory cells which existed during the preceeding lactation period can be carried over to the next lactation period, and if so, how long they can exist or whether they can respond to galactopoietic hormones in a similar manner as can newly-proliferating cells.

Finally, to clarify the mechanism by which continuous suckling adversely affects the next lactation during its early stage, it seems necessary to investigate the changes in the fine structure of the mammary glands in relation to hormone levels in the transitional stage between two consecutive lactations by using concurrently pregnant animals.

SUMMARY

Effects of concurrent pregnancy and continuous suckling on two consecutive lactations were studied in mice. Concurrent pregnancy was established by postpartum mating. To provide continuous suckling, original litters were replaced with foster litters of 5-day-old pups on day 14 of lactation. The duration of the delay in embryo implantation was about 8 to 9 days on the average. The data on litter growth and mammary DNA and RNA contents suggested that concurrent pregnancy did not suppress but rather stimulated the established lactation compared with non-pregnant lactation, possibly due to an increased number of the secretory cells until about one week before the next birth. Towards the end of advancing pregnancy, mammary regression could be effectively retarded. The total mammary cell number (DNA) was maintained at almost the same level as that in the non-pregnant continuously suckled group. On the last day of pregnancy, total mammary DNA content was not different between concurrently pregnant groups and primiparous pregnant groups. However, the secretory activity (RNA and RNA/DNA ratio) decreased markedly and the litters could obtain substantially no milk just before parturition in concurrently pregnant groups while litters continued to gain weight, though at a lower rate, in non-pregnant groups.

On day 1 of the second lactation, a higher mortality among newborn litters was observed in continuously suckled groups. In continuously suckled and naturally-weaning groups, litter growth was depressed during early stages of lactation but recovered gradually and the litter gain between day 5 to day 14 of lactation was not significantly different from that of primiparous normal lactation. The mammary DNA and RNA contents and lactose content were lower on day 2 but these were not different on day 14 of lactation compared with those in the primiparous lactating group. These results indicate that continuous suckling or short dry periods adversely affect the subsequent lactation during early stages, possibly by suppressing cell differentiation and secretory activity which might be enhanced around normal parturition.

Acknowledgment

This work was supported in part by Grants for Scientific Research from the

Ministry of Education, Science and Culture of Japan (Nos. 836021, 111509, and 256196).

REFERENCES

1. Altman, A. D. (1945). Izmeneniya v vimeni korov v protsesse razdoya. *Vest. Zhivot.* **1**, 85–96: Cited from *Dairy Sci. Abstr.* **9**, 287 (1947–1948).
2. Bruce, H. M. and East, J. (1956). Number and viability of young from pregnancies concurrent with lactation in the mouse. *J. Endocrinol.* **14**, 19–27.
3. Burce, H. M. (1958). Suckling stimulus and lactation. *Proc. Roy. Soc. Ser. B* **149**, 421–423.
4. Bruce, H. M. (1961). Observations on the suckling and lactation in the rat. *J. Reprod. Fert.* **2**, 17–34.
5. Dodd, F. H. (1957). Factors affecting the rate of secretion of milk and lactation yield. In *Progress in the Physiology of Farm Animals*, vol. 3, ed. Hammond, J., Chap. 20, pp. 962–1004. London: Butterworths.
6. Enzmann, E. V., Saphin, N. R., and Pincus, G. (1932). Delayed pregnancy in mice. *Anat. Rec.* **54**, 325–338.
7. Ford, J. J. and Melampy, R. M. (1973). Gonadotropin levels in lactating rats: Effect of ovariectomy. *Endocrinology* **93**, 540–547.
8. Guillemin, R., Clayton, G. W., Lipscomb, M. D., and Smith, J. D. (1959). Fluorometric measurement of rat plasma and adrenal corticosterone concentration. A note on technical details. *J. Lab. Clin. Med.* **53**, 830–832.
9. Hollmann, K. H. (1969). Quantitative electron microscopy of subcellular organization in mammary gland cells before and after parturition. In *Lactogenesis: The Initiation* of *Milk Secretion at Parturition*, ed. Reynolds, M. and Folley, S. J., pp. 27–41. Philadelphia, Pa.: Univ. Pennsylvania Press.
10. Hollmann, K. H. (1974). Cytology and fine structure of the mammary gland. In *Lactation: A Comprehensive Treatise*, vol. 1, ed. Larson, B. L. and Smith, V. R., Chap. 1, pp. 3–95. New York, London: Academic Press.
11. Johke, T. (1970). Factors affecting the plasma prolactin level in the cow and the goat as determined by radioimmunoassay. *Endocrinol. Japon.* **17**, 393–402.
12. Koprowski, J. A. and Tucker, H. A. (1973). Serum prolactin during various physiological states and its relationship to milk production in the bovine. *Endocrinology* **92**, 1480–1487.
13. McCarthy, J. C. (1965). Effect of concurrent lactation on litter size and prenatal maturity in an inbred strain of mice. *J. Reprod. Fert.* **9**, 29–39.
14. Mizuno, H. (1960). The effects of administration of prolactin, progesterone or concurrent pregnancy on the mammary gland involution and respiratory activity in the mice. *Endocrinol. Japon.* **7**, 121–131.

15. Mizuno, H. (1960). The effect of concurrent pregnancy on lactation in the mouse. *Endocrinol. Japon.* **7**, 322–326.
16. Mizuno, H. (1961). The changes of nucleic acids content in the mouse mammary glands in the course of involution and the effects of pregnancy, prolactin or progesterone on them. *Endocrinol. Japon.* **8**, 27–34.
17. Nandi, S. and Bern, H. A. (1961). The hormones responsible for lactogenesis in BALB/cCrgl mice. *Gen. Comp. Endocrinol.* **1**, 195–210.
18. Nicoll, C. S. and Tucker, H. A. (1965). Estimates of parenchymal, stromal and lymphnode deoxyribonucleic acid in mammary glands of C3H/Crgl/2 mice. *Life Sci.* **4**, 993–1001.
19. Ôta, K., Harai, Y., Unno, H., Tomogane, H., and Yokoyama, A. (1974). Corticosterone secretion in response to suckling at various stages of normal and prolonged lactation in rats. *J. Endocrinol.* **62**, 679–680.
20. Paape, M. J. and Tucker, H. A. (1969). Mammary nucleic acid, hydroxyproline, and hexosamine of pregnant rats during lactation and post-lactational involution. *J. Dairy Sci.* **52**, 380–385.
21. Paape, M. J. and Tucker, H. A. (1969). Influence of length of dry period on subsequent lactation in the rat. *J. Dairy Sci.* **52**, 518–522.
22. Psychoyos, A. (1967). The hormonal interplay controlling egg-implantation in the rat. In *Advances in Reproductive Physiology*, vol. 2, ed. McLaren, A., Chap. 6, pp. 257–277. London: Longos Press, Academic Press.
23. Reece, R. P. and Warbritton, V. (1953). The rate of cell division in the mammary glands of rats. *J. Dairy Sci.* **36**, 589 (Abstr.).
24. Sachs, B. D. and Rosenblatt, J. S. (1974). Prepartum suckling reduces the survival of newborn in the rat. *Dev. Psychobiol.* **7**, 399–406.
25. Smith, A., Wheelock, J. V., and Dodd, F. H. (1967). The effect of milking throughout pregnancy on milk secretion in the succeeding lactation. *J. Dairy Res.* **34**, 145–150.
26. Swanson, E. W., Pardue, F. E., and Longmire, D. B. (1967). Effect of gestation and dry period on deoxyribonucleic acid and alveolar characteristics of bovine mammary gland. *J. Dairy Sci.* **50**, 1288–1292.
27. Talwalker, P. K., Nicoll, C. S., and Meites, J. (1961). Induction of mammary secretion in pregnant rats and rabbits by hydrocortisone acetate. *Endocrinology* **69**, 802–809.
28. Thatcher, W. W. and Tucker, H. A. (1970). Effect of 9-fluoroprednisolone acetate and transplanted pituitaries on milk synthesis. *Proc. Soc. Exp. Biol. Med.* **134**, 705–710.
29. Thatcher, W. W. and Tucker, H. A. (1970). Lactational performance of rats injected with oxytocin, cortisol-21-acetate, prolactin and growth hormone during prolonged lactation. *Endocrinology* **86**, 237–240.
30. Thompson, L. J. and Anderson, R. R. (1977). Effect of pregnancy on lactation in mice. *J. Dairy Sci.* **60**, 126–128.

31. Tomogane, H., Ôta, K. Unno, H., and Yokoyama, A. (1976). Changes in body weight, milk production, food and water consumptions and vaginal smears in rats during prolonged lactation. *Endocrinol. Japon.* **23**, 129–136.
32. Tomogane, H., Ôta, K., and Yokoyama, A. (1976). Duration of diesterous period and secretion of progestin during prolonged lactation in the rat. *Endocrinol. Japon.* **23**, 137–141.
33. Traurig, H. H. (1967). Cell proliferation in the mammary gland during late pregnancy and lactation. *Anat. Rec.* **157**, 489–504.
34. Tucker, H. A. and Meites, J. (1965). Induction of lactation in pregnant heifers with 9-fluoroprednisolone acetate. *J. Dairy Sci.* **48**, 403–405.
35. Tucker, H. A. and Reece, R. P. (1964). Nucleic acid content of mammary glands of lactating rats simultaneously pregnant. *Proc. Soc. Exp. Biol. Med.* **115**, 885–887.
36. Veomett, M. J. and Daniel, J. C., Jr. (1971). Termination of pregnancy after accerlerated lactation in the rat. *J. Reprod. Fert.* **26**, 415–417.
37 Veomett, M. J. and Daniel, J. C., Jr. (1975). Termination of pregnancy after accelerated lactation in the rat. II. Relationship to number of young, day of pregnancy and length of nursing. *J. Reprod. Fert.* **44**, 513–517.
38. Veomett, M. J. and Daniel, J. C., Jr. (1975). Termination of pregnancy after accelerated lactation in the rat. III. Effects of hormonal treatments. *J. Reprod. Fert.* **44**, 519–527.
39. Veomett, M. J. and Daniel, J. C., Jr. (1975). Termination of pregnancy after accelerated lactation in the rat. IV. Relationship to 20α-hydroxysteroid dehydrogenase activity and plasma progesterone concentration. *J. Reprod. Fert.* **44**, 529–536.
40. Weichert, C. K. (1942). The experimental control of prolonged pregnancy in the lactating rat by means of oestrogen. *Anat. Rec.* **83**, 1–18.
41. Wheelock, J. V. and Dodd, F. H. (1969). Non-nutritional factors affecting milk yield in dairy cattle. *J. Dairy Res.* **36**, 479–493.
42. Whitten, W. K. (1958). Endocrine studies on delayed implantation in lactating mice, role of the pituitary in implantation. *J. Endocrinol.* **16**, 435–440.

II – 7

7 – II

CENTRAL PATHWAYS IN OXYTOCIN AND PROLACTIN RELEASE

J. S. TINDAL

National Institute for Research in Dairying, Shinfield, Reading, England

Despite the known relationship between the suckling stimulus and the release of pituitary hormones concerned with the maintenance of lactation, little was known at the time this work began of the way in which the stimulus achieved this effect. It was decided, therefore, to devote most of our effort to an investigation of the ascending pathways for oxytocin and prolactin release in the brain, and the present chapter represents a personal account of work carried out in this laboratory since 1965. Several comprehensive reviews are available for those who require a wider coverage of the subject (*6*, *8*, *10*, *13*, *42*, *43*).

1. Brainstem Pathways Involved in Oxytocin Release

Although the object of this work was to study the central oxytocin-release pathways which normally are activated by suckling, it was decided to use an electrical stimulation technique in the anesthetized animal, at least for the initial experiments, in preference to blockade of the release of oxytocin in response to suckling by knife cuts or lesions, since it was felt that punctate stimulation would give a more sharply-defined picture. The lactating guinea-pig was chosen for the initial studies, since it had a reasonably large brain for which a stereotaxic atlas had been prepared (*41*) and had two relatively large mammary glands which facilitated the detection of oxytocin release. Work began on exploration of the brain for sites where electrical stimulation caused release of oxytocin, evidenced by a rise in milk-ejection pressure. The brain was transected at the level of the hindbrain to prevent the stimulation triggering sympathetic activation and hence vasoconstriction of the mammary glands. The early experiments were disappointing since, apart from stimulation of such regions as the magnocellular neurosecretory nuclei and the pituitary stalk region, few significant releases of oxytocin occurred, and it began to look as if the ascending pathway for oxytocin release was, in fact, diffuse as had been suggested earlier (*9*). Then, purely by accident, it was found that stimulation of a discrete portion of the far-lateral tegmentum in the caudal midbrain evoked large, repeatable milk-ejection responses. The position led to the conclusion that the spinothalamic system was involved (*8*, *45*, *51*). The brainstem was then explored from the caudal midbrain to the hypothalamus. Responses were obtained from many sites in the brainstem, including the tectum and central grey, but the overall picture was one of a major pathway for milk ejection which ascended through the lateral tegmentum, and which appeared to be coincident with the position of the spinothalamic tract. As the path was traced rostrally to the posterior hypothalamus it appeared to move medially and bifurcate, one part passing forward close to the third ventricle, while the other passed forward in the subthalamus. These were assumed to represent spinothalamic relays with dorsal longitudinal fasciculus and medial forebrain bundle, respectively. Further rostrally, within the hypothalamus, the picture was complicated by the efferent pathways from the neurosecretory nuclei to the neurohypophysis (*16*). The ascending path was shown to be concerned with the preferential release of oxytocin, since stimulation of the path did not lead to detectable release of vasopressin (*52*). In addition, removal of a large part of the forebrain by suction showed that, rostrally, the pathway remained within the brainstem. This rostral portion of the pathway within the hypothalamus was then investigated in detail by stimulation of the path in the midbrain every few minutes while a knife, held transversely in an electrode carrier, was inserted into the brain and lowered progressively into the hypothalamus, one step before each stimulation. This type of experiment was repeated many times until a sufficient number of transverse stereotaxic planes had been explored. It was then possible to conclude, on the basis of blockade of the milk-ejection response following electrical stimulation being attributable to specific knife cuts, that the major portion of the pathway passed forward from the subthalamus to the hypothalamus in the medial forebrain bundle and that the minor portion passed forward close to the third ventricle and then swung out abruptly to rejoin the major path in the lateral hypothalamus. Connection with the paraventricular nuclei appeared to be made by collaterals which sweep dorsomedially from the medial forebrain bundle. Other experiments, which involved forebrain transection or undercutting of the paraventricular nuclei either bilaterally or ipsilaterally to the site of stimulation in the midbrain, indicated that the pathway involved the paraventricular nuclei *en route* to the neurohypophysis. Radiofrequency lesions of these nuclei also indicated that such a connection only had to be made with the extreme lateral tip of each nucleus, and that oxytocin release was only completely abolished if the lesion also included the accessory paraventricular nuclei which lie further laterally in the hypothalamus (*16*, *46*). It was also found that although a large release of oxytocin was evoked by electrical stimulation of the supraoptic nuclei, the same order of release could be achieved by stimulation of either the paraventricular nuclei or the pituitary stalk with the same waveform, frequency, current, and voltage, but for only one tenth of the time, 3 sec instead of 30 sec (*52*). Taking these facts into consideration, therefore, it seems reasonable to assume that, under normal conditions in the guinea-pig, the paraventricular nuclei play the major role in oxytocin release. However, in the rat, it has been reported recently that spherical cuts with a Halasz knife which isolate the paraventricular nuclei do not block the milk-ejection reflex in response to suckling (*58*). Whether this represents a misinterpretation of observations on our part or a genuine species difference, remains to be seen. However, it should be noted that connections have been demonstrated in the rat between the cells of the paraventricular, accessory paraventricular and accessory supraoptic nuclei on the one hand, and those of the supraoptic nuclei on the other, although whether any of the axons of the former group terminates in the supraoptic nucleus or are merely fibers of passage *en route* to the neurohypophysis has not yet been resolved (*5*). If any such synaptic contacts do occur in the supraoptic nucleus then the activation of supraoptic neurons during reflex milk ejection in the rat (*22*, *23*) might represent activation which was, at least in part, relayed by paraventricular neurons. It should also be borne in mind that although the ascending pathway is discrete in the caudal midbrain, as it passes rostrally there are many scattered sites ancillary to the main ascending pathway in the guinea-pig and that alternative pathways may exist which can be called into use when failure of the principal path occurs.

With regard to the spherical cuts around the paraventricular nuclei in the rat (*58*) it should also be pointed out that, in the guinea-pig, lesions of the paraventricular nuclei only abolished the release of oxytocin in response to midbrain stimulation if the lesion also included the accessory paraventricular nuclei (*46*). As mentioned above, these extend some considerable distance from the principal nuclei in the guinea-pig (*16*), as they do in the rat (*5*, *14*). In the absence of any histological information as to whether the accessory nuclei were included within the spherical cuts or not, it is difficult to assess the validity of the findings of Voloschin and Tramezzani (*58*). Indeed, as Bandaranayake (*5*) pointed out, ". . . complete destruction of the 'parent' nucleus (even if this were possible) could still lead to misinterpretation, due to compensatory hyperactivity of the corresponding accessory cells." Electrophysiological studies have demonstrated a complex interaction between cells of the paraventricular and supraoptic nuclei (*61*) so that, quite apart from possible species differences, determination of the relative importance of the roles played by these two pairs of hypothalamic nuclei in reflex milk ejection is not as straightforward as it appears to be.

It is unfortunately true that experiments on the ascending pathways in the brain stem are also subject to misinterpretation. The same group of workers (*57*) have claimed more recently, on the basis of a partial transection technique, that the ascending pathway in the midbrain of the rat is not discrete. However, if the effective stimulation sites at stereotaxic planes A 4.0 and A 4.5 in the guinea-pig (*51*), for instance, are compared with the midbrain cuts made by these workers in the rat, it will be seen that the path is in the form of a vertical band at this level and that the "two thirds dorsal" and "two thirds ventral" cuts would probably, therefore, be ineffective in severing the path totally.

The ascending pathway for oxytocin release was also investigated in the brainstem of the rabbit, and the same general pattern emerged as in the guinea-pig, although the sites were more sparse in the rabbit brain (*54*). Shortly afterwards, B. A. Cross and his group (*56*) reported that they were unable to confirm this pathway in the rabbit and concluded that the ascending pathway was, in fact, diffuse and not discrete in the brainstem. We reinvestigated the rabbit (*48*) and found that although the pathway was where we had reported it to be, we discovered that, unlike the guinea-pig, responses were not repeatable at an effective stimulation site. That is to say, after an initial release of oxytocin in response to electrical stimulation, further periods of stimulation did not elicit a response. This had not been observed in our earlier rabbit studies (*54*), because when we had obtained a response by stimulation of a particular site, the electrode was immediately lowered a step so that the exploration of that particular stereotaxic plane could continue. It also became clear from inspection of the histological material that stimulation of the pathway did not always release oxytocin.

It may be relevant that an oxytocin-release pathway had also been reported in the rabbit to extend from the region of the hippocampal rudiment and nucleus accumbens in the rostral forebrain (*2*) to the paraventricular nuclei, but not directly to the supraoptic nuclei, of the hypothalamus (*60*). However B. A. Cross's group (*56*) were unable to confirm either the extensiveness of the responsive sites or, with one exception, the repeatability of responses, which suggests that some as yet unidentified aspect of experimental technique may be responsible for making the oxytocin-release mechanism refractory to electrical stimulation. It may be, for instance, that if the stimulating current and voltage is accidentally raised above a critical threshold, then this will be sufficient to activate the noradrenergic innervation (*10*, *55*) of the magnocellular nuclei. In our own experiments care was taken to maintain the stimulating voltage at 3 V and the stimulating current only varied between 250–260 μA (*54*).

We felt that the most appropriate proof for the existence of the pathway would be bilateral transection of the pathway in the midbrain of the lactating rabbit, to see whether natural milk ejection was blocked. This was carried out (*48*) and milk ejection was indeed blocked, but returned after a variable period of 7 to 12 days. It should be pointed out that by this time the pups were extremely powerful and assaulted the mother's teats unmercifully during the initial daily test suckling period, after which the mother was injected with oxytocin and the litter gained access to the milk. It would not be surprising, therefore, if other pathways were stimulated into activity at this stage of the experiment. It was clear from the electrical stimulation experiments in the rabbit that there was a powerful central inhibition of the release of oxytocin. This may, of course, be relevant to a species such as the rabbit which feeds its young briefly, once a day, in contrast to a species such as the rat which suckles its young for long periods at a time. The central inhibition of oxytocin release may manifest itself in varying degrees throughout the mammals and may, of course, be concerned with the gating mechanism proposed for oxytocin release in the rat in response to the apparently passive suckling by the litter (*21*). Although it was reported many years ago that spreading cortical depression could overcome pain-induced inhibition of the milk-ejection reflex in the rat (*40*) and, more recently, that stimulation of various sites in the rabbit brainstem could prevent release of oxytocin in response to stimulation of otherwise effective sites (*3*), the neural basis of the normal central inhibition of oxytocin release is not understood and must await further studies.

In addition to studying the oxytocin-release pathways in the guinea-pig and rabbit, we also investigated the goat, since there was evidence that at least the spinal pathways for oxytocin release in ruminants differed from those in laboratory animals (*8*, *10*, *13*, *43*). Two stereotaxic planes were explored in the midbrain at A2 and A4 (*53*) with a stimulating electrode and blood samples which were taken during and immediately after electrical stimulation were extracted and bioassayed for their oxytocin content. Although the effective stimulation sites were clustered most densely in the far-lateral tegmentum, in agreement with the previous findings in other species, there was, nevertheless, a considerable scatter of effective stimulation sites at these levels in the brainstem (*15*). Therefore, although the lateral tegmentum might be expected to carry the burden of sensory information regarding oxytocin release, the more scattered sites may explain the conclusion of Richard (*33*, *34*) that the ascending path of the milk-ejection reflex in the ewe is represented in the midbrain by diffuse spino-reticular fibers. The triggering of milk ejection in the ruminant is also complicated by the fact that, although the spinothalamic fibers of the spinal cord are thought to carry sensory information from the mammary glands with respect to the release of oxytocin, the spinocervicothalamic tract may exert an over-riding control on this mechanism (*35*). However, the picture may be even more complicated in primates since, at least in the rhesus monkey, the dorsal column nuclei receive not only ascending dorsal root fibres but also a more complexly integrated spinal input, which is also ipsilateral (*37*). Cells of origin of the spinocervicothalamic, spinothalamic, and spinal-dorsal column nuclei pathways are to be found in lamina IV of the dorsal horn and although it is not known whether any of the fibers in the three systems have common cells of origin, they share some common functional properties (*37*) and there may be considerably more interplay between these three ascending systems than has been supposed up till now.

In contrast to the afferent pathways involved in oxytocin release, the efferent pathway has been recognized for many years, but it is only recently that the mechanism of action of this section of the neuroendocrine milk-ejection reflex has been explored. Chiefly as a result of the elegant studies of the Bristol and Cambridge groups, the functioning of this part of the reflex is known in great detail (*11*). In the rat, it is the bunching together of action potentials which determines the release of oxytocin, since oxytocin release is controlled at this level by the frequency, and not by the total number, of action potentials reaching the nerve endings in the neural lobe (*20*). It is, therefore, the stages which precede the neurosecretory nuclei which are proving more difficult to interpret, and much more work remains to be done before the functioning of their afferent paths can be described with the same confidence as that of their efferent path. Although the drawbacks and disadvantages of the exploratory stimulation technique in the solution of this problem are fully appreciated, it has, nevertheless, given some insights into the pathways involved in oxytocin release. However, this may be too simplistic an approach and it seems probable that future studies may be directed towards an understanding of the central modulatory and inhibitory mechanisms which appear to impose an overall control over the afferent oxytocin-release pathway itself.

2. *Brainstem Pathways Involved in Prolactin Release*

Our first studies on the control of prolactin release were not, in fact, directly associated with lactation. At the time, there had been considerable argument as to whether the prolactin-releasing action of estrogen was exerted directly on the adenohypophysis or *via* the hypothalamus. We felt that it would be of interest to see whether estrogen could exert its effect even further away from the adenohypophysis, possibly in some portion of the limbic system. Since contemporary neuroanatomical knowledge suggested the amygdala as a possible site of action, we explored this region of the brain with estrogen implants. At the time, the only available means of detecting a raised circulating level of prolactin was the lactogenic response in the pseudopregnant rabbit. The principle of the method is that if a virgin female rabbit is injected once with gonadotrophin, she becomes pseudopregnant and the mammary glands develop, but do not secrete milk. If the animal is either injected with exogenous prolactin or is made to release some of her own endogenous prolactin, milk secretion will commence. At autopsy, after reflection of the overlying skin, the quantity of milk in ducts and secretory tissue can be assessed visually quite easily in the flat, two-dimensional mammary glands, and is roughly proportional to the amount of circulating prolactin. In the context of these experiments, stainless steel tubes which contained a minute quantity of estrogen inside the tip were implanted bilaterally in the amygdalae of rabbits, anesthetized with pentobarbitone, on the 7th day of pseudopregnancy. The mammary glands were assessed for their lactogenic response at autopsy on the 18th day of pseduopregnancy and brains were fixed for histological determination of implant sites. Other animals received blank implants or were injected with prolactin. It was found that lactogenesis occurred, presumably in response to endogenous prolactin release, when estrogen implants were placed in the medial nucleus, the central nucleus and in the basomedial part of the basal nucleus. These three regions of the amygdala had already been reported to project to the preoptic area and/or the hypothalamus *via* the stria terminalis (*4*) and it was concluded that prolactin release had occurred in response to estrogen-sensitive neurons in the amygdala acting *via* the stria terminalis (*50*). Further evidence to support this view came from later studies by others in which it was shown that there is a selective uptake of estrogen not only by the basal hypothalamus and preoptic area but also by these same regions of the amygdala, in the rat and guinea-pig (*30*, *39*, *59*).

It was assumed that the action of estrogen on the amygdala was to modulate the final control mechanism for prolactin release. At the time, this mechanism was not understood and most workers in this field were studying prolactin-inhibiting activity in extracts of basal hypothalamus. We felt that a broader view of the prolactin-release mechanism might be obtained by attempting to find out what pathways and structures would normally be involved in suckling-induced release of prolactin. As in the earlier oxytocin-release studies, we did not utilize the suckling stimulus *per se*, but attempted to mimic the effect by exploration of the brainstem with discrete electrical stimulation.

In the first series of experiments, virgin female rabbits were implanted bilaterally in the midbrain with a pair of monopolar stimulating electrodes. Ten days after surgery they were made pseudopregnant and, starting 1 week later, they received electrical stimulation through the implanted electrodes with a train of square-wave pulses twice daily for 11 days. The stimulated animals were brought from the animal house to the laboratory for their periods of stimulation. They sat quietly in their wicker baskets chewing hay, greenstuff, or preferably the basket itself, and appeared quite untroubled by the stimulation. Control implanted, but unstimulated, animals were also brought into the laboratory at the same time, while another group received injections of exogenous prolactin during the same eleven days of pseudopregnancy. At autopsy on the day following the end of stimulation, the mammary glands were assessed for lactogenic responses

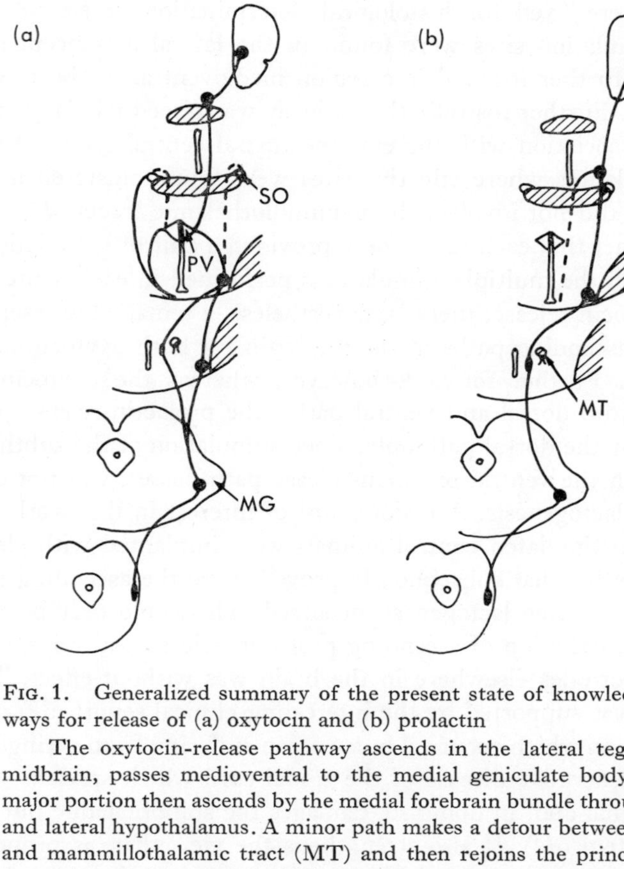

FIG. 1. Generalized summary of the present state of knowledge of the pathways for release of (a) oxytocin and (b) prolactin

The oxytocin-release pathway ascends in the lateral tegmentum of the midbrain, passes medioventral to the medial geniculate body (MG) and the major portion then ascends by the medial forebrain bundle through subthalamus and lateral hypothalamus. A minor path makes a detour between third ventricle and mammillothalamic tract (MT) and then rejoins the principal path in the lateral hypothalamus after which the common pathway makes contact with the tip of the paraventricular nucleus (PV) by collaterals (*16*, *46*, *48*, *51*, *52*, *54*). Another oxytocin-release pathway descends from the region of the hippocampal rudiment in the frontal pole to the PV nucleus (*60*). The question of whether the supraoptic nucleus (SO) is activated directly by suckling or indirectly *via* PV neurones requires investigation. Efferent fibers pass from PV and SO nuclei to the median eminence and thence to the neurohypophysis.

The ascending path for prolactin release follows a similar trajectory in the midbrain, but in the diencephalon it appears to utilize the route between third ventricle and MT on its way to the lateral hypothalamus and preoptic area. A descending path passes from orbitofrontal (sulcal) cortex to preoptic area. The common path then moves medially and briefly caudally before terminating in the medial anterior hypothalamic area. It has been postulated that the stimulus of suckling may switch off a neurone or a short chain of neurones between anterior hypothalamus and median eminence which control dopamine release from arcuate neurons (*44*, *47*, *49*).

and brains were fixed for histological determination of electrode sites. Effective stimulation sites were found in the lateral mesencephalic tegmentum and further forward in a region medioventral to the medial geniculate body. Further rostrally the pathway was traced medially and then rostrally in association with the extreme rostral central grey to the posterior hypothalamus where effective sites were found clustered in the vicinity of, but did not involve, the mammillothalamic tracts (*44*). Bearing in mind the fact that each rabbit only provided a pair of stimulation sites, compared with the multiple stimulations performed in each acute experiment on oxytocin release, there is, nevertheless, a remarkable resemblance between the ascending paths in the midbrain for both oxytocin and prolactin release. Further forward, however, whereas the oxytocin-release path divides into dorsal and ventral paths, the prolactin-release path appears to follow the dorsal path only, since stimulation of the subthalamus, through which the ventral oxytocin-release path passes, was not effective in triggering lactogenesis. A major point of interest in this work was the fact that if unstimulated control animals were implanted with electrodes whose tips lay in what subsequently proved to be the ascending path for prolactin release, then lactogenesis occurred. This could only be attributed to physical irritation of ascending prolactin-release pathways, since insertion of electrodes elsewhere in the brain was without effect. This interpretation was supported by the interesting clinical report (*32*) of spontaneous lactation which occurred in a woman suffering from syringomyelia. This is a degenerative disease of the spinal cord which spreads out from the central canal and, in doing so, damages the spinothalamic but not the lemniscal system (*44*). It also strengthens the view that, as proposed for oxytocin release, the spinothalamic system carries the burden of sensory traffic from the mammary gland to the mesencephalon.

In the second series of experiments carried out on the rabbit, the prolactin-release pathway was traced further rostrally. The technique was also modified slightly, so that each animal was implanted with a single bipolar electrode on one side of the brain only, and the twice-daily periods of stimulation were reduced from 30 to 15 min each. Even so, the electrical stimulation may have been superfluous and simple mechanical irritation may well be a powerful enough tool to investigate prolactin-release pathways in the chronic rabbit preparation (*47*). The position of the pathway which we had found in the earlier work to ascend from the midbrain and enter the posterior hypothalamus between the third ventricle and the mammillothalamic tracts was confirmed, and it was then traced rostrally in the mediodorsal hypothalamus, thence to the far-lateral hypothalamus within the medial forebrain bundle, forward to the lateral preoptic area, medially to the medial preoptic area and the pathway was then traced for a short distance caudally, where it appeared to terminate in the medial anterior hypothalamic area. In addition, a pathway was traced which appeared to descend from the orbitofrontal (sulcal) cortex *via* claustrum and external capsule and to merge with the ascending path in the preoptic area.

By this time, a radioimmunoassay had become available, and we then embarked on a series of experiments on the rat, in which blood samples were assayed for their prolactin content before and after electrical stimulation of the brain (*49*). Initial experiments under urethane anesthesia were uniformly unsuccessful, and it may have been a fortuitous decision to carry out the earlier work in the conscious rabbit, since there is considerable evidence that anesthetics may interfere grossly with studies of prolactin release (*42*). We decided, therefore, not to use anesthesia, and after initial surgery under the short-acting barbiturate methohexitone sodium the rats were decorticated except for frontal cortex, and their brainstems were transected at the mid-collicular level to preclude any possibility of pain. Two stimulation sites were explored in each animal and electrode sites were verified histologically, as before. This more extensive study in the rat permitted exploration of far more stimulation sites than had been possible with the slow and laborious lactogenic assay method and it confirmed our findings in the rabbit, despite the limitations of the earlier technique. Again, the pathway terminated some distance from the median eminence in the mediobasal anterior hypothalamus.

There is now a general concensus that the hypothalamic prolactin-inhibiting factor is, in fact, dopamine (*25*, *43*) and it was concluded (*49*) that the ascending path for prolactin release which had been traced in the brainstem may be activated during suckling-induced release of prolactin, that the descending path from the frontal pole of the brain may be concerned with reinforcing this release and that, at least in the rat, it might play a role in the olfactory-mediated release of prolactin which is known to occur at a particular stage of lactation in this species (*13*, *43*). It was postulated that the mechanism of action of the suckling stimulus in triggering prolactin release was to inhibit, at the mediobasal anterior hypothalamic level, a neuron or short chain of neurones which controlled the function of the arcuate dopaminergic neurons. It was envisaged that the stimulus might temporarily switch off the release of dopamine into the pituitary portal blood vessels, thus allowing a surge release of prolactin to occur. When the effect of the stimulus wears off, after a minute or two in the case of species that suckle for only short periods at a time, then a trickle of dopamine release would be resumed and further prolactin release would be arrested.

As regards the nature of the transmitter involved in the arrest of dopamine release and hence the release of prolactin during suckling, it is known that serotonin (5-hydroxytryptamine) is essential for the suckling-induced release of prolactin in the lactating rat, since inhibition of serotonin synthesis abolishes the release without affecting basal circulating levels of prolactin (*17*) while suckling of the normal animal is accompanied by a fall in hypothalamic content of dopamine and serotonin, and a rise in a product of serotonin metabolism, 5-hydroxyindole acetic acid (*26*). Studies with a specific serotonin uptake inhibitor, fluoxetine, and a serotonin agonist, quipazine, also reinforce the view that serotonin receptor activation leads to release of prolactin (*7*). In this context, the route taken by serotonergic fibers which ascend from the midbrain in the dorsal longitudinal fasciculus to enter the medial forebrain bundle (*28*) has much in common with the ascending path for prolactin release. It could be envisaged, therefore, that some ascending fibers of the spinothalamic system may link up with serotonergic neurons in the mesodiencephalic boundary region which could then transmit the suckling-induced message to the anterior hypothalamus. Serotonin, therefore, would appear to be a neurotransmitter of major importance in the suckling-induced release of prolactin, although acetylcholine (see *43* for references) and histamine (*1*, *18*) may also be involved in the overall control of prolactin secretion. The role of gamma-aminobutyric acid (GABA) is not clear at present. On one hand it has been reported to cause release of prolactin (*27*, *29*) while on the other it has been suggested that GABA may be a prolactin-inhibiting factor, in addition to dopamine (*38*).

The existence of a physiologically-meaningful prolactin-releasing factor (PRF) which can act in its own right on the pituitary has not yet been proved. Although thyrotrophin-releasing hormone (TRH) has the ability to cause the release of prolactin, this may be a pharmacological, rather than a physiological, property of the molecule (see *43* for references). However, even if TRH does not appear to be involved in reflex release of prolactin, it may be concerned in some way with the modulation of prolactin secretion (*31*). The recent discovery of peptides which represent particular amino acid sequences of the β-lipotrophin molecule may yield other candidates for the role of a PRF. In this respect, methionine enkephalin has been shown to raise circulating prolactin levels *in vivo* when administered either subcutaneously, intravenously (*19*) or intraventricularly (*12*) and both methionine enkephalin and leucine enkephalin can evoke release of prolactin *in vitro* from monolayer cultures of rat pituitary. This suggests that each of the enkephalin pentapeptides may possibly be a natural PRF. In addition, β-endorphin, which represents the entire 61–91 sequence of the C-terminal fragment of β-lipotrophin, not only causes release of prolactin when given by the intraventricular (*12*), intravenous or intracisternal routes (*36*), but is ineffective *in vitro* on cultured rat pituitary cells (*36*) and also inhibits striatal dopamine release (*24*). This suggests that the ability of β-endorphin to evoke prolactin release might be attributable to inhibition of arcuate dopamine release.

The other major problem is to determine precisely how and why particular stimuli trigger prolactin release. The final sorting center would appear to be the preoptic-anterior hypothalamic region, but whether it is purely a question of connectivity, such that prolactin-releasing stimuli happen to be correctly wired to the appropriate mechanism, or whether a sophisticated decision-making mechanism exists at this level, should keep workers in this field gainfully occupied for the foreseeable future.

SUMMARY

In the guinea-pig and rabbit the central afferent pathway for release of oxytocin in the midbrain appears to be coexistent with the spinothalamic system. Further rostrally the main pathway was traced through the subthalamus to the medial forebrain bundle in the hypothalamus, from which collaterals are believed to make contact with the magnocellular neurosecretory nuclei. A minor path reaches the hypothalamus *via* the dorsal longitudinal fasciculus and rejoins the medial forebrain bundle. The afferent pathway in the rabbit is subject to intense central inhibition. The afferent path was explored in the midbrain of the goat where, although the path appears to be concentrated in the lateral tegmentum in the region of the spinothalamic system, it is more diffuse than in the other species studied.

Afferent pathways for release of prolactin were studied in the midbrain of the rabbit where a pathway could be distinguished in the lateral tegmentum, suggesting involvement of the spinothalamic system. The pathway was investigated further rostrally into the forebrain in both the rabbit and rat and was shown to enter the hypothalamus in the region between the third ventricle and the mammillothalamic tract. Further rostrally the path was traced to the mediodorsal hypothalamus and then to the medial forebrain bundle in the lateral hypothalamus in which it travelled to the lateral preoptic region. Here, the path appeared to move medially, and then, briefly, caudally to terminate in the medial anterior hypothalamus. Another pathway was traced which descended from orbitofrontal (sulcal) cortex to the preoptic area, where it merged with the ascending path. It has been postulated that the effect of suckling in evoking prolactin release is mediated by the stimulus inhibiting a neuron or a short chain of neurons which control dopamine release from the arcuate neurons into the portal vessels of the median eminence.

REFERENCES

1. Arakelian, M. C. and Libertun, C. (1977). H_1 and H_2 histamine receptor participation in the brain control of prolactin secretion. *Endocrinology* **100**, 890–895.
2. Aulsebrook, L. H. and Holland, R. C. (1969). Central regulation of oxytocin release with and without vasopressin release. *Am. J. Physiol.* **216**, 818–829.
3. Aulsebrook, L. H. and Holland, R. C. (1969). Central inhibition of oxytocin release. *Am. J. Physiol.* **216**, 830–842.
4. Ban, T. and Omukai, F. (1959). Experimental studies on the fiber connections of the amygdaloid nuclei in the rabbit. *J. Comp. Neurol.* **113**, 245–279.
5. Bandaranayake, R. C. (1971). A morphology of the accessory neurosecretory nuclei and of the retrochiasmatic part of the supraoptic nucleus of the rat. *Acta Anat.* **80**, 14–22.
6. Bisset, G. W. (1974). Milk ejection. In *Handbook of Physiology*, sect. 7, vol. IV, Part 1, pp. 493–520. Washington, D. C.: American Physiol. Soc.
7. Clemens, J. A., Sawyer, B. D., and Cerimele, B. (1977). Further evidence that serotonin is a neurotransmitter involved in the control of prolactin secretion. *Endocrinology* **100**, 692–698.
8. Cowie, A. T. and Tindal, J. S. (1971). *The Physiology of Lactation.* London: Edward Arnold.
9. Cross, B. A. (1961). Neural control of lactation. In *Milk: the Mammary Gland and Its Secretion*, vol. 1, ed. Kon, S. K. and Cowie, A. T., pp. 229–277. New York, London: Academic Press.
10. Cross, B. A. and Dyball, R.E.J. (1974). Central pathways for neurohypophysial hormone release. In *Handbook of Physiology*, sect. 7, vol. IV, Part 1, pp. 269–285. Washington, D. C.: American Physiol. Soc.
11. Cross, B. A., Dyball, R.E.J., Dyer, R. G., Jones, C. W., Lincoln, D. W.,

Morris, J. F., and Pickering, B. T. (1975). Endocrine neurons. *Recent Prog. Horm. Res.* **31**, 243–294.

12. Dupont, A., Cusan, L., Labrie, F., Coy, D. H., and Li, C. H. (1977). Stimulation of prolactin release in the rat by intraventricular injection of beta-endorphin and methionine-enkephalin. *Biochem. Biophys. Res. Commun.* **75**, 76–82.
13. Grosvenor, C. E. and Mena, F. (1974). Neural and hormonal control of milk secretion and milk ejection. In *Lactation*, vol. 1, ed. Larson, B. L. and Smith, V. R., pp. 227–276. New York, London: Academic Press.
14. Holmes, R. L. and Ball, J. N. (1974). *The Pituitary Gland. A Comparative Account.* Cambridge: Cambridge University Press.
15. Knaggs, G. S., McNeilly, A. S., and Tindal, J. S. (1972). The afferent pathway of the milk-ejection reflex in the mid-brain of the goat. *J. Endocrinol.* **52**, 333–341.
16. Knaggs, G. S., Tindal, J. S., and Turvey, A. (1971). Paraventricular-hypophysial neurosecretory pathways in the guinea-pig. *J. Endocrinol.* **50**, 153–162.
17. Kordon, C., Blake, C. A., Terkel, J., and Sawyer, C. H. (1973/74). Participation of serotonin-containing neurons in the suckling-induced rise in plasma prolactin levels in lactating rats. *Neuroendocrinology* **13**, 213–223.
18. Libertun, C. and McCann, S. M. (1976). The possible role of histamine in the control of prolactin and gonadotropin release. *Neuroendocrinology* **20**, 110–120.
19. Lien, E. L., Fenichel, R. L., Garsky, V., Sarantakis, D., and Grant, N. H. (1976). Enkephalin-stimulated prolactin release. *Life Sci.* **19**, 837–840.
20. Lincoln, D. W. (1974). Dynamics of oxytocin secretion. In *Neurosecretion—the Final Neuroendocrine Pathway*, ed. Knowles, F. and Vollrath, L., pp. 129–133. Berlin: Springer-Verlag.
21. Lincoln, D. W., Hill, A., and Wakerley, J. B. (1973). The milk-ejection reflex of the rat: An intermittent function not abolished by surgical levels of anaesthesia. *J. Endocrinol.* **57**, 459–476.
22. Lincoln, D. W. and Wakerley, J. B. (1974). Electrophysiological evidence for the activation of supraoptic neurones during the release of oxytocin. *J. Physiol.* **242**, 533–554.
23. Lincoln, D. W. and Wakerley, J. B. (1975). Factors governing the periodic activation of supraoptic and paraventricular neurosecretory cells during suckling in the rat. *J. Physiol.* **250**, 443–461.
24. Loh, H. H., Brase, D. A., Sampath-Khanna, S., Mar, J. B., Way, E. L., and Li, C. H. (1976). β-Endorphin *in vitro* inhibition of striatal dopamine release. *Nature* **264**, 567–568.
25. MacLeod, R. M. (1976). Regulation of prolactin secretion. In *Frontiers in*

Neuroendocrinology, vol. 4, ed. Martini, L. and Ganong, W. F., pp. 169–194. New York: Raven Press.

26. Mena, F., Enjalbert, A., Carbonell, L., Priam, M., and Kordon, C. (1976). Effect of suckling on plasma prolactin and hypothalamic monoamine levels in the rat. *Endocrinology* **99**, 445–451.
27. Mioduszewski, R., Grandison, L., and Meites, J. (1976). Stimulation of prolactin release in rats by GABA. *Proc. Soc. Exp. Biol. Med.* **151**, 44–46.
28. Pasquier, D. A. and Reinoso-Suarez. F. Unpublished work quoted by Pasquier, D. A. and Reinoso-Suarez, F. (1976). Direct projections from hypothalamus to hippocampus in the rat demonstrated by retrograde transport of horseradish peroxidase. *Brain Res.* **108**, 165–169.
29. Pass, K. A. and Ondo, J. G. (1977). Effects of gamma-aminobutyric acid on prolactin and gonadotropin secretion in unanesthetized rat. *Endocrinology* **100**, 1437–1442.
30. Pfaff, D. W. and Keiner, M. (1973). Estradiol-concentrating cells in the rat amygdala as part of a limbic-hypothalamic hormone-sensitive system. In *The Neurobiology of the Amygdala*, ed. Eleftheriou, B. E., pp. 775–785. New York: Plenum.
31. Reichlin, S., Saperstein, R., Jackson, I.M.D., Boyd, A. E., III, and Patel, Y. (1976). Hypothalamic hormones. *Ann. Rev. Physiol.* **38**, 389–424.
32. Relkin, R. (1967). Neurologic pathways involved in lactation. *Dis. Nerv. Syst.* **28**, 94–97.
33. Richard, P. (1970). An electrophysiological study in the ewe of the tracts which transmit impulses from the mammary glands to the pituitary stalk. *J. Endocrinol.* **47**, 37–44.
34. Richard, P. (1972). The reticulo-hypothalamic pathway controlling the release of oxytocin in the ewe. *J. Endocrinol.* **53**, 71–83.
35. Richard, P., Urban, I., and Denamur, R. (1970). The role of the dorsal tracts of the spinal cord and of the mesencephalic and thalamic lemniscal system in the milk-ejection reflex during milking in the ewe. *J. Endocrinol.* **47**, 45–53.
36. Rivier, C., Vale, W., Ling, N., Brown, M., and Guillemin, R. (1977). Stimulation *in vivo* of secretion of prolactin and growth hormone by beta-endorphin. *Endocrinology* **100**, 238–241.
37. Rustioni, A. (1977). Spinal neurons project to the dorsal column nuclei of rhesus monkeys. *Science* **196**, 656–658.
38. Schally, A. V., Redding, T. W., Arimura, A., Dupont, A., and Linthicum, G. L. (1977). Isolation of gamma-aminobutyric acid from pig hypothalami and demonstration of its prolactin release-inhibiting (PIF) activity *in vivo* and *in vitro*. *Endocrinology* **100**, 681–691.
39. Stumpf, W. E. and Sar, M. (1971). Estradiol concentrating neurons in the amygdala. *Proc. Soc. Exp. Biol. Med.* **136**, 102–106.

40. Taleisnik, S. and Deis, R. P. (1964). Influence of cerebral cortex in inhibition of oxytocin release induced by stressful stimuli. *Am. J. Physiol.* **207**, 1394–1398.

41. Tindal, J. S. (1965). The forebrain of the guinea-pig in stereotaxic coordinates. *J. Comp. Neurol.* **124**, 259–266.

42. Tindal, J. S. (1974). Hypothalamic control of secretion and release of prolactin. *J. Reprod. Fert.* **39**, 437–461.

43. Tindal, J. S. (1978). Neuroendocrine control of lactation. In *Lactation*, vol. IV, ed. Larson, B. L. New York, London: Academic Press (in press).

44. Tindal, J. S. and Knaggs, G. S. (1969). An ascending pathway for release of prolactin in the brain of the rabbit. *J. Endocrinol.* **45**, 111–120.

45. Tindal, J. S. and Knaggs, G. S. (1970). Environmental stimuli and the mammary gland. *Mem. Soc. Endocrinol.* **18**, 239–258.

46. Tindal, J. S. and Knaggs, G. S. (1971). Determination of the detailed hypothalamic route of the milk-ejection reflex in the guinea-pig. *J. Endocrinol.* **50**, 135–152.

47. Tindal, J. S. and Knaggs, G. S. (1972). Pathways in the forebrain of the rabbit concerned with the release of prolactin. *J. Endocrinol.* **52**, 253–262.

48. Tindal, J. S. and Knaggs, G. S. (1975). Further studies on the afferent path of the milk-ejection reflex in the brainstem of the rabbit. *J. Endocrinol.* **66**, 107–113.

49. Tindal, J. S. and Knaggs, G. S. (1977). Pathways in the forebrain of the rat concerned with the release of prolactin. *Brain Res.* **119**, 211–221.

50. Tindal, J. S., Knaggs, G. S., and Turvey, A. (1967). Central nervous control of prolactin secretion in the rabbit: Effect of local oestrogen implants in the amygdaloid complex. *J. Endocrinol.* **37**, 279–287.

51. Tindal, J. S., Knaggs, G. S., and Turvey, A. (1967). The afferent path of the milk-ejection reflex in the brain of the guinea-pig. *J. Endocrinol.* **38**, 337–349.

52. Tindal, J. S., Knaggs, G. S., and Turvey, A. (1968). Preferential release of oxytocin from the neurohypophysis after electrical stimulation of the afferent path of the milk-ejection reflex in the brain of the guinea-pig. *J. Endocrinol.* **40**, 205–214.

53. Tindal, J. S., Knaggs, G. S., and Turvey, A. (1968). The forebrain of the goat in stereotaxic coordinates. *J. Anat.* (*London*) **103**, 457–469.

54. Tindal, J. S., Knaggs, G. S., and Turvey, A. (1969). The afferent path of the milk-ejection reflex in the brain of the rabbit. *J. Endocrinol.* **43**, 663–671.

55. Ungerstedt, U. (1971). Stereotaxic mapping of the monoamine pathways in the rat brain. *Acta Physiol. Scand.* **82**, Suppl. **367**.

56. Urban, I., Moss, R. L., and Cross, B. A. (1971). Problems in electrical stimulation of afferent pathways for oxytocin release. *J. Endocrinol.* **51**, 347–358.

57. Voloschin, L. M. and Dottaviano, E. J. (1976). The channeling of natural stimuli that evoke the ejection of milk in the rat. Effect of transections in the midbrain and hypothalamus. *Endocrinology* **99**, 49–58.
58. Voloschin, L. M. and Tramezzani, J. H. (1973). The neural input of the milk ejection reflex in the hypothalamus. *Endocrinology* **92**, 973–983.
59. Warembourg, M. (1977). Radioautographic localization of estrogen-concentrating cells in the brain and pituitary of the guinea pig. *Brain Res.* **123**, 357–362.
60. Woods, W. H., Holland, R. C., and Powell, E. W. (1969). Connections of cerebral structures functioning in neurohypophysial hormone release. *Brain Res.* **12**, 26–46.
61. Yamashita, H., Koizumi, K., and Brooks, C. McC. (1970). Electrophysiological studies of neurosecretory cells in the cat hypothalamus. *Brain Res.* **20**, 462–466.

II – 8

8-II

HORMONE SECRETION AT LACTOGENESIS AND DURING LACTATION IN DAIRY FARM ANIMALS

Tetsu Johke

Department of Physiology, National Institute of Animal Industry, Chiba, Japan

It has been well established that hormones control mammary growth, initiation and maintenance of lactation (*17*, *19*). The essential hormones for lactogenesis in mice and rats observed *in vivo* are prolactin (PRL) and glucocorticoids (*19*). PRL, glucocorticoid, and insulin are also required *in vitro* (*19*). In goats and sheep, a combination of PRL, glucocorticoids, growth hormone (GH), and thyroid horomone is essential for restoration of milk secretion after pituitary ablation (*15–17*, *19*). Such experiments with cows have not yet been carried out *in vivo*.

In the last decade, the changes of hormone concentration in the blood during mammary growth, lactogenesis, and lactation in ruminants have been studied using radioassay techniques.

In this paper, our studies on the concentration of PRL, GH, thyrotropin (TSH) and triiodothyronine (T3) in the blood during lactogenesis and lactation in dairy cows and goats, as well as related studies by other investigators are described. For recent comprehensive reviews on hormonal control of the mammary gland function, the readers are referred to numerous reviews (*2*, *14*, *17*, *19*, *23*, *29*, *63*, *92*).

1. Methods of Radioimmunoassay

Introduction of the radioimmunoassay into the field of endocrinology has revolutionized techniques for assay of hormones in the blood (*3*, *98*). With this technique, it has become possible to assay a series of pg to ng levels of immunoreactive proteins and steroid hormones in the blood (*39*). The methods are all based on the same fundamental principle: the highly-specific reaction between a radioisotope labeled or non-labeled hormone and its corresponding antibodies. In recent years, developments of the radioimmunoassay technique for PRL, GH, and TSH in ruminants have been studied in our laboratory. Contrary to steroid hormones or thyroid hormones, pituitary PRL, GH, and TSH show more or less immunological species specificities. Furthermore, it has not always been easy to obtain antisera to these hormones which have specific reaction and high affinity. There have been no commercial sources for antisera to these hormones. Therefore, the successful development of radioimmunoassay for these anterior pituitary hormones mainly depended on production of suitable antisera.

1) *PRL*

A specific and sensitive radioimmunoassay for bovine PRL has been developed (*41*, *42*, *47*). Antisera to PRL were obtained from guinea pigs immunized with bovine PRL emulsified with Freund's complete adjuvant. Purified bovine or ovine PRL was iodinated with ^{131}I or ^{125}I by the chloramine T method. The separation of free and antibody-bound radioiodinated PRL was accomplished by the double antibody method. This assay method was able to determine PRL concentration in as little as 1 ng/ml of plasma or serum. Bovine PRL in plasma and pituitary extracts produced an identical dose response curve obtained by the purified bovine PRL preparation. Caprine PRL in plasma and pituitary extract can also be estimated using ovine PRL as the standard hormone. The binding of the antibody to radioiodinated PRL was not inhibited by other pituitary hormones. Neither was a change in the immunoreactive PRL concentration observed during storage for a year at −20°C, nor was a difference in PRL concentration in plasma and serum from the same blood sample detected. PRL concentrations in blood from cattle and goats were determined with bovine PRL (NIH-P-B2) and ovine PRL (NIH-P-S8), respectively, as the standard hormones.

2) *GH*

Antisera to bovine GH were prepared in monkeys (crab-eating macaque). The separation of free and antibody-bound ^{125}I-bovine GH was accomplished by the double antibody method (*47*). In the homologous radioimmunoassay for bovine GH, bovine plasma and pituitary extract inhibited the reaction between ^{125}I-GH and the antibody to GH in the same way as standard bovine or ovine GH. Caprine plasma and pituitary extracts also inhibited the reaction identically with purified ovine or bovine GH. Pituitary hormones other than GH up to 100 ng did not show any significant change in the percentage of antibody-bound ^{125}I-GH. The maximum sensitivity was 1 ng/ml in plasma (*47*). GH concentration in blood from cows and goats were determined with bovine GH (NIH-GH-B16) and ovine GH (NIH-GH-S9), respectively, as the standard hormones.

3) *TSH and T3*

TSH was determined by the double antibody method (*37*). Plasma TSH concentrations in cattle and goats were determined with NIH-TSH-B7 as the standard hormone. Plasma T3 was determined by T3 radioimmunoassay kits (Dinabot Radioisotope Laboratory).

2. *Serum Hormone Levels during Late Pregnancy and Early Lactation in Dairy Cows and Goats*

During the late stage of pregnancy, bovine serum PRL was maintained at a relatively low level (*44*, *48*). A conspicuous rise in circulating PRL levels occurred at the end of pregnancy. Peak values were observed from one day before the day of parturition (*44*, *48*). The PRL surge around parturition continued for 2 to 3 days (Fig. 1). Basal bovine plasma PRL levels in the early stage of lactation were not different from those in the late stage of pregnancy. Similar changes in bovine PRL in the blood around calving have been reported by other researchers (*22*, *38*, *76*). Bovine serum GH levels during late pregnancy were also low until the end of pregnancy (Fig. 1). The highest levels were observed on the day of parturition (*38*, *48*, *69*). Postpartum, the mean serum GH level was higher than that during late pregnancy, though considerable day to day variation was observed (*48*). Plasma T3 concentrations decreased postpartum (*48*), while no marked change in serum TSH level was observed around parturition (Johke and Hodate, unpublished). A low serum thyroxine level during late stage of pregnancy was also reported (*83*).

In goats, serum PRL levels were low during late pregnancy and increased 2 to 3 days before parturition (*9*, *31*, *44*, *50*). A peak value of PRL was usually obtained on the day before parturition. A marked elevation of PRL concentration in the blood near parturition has also

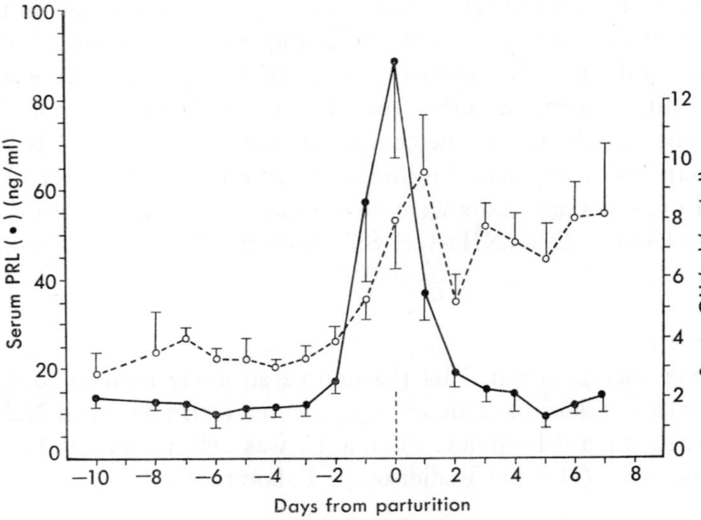

FIG. 1. Serum PRL and GH concentrations in dairy cows during late pregnancy and early lactation

The cows calved in September. Mean±SE. (From Johke, T. and Hodate, K. (1977). *Japan. J. Zootech. Sci.* **48**, 772–776).

been observed in sheep (*18*, *25*). Serum GH concentration increased 1 to 2 days before parturition and reached a peak on the day of kidding (*50*). Postpartum, a marked day to day variation was observed. A transient decrease in serum T3 concentration occurred on the day before parturition (*50*). During later stages of pregnancy, high placental lactogen concentration in the blood may suppress PRL and GH secretion of the pituitary gland in cows and goats. Bovine and caprine placental lactogen have both PRL-like and GH-like activities (*5*, *10*, *54*).

Recent determinations by radioassay also revealed changes in several circulating steroid hormones during pregnancy and lactation in ruminants (*14*, *23*). Peripheral estrogen concentrations in bovine plasma increased linearly during the last 3 weeks of pregnancy (*12*, *14*, *35*, *36*, *74*, *85*). Peak values were observed immediately before parturition (*12*, *14*). Precipitous drops in plasma progesterone levels occurred at the end of pregnancy (*14*, *23*, *24*, *85*). A transient increase (*85*) or no increase (*12*) in maternal peripheral plasma glucocorticoid was observed around parturition. Concentration of prostaglandin F (PGF) in the uterine vein increased markedly near parturition (*24*).

In goats, similar changes in concentrations of estrogen and progesterone in peripheral plasma at the end of pregnancy have been observed (*87*, *95*). Caprine PGF concentration in the vena caval plasma near parturition paralleled that in the uterine vein (*95*).

Although many factors in the elevation of serum PRL and GH in ruminants have been studied, the factor or factors which enhance PRL and GH secretion around parturition in cows and goats have not been well established. One of the possibilities is the conspicuous increase in circulating levels of estrogen and the precipitous drop in progesterone. Administration of estrogen elevated plasma concentrations of PRL (*78*) and GH (*89*) in cows. Another possibility is the effect of stress associated with parturition. It has been found that stressful stimuli enhanced PRL release in cattle and goats (*41*, *43*, *90*). Bovine GH did not respond to stress such as venipuncture (*47*, *90*). However, there is the possibility that GH responds to "severe" stress such as parturition. Removal of the fetus by caesarian section induced a marked increase in plasma concentrations of PRL and GH in cows (*81*). Although $PGF_{2\alpha}$ administration induced a marked increase in plasma concentrations of PRL and GH in heifers (*64*), the physiological significance of circulating PGF for enhanced secretion of both hormones near parturition has not been elucidated. The elevated circulating levels of PRL and GH around parturition may accelerate lactogenesis. It has been demonstrated that the decrease in PRL secretion during late pregnancy and postpartum by 2-Br-α-ergocryptine administration depressed lactogenesis (*46*, *49*, *79*).

3. Effect of 2-Br-α-Ergocryptine on Serum Hormone Concentration and Lactogenesis in Cows and Goats

Subcutaneous administration of a potent PRL inhibitor, 2-Br-α-ergocryptine methane sulfonate (CB154: Sandoz Co., Basel) to multiparous Holstein cows during the 2 weeks before parturition induced a decrease in basal serum PRL levels and complete disappearance of the PRL surge around parturition (*46*, *49*). Serum PRL concentration during 2 weeks postpartum was less than 2 ng/ml. In all cases, lactogenesis was not completely but partially inhibited (*49*). The mean milk production of three cows during the week postpartum was 58.5% (33.6–72.7%) of that obtained in the previous lactation. It needed 30 to 50 days to regain the milk production of the previous lactation (Fig. 2). Simultaneous administration of an antiserum to bovine PRL to a CB154-treated cow near parturi-

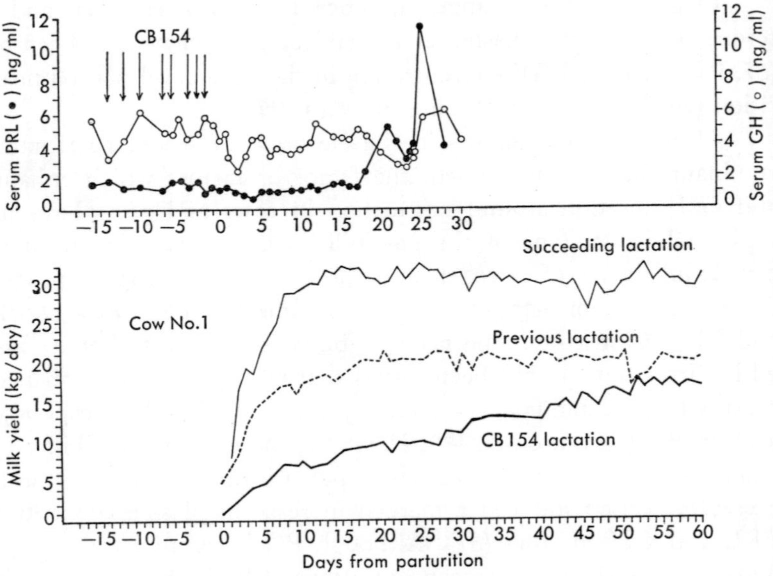

FIG. 2. Effects of CB154 on serum PRL, GH, and milk production during lactogenesis in a cow

One hundred mg of CB154 was administered 8 times s.c. to the cow from the 2nd to 14th day prepartum. The milk yield after CB154 is compared to those of previous and subsequent lactations. (From Johke, T. and Hodate, K. (1978). *Endocrinol. Japon.* **25**, 67–74).

tion induced a 93% decrease in milk production immediately after parturition as compared to the previous lactation (*49*). Milk production during the week postpartum was 43.7% of that of the previous lactation. Previous milk production levels were not regained even 50 days after parturition. Schams *et al.* (*79*), reported a greater depression of lactogenesis (5–53.1% of milk production of the previous lactation) in CB154-treated Brown Swiss cows. Milk yield in two cows decreased to 72–78% of that of the previous lactation after CB154 administration immediately before parturition (*26*).

The concentrations of total milk protein, IgG, and β-lactoglobulin in colostrum from CB154-administered cows were significantly higher than those from untreated cows (*49*). On the contrary, concentration of α-lactalbumin in colostrum from cows administered a PRL inhibitor was 40% of that of the untreated cows (*49*). Concentrations of lactose and α-lactalbumin on the 6th day postpartum were also significantly lower than those of normal cows (*49*). A significant decrease in the concentration of caseins was also detected (*55*).

In contrast to the uniform decrease in circulating levels of PRL, a marked individual difference in suppression of lactogenesis was observed (*49*, *79*). Several possibilities exist which could cause different responses in lactogenesis to PRL-inhibitor administration. One of the possibilities is the individual difference in the commencement of milk synthesis before parturition. The cow mammary gland can synthesize milk before parturition and the milk yield obtained by prepartum milking varied markedly from cow to cow (*75*, *100*). There was also a marked individual difference in the contents of acid-soluble phosphates and lactose in mammary secretions during the month prepartum in cows (*40*).

In mice and rats, progesterone directly inhibited lactose synthesis in the mammary gland during pregnancy (*66*, *94*). The precipitous decrease in the circulating levels of progesterone immediately before parturition has been considered to be the trigger to lactogenesis (*59*, *66*, *94*). The difference in the levels of progesterone and estrogen in the blood or activity of the hormone receptor of the mammary gland epithelial cells might affect prepartum milk synthesis in the cow. It seems likely that estrogen and progesterone have key roles in mammogenesis and lactogenesis in cows (*14*, *23*). Another possibility is the effect of galactopoietic hormones other than PRL. It has been established that GH and the thyroid hormone have potent galactopoietic activities in lactating cows (*65*). Administration of CB154 did not depress serum GH and T3 levels (*49*). Placental lactogen may also participate in lactogenesis in cows. Serum placental lactogen levels in CB154-administered cows during late pregnancy (determined by radioreceptor assay) were not low as compared with untreated cows (*49*). Turkington and Hill (*94*) demonstrated that the human placental lactogen can replace ovine PRL in lactogenesis in the mouse mammary gland *in vitro*. Unlike placental lactogen in humans, rats or sheep (*54*), the PRL-like activity of bovine placental lactogen was only 5% that of bovine PRL (*5*). Such low PRL-like activity of bovine placental lactogen may participate only in a small way in lactogenesis. Depression of feed intake was not detected in CB154-administered cows. Therefore, it seems likely that the depression or retardedness of lactogenesis in the cows treated with CB154 is caused mainly by a decrease in circulating PRL levels around parturition. As in the case of small laboratory animals, PRL or PRL-like activity seems to be essential for lactogenesis in the cow mammary gland *in vitro* (*11*, *20*). Lactose synthesis is considered to be the rate-limiting factor in milk secretion. The control of lactose biosynthesis seems to be directly related to the concentration and rate of flow of α-lactalbumin (B protein of lactose synthetase) through the Golgi bodies of mammary epithelial cells (*21*). The concentration of α-lactalbumin in mammary secretions from untreated cows increased around parturition (Johke and Hodate, unpublished). PRL stimulates the formation of α-lactalbumin in the mouse mammary gland *in vitro* (*96*). The increase of the concentration of bovine IgG result from the depression in milk secretion. The transfer of bovine IgG from the blood serum to mammary secretions has been considered to be controlled mainly by estrogen and progesterone (*84*). The marked increase of β-lactoglobulin concentration in colostrum was rather unexpected and the reason for it is not clear. As in the case of α-lactalbumin, β-lactoglobulin is synthesized in the mammary gland (*62*).

These results suggest that depression of PRL secretions around parturition induced a decrease in α-lactalbumin and hence lactose synthesis in the cow mammary gland. Although low circulating PRL levels continued for more than 2 weeks postpartum, milk production progressively increased with repeated milking. Removal of milk from the mammary gland by milking and galactopoietic hormones including GH and thyroid hormone may favor the restoration of milk production in the cow. No trouble in calving nor abnormality of calves was observed after CB154 administration (*49*).

In goats, CB154 treatment during the 2 weeks prepartum depressed PRL secretion (*50*). The mean serum PRL level on the day before parturition was less than 3% (6.4 ng/ml) of the value in untreated goats (*50*). No effect of CB154 on serum concentrations of GH and T3 was observed (*50*). As compared to milk production in untreated goats, a marked depression of milk production was not detected in CB154-treated goats. One of the possible reasons for no marked depression of lactogenesis in the CB154-treated goats may be incomplete suppression of PRL secretion. Even with high doses of CB154 (3 times the dose per kg of body weight in cows), suppression of circulating PRL concentration was not complete and the duration of depression of PRL secretion postpartum was relatively short when compared to cows. Another possibility is the effect of hormones other than PRL. PRL-like activity in caprine placental lactogen was at least 3 times higher than that of cow (*50*, *54*). Placental lactogen may substitute for PRL in lactogenesis in goats. Although GH did not show any favorable direct effect on lactogenesis in the goat's mammary gland *in vitro* (*82*), there is a possibility that GH may act on the mammary gland *in vivo* through a mediator such as the somatomedins. No difference in maternal behavior was observed between the CB154-treated and untreated goats (*50*).

4. *Milking Stimulus and Release of Hormones*

A precipitous fall in the pituitary PRL store due to suckling stimulus has been demonstrated in lactating rats by bioassay (*28*). However, the effect of suckling or milking stimulus on circulating levels of PRL had not been assessed until application of the radioimmunoassay method. Using radioimmunoassay and cannulated animals, it has been demonstrated that milking stimulus induces a rapid and conspicuous rise in plasma PRL levels in lactating cows (*41*, *43*, *90*, *91*) and goats (*7*, *41*, *43*). In early lactation, plasma PRL rose within 2 min and reached a peak around 10 min after the start of milking (Figs. 3 and 4). The stage of

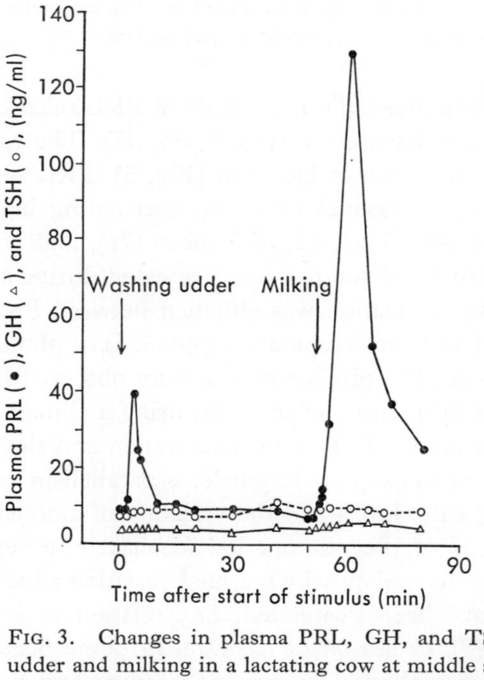

FIG. 3. Changes in plasma PRL, GH, and TSH concentrations by washing udder and milking in a lactating cow at middle stage of lactation

The cow's udder was washed for 1 min with warm water or milked for 5 min by machine. Blood samples were taken from a jugular venous catheter in May.

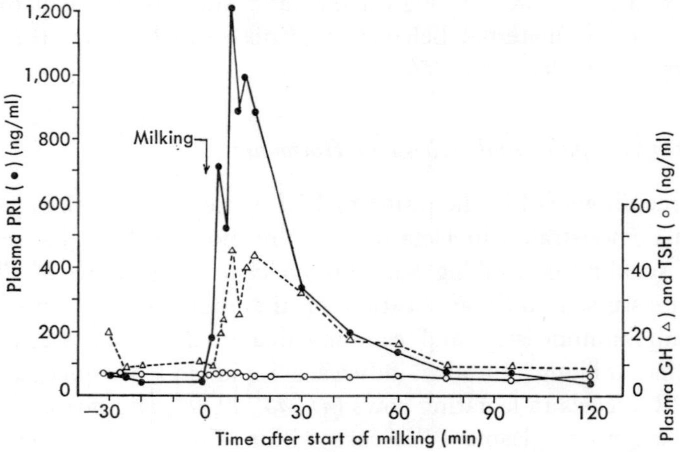

FIG. 4. Changes in plasma concentrations of PRL, GH, and TSH in a lactating goat due to milking

The goat was milked for 4 min by hand. Blood samples were taken from a jugular venous catheter in September, 2 months postpartum.

lactation as well as the season affect the magnitude of PRL release in response to milking stimulus in lactating cows (*45*, *46*, *57*). The response diminished markedly in later stages of lactation (Fig. 5). PRL secretion in ruminants shows a marked seasonal variation. Circulating basal and stimulated PRL level in cattle (*45–47*, *52*, *57*,) sheep (*71*), and goats (*8*, *45*, *46*) increased during spring and summer and decreased during autumn and winter. A high positive correlation was obtained between PRL concentration in the blood and ambient temperature (+0.835) or photoperiod (+0.764) in Holstein heifers (*46*). Similar results were observed in male (*8*) and non-lactating goats (*46*). In an experiment using a climate chamber, a parallelism of the variation of plasma concentration and the photoperiod was demonstrated in rams (*71*). In cattle, a parallelism between the variation of circulating PRL levels and the variation of ambient temperature (*93*, *97*) as well as of the photoperiod (*6*) has been reported. Though several possibilities to explain why seasonal variation affects PRL secretion in ruminants have been postulated, *i.e.*, relation to breeding season (*8*), salt retention (*8*), or season of lactation in domesticated and wild ruminants (*45*), its physiological significance remains to be elucidated.

A significant positive correlation (+0.460–+0.676) was obtained be-

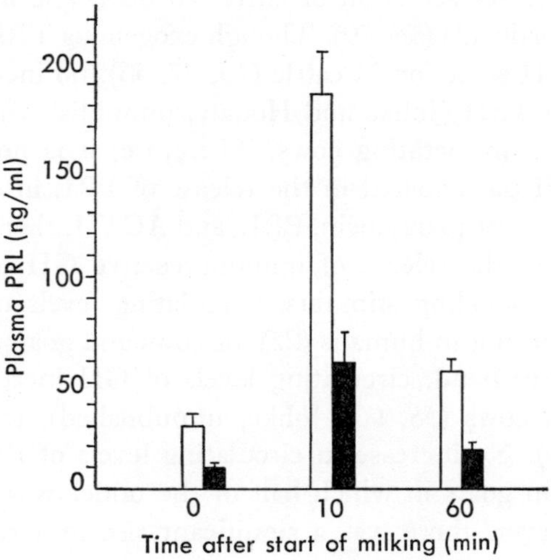

FIG. 5. Effect of season on the magnitude of PRL release due to milking in dairy cows

The peak value of plasma PRL was obtained 10 min after the commencement of milking. The peak value obtained in April–August was 4.7 times that in October–January. On the other hand, the increase rate of PRL after milking was approximately equal. Mean±SE. □ April–August (n=19); ■ October–January (n=8)

tween the peak plasma PRL level and milk production in cows, but not for the level immediately before milking within one season (*46*, *57*). Suckling stimulus caused a marked elevation in serum PRL in humans (*27*, *68*), rats (*1*, *4*, *30*, *99*), mice (*80*), and sheep (*61*).

PRL release due to tactile stimulus to the udder is often observed in non-lactating animals. Teat manipulation or sham-milking for 5 min can induce PRL release in non-lactating heifers and virgin goats (*43*). The pattern of PRL discharge in non-lactating heifers was similar to that in lactating cows (*43*, *73*). These results suggest that PRL release in response to udder manipulation is evoked by activation of the sensory nerve-hypothalamus-anterior pituitary reflex. It has been well established that milking stimulus discharges oxytocin from the posterior pituitary gland (*17*). On the other hand, administration of oxytocin to cows (*43*, *56*, *77*), goats (*43*; Johke, unpublished), and rats (*60*) did not stimulate PRL secretion markedly. Accordingly, it seems likely that oxytocin and PRL are independently discharged from the pituitary gland by milking. Suckling or milking stimulus also increases secretion of adrenocorticotropic hormone (ACTH) (*17*) and glucocorticoids (*58*, *70*). Though exogenous TRH stimulates TSH, PRL, and GH secretion in cattle (*13*, *47*, *53*), no increase in plasma GH (*46*, *90*) or in TSH (Johke and Hodate, unpublished) due to milking has been observed in lactating cows. Therefore, it is not likely that the endogenous TRH participated in the release of PRL in cows in response to milking. In contrast to oxytocin, PRL, and ACTH, there seems to be species differences in the release of immunoreactive GH or TSH in response to milking or suckling stimulus. Circulating levels of TSH rose in lactating rats (*4*) but not in humans (*27*), or cows and goats (Johke, unpublished). On the other hand, circulating levels of GH increased in goats (*32–34*), but not in cows (*58*, *90*; Johke, unpublished), rats (*80*), mice (*80*), or humans (*68*). No increase in circulating levels of PRL due to milking was observed in goats in which half of the udder was grafted onto the neck (*34*). However, there was a significant rise in circulating levels of GH.

5. *Effects of 2-Br-α-Ergocryptine on Hormone Secretion and Lactation*

Administration of CB154 to lactating cows and goats depressed the basal levels of plasma PRL and inhibited the release of PRL in response to milking (*26*, *32*, *51*, *86*). However, the resultant decrease in milk production varied from 0 to 30% of pretreatment milk yields. On the other hand, CB154 depressed lactation as well as circulating PRL in humans (*72*) and mice (*67*). Administration of antiserum to PRL also depressed lactation in rats (*88*). No decrease in circulating GH concentration was observed after CB154 treatment in lactating cows (*86*) and goats (*32*). These results indicate that once lactation is established, lactation can be maintained with very low circulating PRL concentration (less than 2 ng/ml). In hypophysectomized lactating goats, Cowie has already found that once milk production was restored by the administration of a combination of hormones including PRL, full lactation was maintained for over 3 weeks with GH, T3, and dexamethasone (*16*). It has also been known that GH shows potent galactopoietic effects, but PRL does not, in lactating cows and goats (*65*). The biochemical mechanism by which the mammary glands of cows and goats are able to maintain milk secretion with very low circulating levels of PRL remains to be elucidated. The physiological significance of PRL release in response to milking or suckling stimulus in lactating ruminants has also not been clarified. However, high circulating levels of PRL after milking or suckling may act to establish full lactation after parturition.

SUMMARY

Bovine and caprine serum concentrations of PRL, GH, and TSH during lactogenesis and lactation were determined by radioimmunoassay. Serum PRL was maintained low levels during the month prepartum in cows and goats. A conspicuous rise in circulating PRL levels occurs at the end of pregnancy. The peak values were observed from the day before to the day of parturition. Serum GH levels during late pregnancy remained low until the end of pregnancy. The concentration of serum GH rose around parturition. Elevation of serum TSH and T3 levels was not observed near parturition. Administration of 2-Br-α-ergocryptine (CB154) during the 2 weeks prepartum depressed circulating PRL levels and lactogenesis in cows. The mean milk production of four cows during the week postpartum was 54.8% of that obtained in previous lactations. Concentrations of α-lactalbumin and lactose also decreased significantly in milk from CB154-treated cows.

Milking stimulus induced a conspicuous but temporal increase in plasma PRL levels in lactating cows and goats. The response was greater in earlier stages of lactation than in later stages. Sham-milking also caused a PRL release in non-lactating animals. Rises in circulating TSH and T3 levels caused by milking were not observed in either cows or goats. Plasma GH levels in lactating goats increased due to milking but bovine GH levels did not. A marked seasonal variation in circulating PRL levels was observed in cattle and goats. Basal and stimulated plasma PRL concentrations were highest in summer and lowest in winter. Studies using CB154 indicate that cows and goats can maintain lactation with a very low circulating PRL level.

REFERENCES

1. Amenomori, Y., Chen, C. L., and Meites, J. (1970). Serum prolactin levels in rats during different reproductive states. *Endocrinology* **86**, 506–510.
2. Anderson, R. R. (1974). Endocrinological control. In *Lactation: A Comprehensive Treatise*, vol. 1, ed. Larson, B. L. and Smith, V. R., pp. 97–140. New York, London: Academic Press.
3. Berson, S. A. and Yalow, R. S. (1964). Immunoassay of protein hormones.

In *The Hormones*, vol. 4, ed. Pincus, G., Thimann, K. V., and Astwood, E. B., pp. 557–630. New York, London: Academic Press.
4. Blake, C. A. (1974). Stimulation of pituitary prolactin and TSH release in lactating and proestrus rats. *Endocrinology* **94**, 503–508.
5. Bolander, F. F., Jr., Ulberg, L. C., and Fellows, R. E. (1976). Circulating placental lactogen levels in dairy and beef cattle. *Endocrinology* **99**, 1273–1278.
6. Bourne, A. and Tucker, H. A. (1975). Serum prolactin and LH responses to photoperiod in bull calves. *Endocrinology* **97**, 435–475.
7. Bryant, G. D., Linzell, J. L., and Greenwood, F. C. (1970). Plasma prolactin in the blood of goats measured by radioimmunoassay: The effect of teat stimulation, mating behaviour, stress, fasting, oxytocin, insulin and glucose injections. *Hormones* **1**, 26–35.
8. Buttle, H. L. (1974). Seasonal variation of prolactin in plasma of male goats. *J. Reprod. Fert.* **37**, 95–99.
9. Buttle, H. L., Forsyth, I. A., and Knaggs, G. S. (1972). Plasma prolactin measured by radioimmunoassay and bioassay in pregnant and lactating goats and the occurrence of a placental lactogen. *J. Endocrinol.* **53**, 483–491.
10. Buttle, H. L. and Forsyth, I. A. (1976). Placental lactogen in the cow. *J. Endocrinol.* **68**, 141–146.
11. Collier, J. R., Bauman, D. E., and Hays, R. L. (1977). Lactogenesis in explant cultures of mammary tissue from pregnant cows. *Endocrinology* **100**, 1192–1200.
12. Comline, R. S., Hall, L. W., Labelle, R. B., Nathanielsz, P. W., and Silber, M. Parturition in the cow: Endocrine changes in animals with chronically implanted catheters in the foetal and maternal circulations. *J. Endocrinol.* **63**, 451–472.
13. Convey, E. M., Tucker, H. A., Smith, V. G., and Jolman, J. (1973). Bovine prolactin, growth hormone, thyroxine and corticoid response to thyrotropin releasing hormone. *Endocrinology* **92**, 471–476.
14. Convey, E. M. (1974). Serum hormone concentrations in ruminants during mammary growth, lactogenesis and lactation: A review. *J. Dairy Sci.* **57**, 905–917.
15. Cowie, A. T., Knaggs, G. S., and Tindal, J. S. (1964). Complete restoration of lactation in the goat after hypophysectomy. *J. Endocrinol.* **40**, 243–252.
16. Cowie, A. T. (1969). General hormonal factors involved in lactogenesis. In *Lactogenesis: The Initiation of Milk Secretion at Parturition*, ed. Reynolds, M. and Folley, S. J., pp. 157–169. Philadelphia, Pa.: Univ. Pennsylvania Press.
17. Cowie, A. T. and Tindal, J. S. (1971). The Physiology of Lactation. London: Edward Arnold.
18. Davis, S. L., Reichert, L. E., Jr., and Niswender, G. D. (1971). Serum level

of prolactin in sheep as measured by radioimmunoassay. *Biol. Reprod.* **4**, 145–153.

19. Denamur, R. (1971). Hormonal control of lactogenesis. *J. Dairy Res.* **38**, 237–264.
20. Djiane, J., Delouis, C., and Denamur, R. (1975). Lactogenesis in organ cultures of heifer's mammary tissue. *J. Endocrinol.* **65**, 453–454.
21. Ebner, K. E. and Schanbacher, F. S. (1974). Biochemistry of lactose and related carbohydrates. In *Lactation: A Comprehensive Treatise*, vol. 2, ed. Larson, B. L. and Smith, V. R., pp. 77–113. New York, London: Academic Press.
22. Edgerton, L. A. and Hafs, H. D. (1973). Serum LH, prolactin, glucocorticoid and progestin in dairy cows from calving to gestation. *J. Dairy Sci.* **56**, 451–458.
23. Erb, R. E. (1977). Hormonal control of mammogenesis and onset of lactation in cows—A review. *J. Dairy Sci.* **60**, 155–169.
24. Fairclough, R. J., Hunter, J. J., and Welch, R.A.S. (1975). Peripheral plasma progesterone and utero-ovarian prostaglandin F concentrations in the cow around parturition. *Prostaglandins* **9**, 901–914.
25. Fell, L. R., Beck, C., Brown, J. M., Catt, K. J., Cumming, I. A., and Goding, J. R. (1972). Solid-phase radioimmunoassay of ovine prolactin in antibody-coated tubes, prolactin secretion during estradiol treatment, at parturition and during milking. *Endocrinology* **91**, 1329–1336.
26. Fell, L. R., Chandler, N. J., and Goding, J. R. (1974). Effect of inhibition of prolactin secretion by 2-Br-α-ergocryptine at parturition and during lactation in dairy cows. *J. Reprod. Fert.* **36**, 480–481.
27. Gautvik, K. M., Weintraub, B. D., Graeber, C. T., Maloof, F., Zuckerman, J. E., and Tashjian, A. H., Jr. (1973). Serum prolactin and TSH: Effects of nursing and pyroGlu-His-ProNH_2 administration in postpartum women. *J. Clin. Endocrinol. Metab.* **36**, 135–139.
28. Grosvenor, C. E. and Turner, C. W. (1958). Pituitary lactogenic hormone concentration and milk secretion in lactating rats. *Endocrinology* **63**, 535–539.
29. Grosvenor, C. E. and Mena, F. (1974). Neural and hormonal control of milk secretion and milk ejection. In *Lactation: A Comprehensive Treatise*, vol. 1, ed. Larson, B. L. and Smith, V. R., pp. 227–276. New York, London: Academic Press.
30. Grosvenor, C. E. and Whitworth, N. (1974). Evidence for a steady rate of secretion of prolactin following suckling in the rat. *J. Dairy Sci.* **57**, 900–904.
31. Hart, I. C. (1972). A solid phase radioimmunoassay for ovine and caprine prolactin using Sepharose 6B: Its application to the measurement of circulating level of prolactin before and during parturition. *J. Endocrinol.* **55**, 51–62.

32. Hart, I. C. (1973). Effect of 2-Br-α-ergocryptine on milk yield and growth hormone in the blood of the goat at milking. *J. Endocrinol.* **57**, 179–180.
33. Hart, I. C. and Flux, D. S. (1973). The release of growth hormone in response to milking in the goat during early and late lactation. *J. Endocrinol.* **57**, 177–178.
34. Hart, I. C. (1974). The relationship between lactation and the release of prolactin and growth hormone in the goat. *J. Reprod. Fert.* **39**, 485–499.
35. Henricks, D. M., Dickey, J. F., Hill, J. R., and Johnston, W. E. (1972). Plasma estrogen and progesterone levels after mating, and during late pregnancy and postpartum in cows. *Endocrinology* **90**, 1336–1342.
36. Hoffman, B., Schams, D., Giménez, E.M.L., Hermann, Ch., and Karg, H. (1973). Changes of progesterone, total estrogens, corticoids, prolactin and LH in bovine peripheral plasma around parturition with special reference to the effect of exogenous corticoids and a prolactin inhibitor respectively. *Acta Endocrinol.* **73**, 385–395.
37. Hodate, K. and Johke, T. (1977). Radioimmunoassay for bovine thyrotropin. Proc. 67th Ann. Meet. Japan Zootech. Sci. Assoc. (Abstr. in Japanese).
38. Ingalls, W. G., Convey, E. M., and Hafs, H. D. (1973). Bovine serum LH, GH, and prolactin during late pregnancy, parturition and early lactation. *Proc. Soc. Exp. Biol. Med.* **143**, 161–164.
39. Jaffe, B. and Behrman, H. R. (eds.) (1974). *Methods of Hormone Radioimmunoassay*. New York: Academic Press.
40. Johke, T. and Goto, T. (1961). Phosphorus metabolism of the mammary gland. 1. Studies of phosphorus compounds of the lacteal secretion during late pregnancy of the colostrum and milk during early lactation in cows and goats. *Bull. Natl. Inst. Agric. Sci.* **G20**, 211–224.
41. Johke, T. (1969). Prolactin release in response to milking stimulus in the cow and goat estimated by radioimmunoassay. *Endocrinol. Japon.* **16**, 179–185.
42. Johke, T. (1969). Radioimmunoassay for bovine prolactin in plasma. *Endocrinol. Japon.* **16**, 581–589.
43. Johke, T. (1970). Factors affecting the plasma prolactin level in the cow and the goat as determined by radioimmunoassay. *Endocrinol. Japon.* **17**, 393–401.
44. Johke, T., Fuse, H., and Oshima, M. (1971). Changes of plasma prolactin level during late pregnancy and early lactation in the goat and the cow. *Japan. J. Zootech. Sci.* **42**, 173–179.
45. Johke, T. (1974). Prolactin secretion in farm animals. *Hormone to Rinsho* **22**, 343–351 (in Japanese).
46. Johke, T. (1974). Studies of prolactin secretion in dairy farm animals by radioimmunoassay. *Japan. J. Zootech. Sci.* **47**, 183–191.
47. Johke, T. (1978). Effects of TRH on growth hormone, prolactin, and triiodothyronine secretions in the bovine. *Endocrinol. Japon.* **25**, 19–26.

48. Johke, T. and Hodate, K. (1977). Bovine serum prolactin, growth hormone, and triiodothyronine during late pregnancy and early lactation. *Japan. J. Zootech. Sci.* **48**, 772–776.
49. Johke, T. and Hodate, K. (1978). Effects of CB154 on serum hormone level and lactogenesis in dairy cows. *Endocrinol. Japon.* **25**, 67–74.
50. Johke, T. and Hodate, K. (1978). Effects of CB154 on serum hormone levels and lactogenesis in dairy goats. *Endocrinol. Japon.* (in press).
51. Karg, H., Schams, D., and Reinhardt, V. (1972). Effects of 2-Br-α-ergocryptine in plasma prolactin level and milk yield in cows. *Experientia* **28**, 574–576.
52. Karg, H. and Schams, D. (1974). Prolactin release in cattle. *J. Reprod. Fert.* **39**, 463–472.
53. Kelly, P. A., Bedirian, K. N., Baker, R. P., and Friesen, H. G. (1973). Effect of synthetic TRH on serum prolactin, TSH, and milk production in the cow. *Endocrinology* **92**, 1289–1293.
54. Kelly, P. A., Tsushima, T., Shiu, R.P.C., and Friesen, H. G. (1976). Lactogenic and growth hormone like activities in pregnancy determined by radioreceptor assays. *Endocrinology* **99**, 765–773.
55. Komatsu, M., Johke, T., Abe, T., and Hodate, K. (1976). Postpartum changes in milk protein fractions of cows determined by starch-urea-gel electrophoresis. *Bull. Natl. Inst. Anim. Ind.* No. 30, 21–26.
56. Koprowski, J. A. and Tucker, H. A. (1971). Failure of oxytocin to initiate prolactin or luteinizing hormone release in lactating dairy cows. *J. Dairy Sci.* **54**, 1675–1680.
57. Koprowski, J. A. and Tucker, H. A. (1973). Serum prolactin during various physiological states and its relationship to milk production in the bovine. *Endocrinology* **92**, 1480–1487.
58. Koprowski, J. A. and Tucker, H. A. (1973). Bovine serum growth hormone, corticoids and insulin during lactation. *Endocrinology* **93**, 645–651.
59. Kuhn, N. J. (1971). Control of lactogenesis and lactose biosynthesis. In *Lactation*, ed. Falconer, I. R., pp. 161–176. London: Butterworths.
60. Kühn, E. R., Krulich, L., and MacCann, S. M. (1973). Influence of exogenously administered oxytocin on prolactin release in the lactating rat. *Neuroendocrinology* **11**, 11–21.
61. Lamming, G. E., Moseley, S. R., and McNeilly, J. R. (1974). Prolactin release in the sheep. *J. Reprod. Fert.* **40**, 151–168.
62. Larson, B. L. and Jorgensen, G. N. (1974). Biosynthesis of the milk proteins. In *Lactation: A Comprehensive Treatise*, vol. 2, ed. Larson, B. L. and Smith, V. R., pp. 115–146. New York, London: Academic Press.
63. Larson, B. L. (ed.) (1978). *Lactation: A Comprehensive Treatise*, vol. 4. New York, London: Academic Press (in press).
64. Louis, T. M., Stellflug, N., Tucker, H. A., and Hafs, H. D. (1974). Plasma

prolactin, growth hormone, luteinizing hormone and glucocorticoids after prostaglandin $F_{2\alpha}$ in heifers. *Proc. Soc. Exp. Biol. Med.* **147**, 128–133.

65. Meites, J. (1961). Farm animals: Hormonal induction of lactation and galactopoiesis. In *Milk: The Mammary Gland and Its Secretion*, ed. Kon, S. K. and Cowie, A. T., pp. 321–367. New York, London: Academic Press.
66. Murphy, G., Ariyanayagam, A. D., and Kuhn, N. J. (1973). Progesterone and the metabolic control of the lactose biosynthetic pathway during lactogenesis in the rat. *Biochem. J.* **136**, 1105–1116.
67. Nagasawa, H. and Yanai, R. (1973). Effects of adrenalectomy and/or deficiency of pituitary prolactin secretion on initiation and maintenance of lactation in mice. *J. Endocrinol.* **58**, 67–73.
68. Noel, G. L., Suh, H. K., and Frantz, A. G. (1974). Prolactin release during nursing and breast stimulation in postpartum and non-postpartum subjects. *J. Clin. Endocrinol. Metab.* **38**, 413–423.
69. Olsen, J. D., Trenkle, A., Witzel, D. A., and McDonald, J. S. (1974). Plasma growth hormone concentrations in cows before, during and after parturition. *Am. J. Vet. Res.* **35**, 1131–1134.
70. Ôta, K., Harai, Y., Unno, H., Tomogane, H., and Yokoyama, A. (1974). Corticosterone secretion in response to suckling at various stages of normal and prolonged lactation in rats. *J. Endocrinol.* **62**, 679–680.
71. Pelletier, J. (1973). Evidence for photoperiodic control of prolactin release in rams. *J. Reprod. Fert.* **35**, 143–147.
72. del Pozo, E. and Flückiger, E. (1973). Prolactin inhibition: Experimental and clinical studies. In *Human Prolactin*, ed. Pasteels, J. L. and Robyn, C., pp. 291–301. New York: Excerpta Medica, American Elsevier.
73. Reinhardt, V. and Schams, D. (1974). Analysis of teat stimulation as specific stimulus for prolactin in cattle. *Neuroendocrinology* **14**, 289–296.
74. Robertson, H. A. (1974). Changes in the concentration of unconjugated oestrone, oestradiol-17α, and oestradiol-17β in the maternal plasma of the pregnant cow in relation to the initiation of parturition and lactation. *J. Reprod. Fert.* **36**, 1–7.
75. Rowland, S. J., Roy, J.H.B., Sears, H. J., and Thompson, S. Y. (1953). The effect of prepartum milking on the composition of the prepartum and postpartum secretions of the cow. *J. Dairy Res.* **20**, 16–28.
76. Schams, D. and H. Karg (1970). Untersuchungen über Prolaktin im Rinderblut mit einer radioimmunologischen Bestimmungsmethode. *Zentralbl. Vet. Med., Reihe A* **17**, 193–212.
77. Schams, D. (1972). Prolactin levels in bovine blood, influenced by milking manipulation, genital stimulation and oxytocin administration with specific consideration of the seasonal variations. *Acta Endocrinol.* **71**, 684–696.
78. Schams, D. and Karg, H. (1972). The immediate response of the plasma prolactin level to oestrogen infusions in dairy cows. *Acta Endocrinol.* **69**, 47–52.

79. Schams, D., Reinhardt, V., and Karg, H. (1972). Effects of 2-Br-α-ergocryptine on plasma prolactin level during parturition and onset of lactation in cows. *Experientia* **28**, 697–699.
80. Shina, Y. N., Salocks, C. B., Lewis, U. S., and Vanderlaan, W. P. (1974). Influence of nursing on the release of prolactin and GH in mice with high and low incidence of mammary tumors. *Endocrinology* **95**, 947–954.
81. Schirley, J. E., Emery, R. S., Convey, E. M., and Oxender, W. D. (1973). Enzymic changes in bovine adipose tissue, serum and mammary tissue, hormonal changes with initiation of lactation. *J. Dairy Sci.* **56**, 569–574.
82. Skarda, J. and Bliek, J. (1975). Response of mammary tissue from pregnant goats to prolactin and growth hormone in organ culture. *J. Endocrinol.* **67**, 129–130.
83. Shoda, Y. and Ishi, T. (1976). Effects of season, pregnancy and lactation on serum thyroxine level in dairy cattle. *Japan. J. Zootech. Sci.* **47**, 659–664.
84. Smith, K. L., Muir, L. A., Ferguson, L. C., and Conrad, H. R. (1971). Selective transport of IgG into the mammary gland: Role of estrogen and progesterone. *J. Dairy Sci.* **54**, 1886–1894.
85. Smith, V. G., Edgerton, L. A., Hafs, H. D., and Convey, E. M. (1973). Bovine serum estrogens, progestins and glucocorticoid during late pregnancy and early lactation. *J. Anim. Sci.* **36**, 391–396.
86. Smith, V. G., Beck, T. W., Convey, E. M., and Tucker, H. A. (1974). Bovine serum prolactin, growth hormone, cortisol and milk yield after ergocryptine. *Neuroendocrinology* **15**, 172–181.
87. Thorburn, G. D., Nicol, D. H., Bassett, J. M., Shutt, D. A., and Cox, R. I. (1972). Parturition in the goat and sheep: Changes in corticoids, progesterone, oestrogens and prostaglandin F. *J. Reprod. Fert.* Suppl. **16**, 61–84.
88. Tomogane, H., Ôta, K., and Yokoyama, A. (1976). Decrease in litter weight gain and progesterone secretion in lactating rats treated with antiserum to rat prolactin. *J. Reprod. Fert.* **47**, 347–349.
89. Trenkle, A. (1970). Plsama levels of growth hormone, insulin and plasma protein-bound iodine in finishing cattle. *J. Anim. Sci.* **31**, 389–393.
90. Tucker, H. A. (1971). Hormonal response to milking. *J. Anim. Sci.* Suppl. **1**, 137–141.
91. Tucker, H. A., Convey, E. M., and Koprowski, J. A. (1973). Milking-induced release of endogenous prolactin in cows infused with exogenous prolactin. *Proc. Soc. Exp. Biol. Med.* **142**, 72–75.
92. Tucker, H. A. (1974). General endocrinological control of lactation. In *Lactation: A Comprehensive Treatise*, vol. 1, ed. Larson, B. L. and Smith, V. R., pp. 277–326. New York, London: Academic Press.
93. Tucker, H. A. and R. P. Wetteman (1976). Effect of ambient temperature and relative humidity on serum prolactin and growth hormone in heifers. *Proc. Soc. Exp. Biol. Med.* **151**, 623–626.

94. Turkington, R. W. and Hill, R. L. (1969). Lactose synthetase: Progesterone inhibition of the induction of α-lactalbumin. *Science* **163**, 1458–1460.
95. Umo, I., Fitzpatrick, R., and Ward, W. R. (1976). Parturition in the goat: Plasma concentration of prostaglandin F and steroid hormones and uterine activity during late pregnancy and parturition. *J. Endocrinol.* **68**, 383–389.
96. Vonderhear, B. K., Owens, I. S., and Topper, Y. J. (1973). An early effect of prolactin on the formation of α-lactalbumin by mouse mammary epithelial cells. *J. Biol. Chem.* **248**, 467–471.
97. Wettemann, R. P. and Tucker, H. A. (1974). Relationship of ambient temperature to serum prolactin in heifers. *Proc. Soc. Exp. Biol. Med.* **146**, 908–911.
98. Wright, A. D. and Taylor, K. W. (1967). Immunoassay of hormones. In *Hormones in Blood*, vol. 1, ed. Gray, C. H. and Bacharach, A. L., pp. 23–45. New York, London: Academic Press.
99. Yanai, R. and Nagasawa, H. (1973). Effect of non-suckling period on pituitary prolactin secretory activity in rats. *Horm. Res.* **4**, 169–176.
100. Zeliger, Y., Volcani, R., and Sklan, D. (1973). Yield and protein composition in cows milked prepartum. *J. Dairy Sci.* **56**, 869–872.

II – 9

ROLE OF MILKING IN INITIATION AND MAINTENANCE OF LACTATION IN THE DAIRY ANIMALS

YOZO SHINDE

Department of Dairy Science, Obihiro Zootechnical University, Obihiro, Hokkaido, Japan

The importance of milking in the maintenance of lactation has been well established. For example, if milking is stopped, milk synthesis stops and the secretory cells of the udder disappear rapidly. Two concepts have been proposed to explain how mammary function and lactation in dairy animals are maintained by the milking process. The first concept states that milking stimulus results in the release of prolactin, adrenocorticotropic hormone (ACTH) and oxytocin from the pituitary gland, which is responsible for the maintenance of the mammary function and lactation. Many findings supporting this concept have been reported (*17*). The other concept states that the removal of the milk from the udder, which is the primary reason for milking, is indispensable for maintenance of the mammary function and lactation. Milking stimuli without accompanying milk removal cannot maintain lactation. Goats continued to secrete normal amounts of milk when they were milked under anesthesia (*19*). However, the experimental evidence supporting the latter concept is relatively scarce compared with that of the former. Therefore, the present paper deals with experiments in which effects of milk removal on lactation in the goat and cow were studied by the half-udder milking procedure.

1. The Effects of Milk Removal on the Mammary Function and Induction of Lactation in the Goat

Seventeen Japanese Saanen virgin goats were used. The goats were

33–48 months old, and weighed 35–45 kg when the first injection of hormones was given. Hormonal treatment carried out was similar to that described by Cowie *et al.* (*1*). Hexestrol administered was dissolved in arachis oil at a concentration of 0.5 mg/ml and progesterone in a 4: 1 mixture of arachis oil and benzyl alcohol at a concentration of 70 mg/ml. The goats were subcutaneously injected once daily with 0.5 mg of hexestrol and 70 mg of progesterone. Duration of the treatment (107–121 days) corresponds approximately to the normal gestation period in the goat. During the hormonal treatment, the left half (experimental half) of the udder was milked twice a day at about 9.00 a.m. and 4.00 p.m. by hand. The right half (control half) was kept intact during the hormonal treatment. After the hormonal treatment was finished, both halves of the udder were milked twice a day. For the first 3 weeks of the treatment, only a few milliliters of lymph-like fluid was obtained from the left half at each milking. The secretion, thereafter, gradually became more milky in appearance and looked like milk at the end of the 7th week, although the yield was still about 10 g/day. The time of onset of milk secretion was

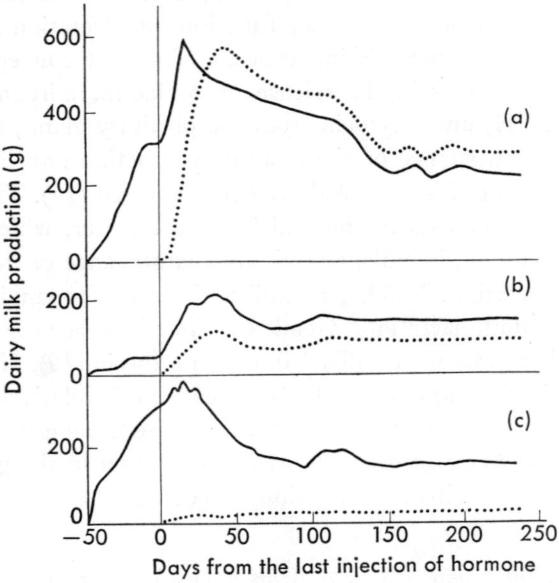

FIG. 1. Lactation curves for induced lactation
(a) Group I (goat 1), (b) Group II (goat 5), (c) Group III (goat 10). —— left quarter; ······ right quarter.

TABLE I. Milk Production during Hormone Treatments in Induced Lactation

Group	No. of animals	Duration of hormone treatments (days)	Total milk yield (g)
I	5	115±1.8	9,998±574[a]
II	9	118±1.5	3,016±998[b]
III	3	116±1.8	14,236±982[c]

Values presented are means±standard deviation (SD). [a,b,c] Dissimilar superscripts indicate significant differences ($p<0.05$).

not different from animal to animal. After lactation was initiated the goats could be divided into 3 groups on the basis of the lactational response, as shown in Fig. 1 and Table I. In Group I (5 animals) and in Group III (2 animals) daily milk yield increased steadily during the last 7 weeks of the hormone treatment. Daily milk yield of the remaining 9 animals did not increase linearly during the period of hormone treatment and the total milk obtained during this period was significantly less than that obtained from animals in other groups (Table I). Total milk yield of Group III during the period of the treatments was significantly higher than that of the two other groups ($p<0.05$). These differences in lactational performance obtained during the hormone treatment seemed to affect the yield of milk obtained after the hormone treatments. Lactation curves of representative animals in each group and the peak production and total yield are shown in Table II and Fig. 1, respectively. The daily yields of milk from the milking (experimental) halves of each group rapidly increased immediately after the end of the hormone treatment and reached a maximum at 21, 42, and 14 days in Groups I, II, and III, respectively. The number of days required to reach maximum production and the yield

TABLE II. Milk Production after the Last Injection of Hormones in Induced Lactation

Group	Udder half	Duration of lactation (days)	Days to peak	Peak production (g)	Total yield (g)
I	Left	302±2.2	21±1.2*	568±22	81,457±4,025*
	Right		36±1.8	554±18	91,335±4,211
II	Left	212±2.5	42±2.1	310±25*	32,185±3,164*
	Right		43±1.8	152±18	20,103±2,906
III	Left	211±2.1	14±1.4	426±30	47,420±3,690*
	Right		—	—	3,798± 358

Values presented are means±SD. Peak lactation is not clear in right half of Group III. * Left half *versus* right half: $p<0.05$.

TABLE III. Comparison of Nucleic Acids in Left and Right Halves of Udders on the Last Day of Hormone Treatments (Groups I and II)

Items	Left half	Right half
Mammary wt. (wet, g)	168 ±41**	68 ±11
DNA (mg/wet tissue)	2.74± 0.18**	1.34± 0.09
RNA (mg/wet tissue)	20.48± 0.86**	1.38± 0.10
RNA/DNA	7.48± 0.25**	0.98± 0.08

Values presented are means±standard deviation.
** Left half *versus* right half: $p<0.01$.

at the peak were closely related to the extent of lactational performance attained during the hormone treatment. The daily yields of milk from control halves which had not been milked during the treatment were low in all groups until 4 days after the start of milking. The increase in the daily yield was steep in Group I and the peak production and total milk obtained from the control half were almost the same as, or greater than, that from the experimental half. In Groups II and III, the increase was gradual and the total yield of the control was much less than that of the experimental half (Table II). The nucleic acid contents of both halves of the udder in Groups I and II on the last day of hormone treatments are listed in Table III. As expected, the average mammary DNA and RNA content and RNA/DNA ratio were significantly higher in the milked halves than in the non-milked halves. These results clearly show that removal of mammary secretions twice daily from a half udder throughout the hormonal treatments activates proliferation of the mammary tissue and increases the synthetic activity of a mammary cell. These findings are in close agreement with the findings of Shinde (*11*) in cows in which the left-hand quarter was milked shortly before and after parturition.

About 16 hr after the last injection of hormones, there was second rapid increase in the milk production in the experimental half in Groups I and II. This second rapid increase in milk production appears to correspond to the precipitous fall in the concentrations of progesterone and estrogen in the peripheral blood, which resulted from the termination of hormone treatments. These observations agree well with the finding that in rats copious milk secretion results from the withdrawal of the suppressing effect of hormones (*7*, *20*). In the present study, since the comparison was made between halves within one goat, hormonal conditions are common to both halves. Therefore, a considerable variation in the milk yields obtained in two halves within one goat might be ascribed either to direct stimulation or to the indirect—by removing the accumulated milk—stimulation of milking to the mammary cells. Although it has been generally assumed that milk secretion is controlled by hormones, the results described above clearly indicate that factors other than hormones can influence the secretory activity of the goat mammary gland.

In the animals in Group III induction of lactation was most successful during the hormone treatments, and a steady increase in daily milk yield was obtained from the milked halves from the last 9th week of hormone treatments to 14 days after the hormone treatments. On the other hand, only a small amount of milk could be obtained from the control halves, although these halves were free of mastitis. During the hormone treatments the control halves of these animals engorged with milk. It appears that accumulation of secretions in the mammary glands during hormone treatments might cause irreversible damage to the mammary cells. These results also suggest that optimum hormonal conditions for lactogenesis fail to stimulate mammary proliferation and milk synthesis of involuted mammary cells. Therefore, lactogenesis takes place only when a sufficient hormone complex acts on the competent mammary gland cells.

Using twins, Swanson (*13*) demonstrated that milking throughout the whole period of pregnancy caused a decrease in milk yield during the succeeding lactation. In a similar type of experiment Smith *et al.* (*12*) made a treatment comparison between quarters of the same mammary gland. They obtained results similar to those of Swanson and suggested that continued removal of secretions probably prevents the regeneration of the mammary tissue and depressed the yield of the following lactation. It has also been shown that the administration of oxytocin in the dry period (*5*, *14*) would retard involution and depress the milk yield. These findings could also be explained by continued removal retarding the involution and thus causing a decrease in the yield.

It has been generally accepted that milk secretion is initiated by hormonal changes which occur at parturition. However, the alveolar cells of the mammary gland may acquire secretory activity several weeks before parturition, since high yields of milk of normal composition can be obtained from prepartum milking. Experiments with prepartum milking demonstrated that there was considerable variation among cows as to times when copious milk was obtained (*6*, *9*, *11*), *i.e.*, some cows began to secrete copious milk several weeks before parturition and other cows at parturition.

As described above, a sufficient amount and an appropriate combination of hormones and a responsiveness of mammary gland are prerequisite for lactogenesis. If these prerequisites are fully provided in dairy animals well in advance of parturition, lactogenesis might occur during prepartum milking before parturition. This means that the time of initiation of lactation merely shifts from parturition to the middle stages of pregnancy. When the prerequisite for lactogenesis are not met, secretory activity of the mammary gland is inhibited by prepartum milking, as shown in the experimental halves in Group I. Prepartum milking is recommended only for the cow suffering pain from extensive swelling and congestion, since the accumulation of milk causes an irreversible change in the mammary cells, as can be seen in Group III of the present experiment. The basic objection to prepartum milking is the loss of colostrum, which is valuable to the calf. However, swelling in the udder is most common in heifers in which prepartum milking rarely satisfactory.

2. The Effect of Milk Removal from the Udder of the Dairy Cow upon Milk Secretion

It has been known for many years that cows milked 3 or 4 times daily produce higher milk yields than those milked twice daily (*2*, *10*, *18*, *21*). This increase has been generally ascribed to the relief of udder pressure by frequent emptying of the udder. However, Elliott *et al.* (*4*) found that the milk and solids other than fat secretion rates were linear with the duration of milking intervals up to 16 hr. To explain this inconsistency it is necessary to determine whether an increase in the rate of secretion does occur during the milking interval.

Of the 12 lactating Holstein cows used, 10 were in the first lactation and 2 were in the second lactation in Experiment I. Using an experimental

TABLE IV. Experimental Design in Experiment 1

Group	Lactation stage at the beginning of experiment	Experimental periods		
		I (5 days)	II (50 days)	III (10 days)
I	6–7 th day	A	B	A
II	98–117 th day	A	B	A
III	127–168 th day	A	B	A

A: Both udder halves were milked 2× daily (7.00, 21.00). B: Right udder half was milked 2× and left half milked 3× daily (7.00, 14.00, 21.00). Each group contained 4 animals.

method of half udder comparison, the effects of frequency of milking on milk secretion were assessed. The yield of milk produced by the individual quarters of the mammary gland of each cow was determined in the various stages of lactation by milking with a milking machine designed to collect milk from each quarter separately. Experimental procedures are detailed in Table IV.

The results are summarized in Fig. 2 and Table V. The milk yields

TABLE V. Comparative Milk Yields of Left and Right Half of Udder in Dairy Cows in Experiment 1

Group	Experimental periods			
	II		III	
	Difference in daily milk yield (left − right)	Milk yield ratio (left/right)	Difference in daily milk yield (left − right)	Milk yield ratio (left/right)
I	2.38 ± 0.18 kg[a]	1.24 ± 0.05[a]	2.10 ± 0.10 kg[a]	1.24 ± 0.04[a]
II	1.20 ± 0.09[b]	1.15 ± 0.04[b]	0.80 ± 0.05[b]	1.09 ± 0.03[b]
III	0.60 ± 0.04[c]	1.11 ± 0.04[b]	0.30 ± 0.03[c]	1.06 ± 0.03[b]

Values presented are means ± SD. [a,b,c] Dissimilar superscripts indicate significant differences ($p < 0.05$). Each group contains 4 animals. Lactation stage at the beginning of experiment is 6–7 th day for Group I, 98–117 th day for Group II, and 127–168 th day for Group III.

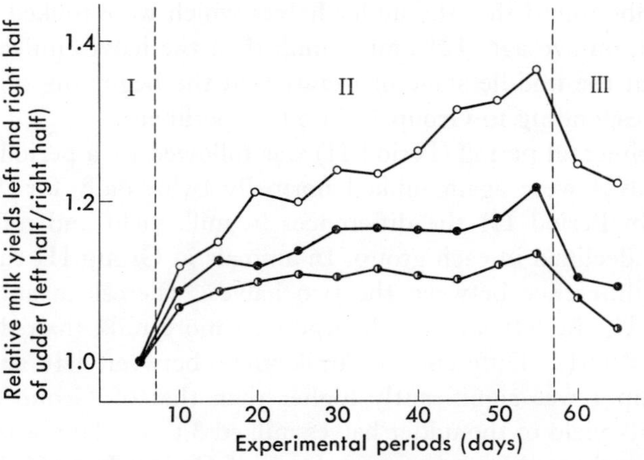

FIG. 2. Effect of lactation stage at beginning of experiment on milk yield of cows ○ Group I, 6–7th day; ● Group II, 98–117th day; ◑ Group III, 127–168th day.

of the udder halves milked 3 times a day have been corrected by the pretreatment differences in the yield between the udder halves. The difference in yields appeared on the first day of the experimental period (Period II), it increased very quickly over the next few days, and then gradually during the rest of the experimental period (Period II). The difference in yields was the highest in Group I which consisted of cows at 6–7th day of lactation at the beginning of the experiment. In this group the ratio of daily milk yield of the left udder half (experimental udder half) to that of the right udder half (control udder half) increased progressively until the end of Period II. Total milk yield from the experimental half was 24% more than that from the control half. On the other hand, in cows at 98–117th day of lctation (Group II) daily milk yield from the left udder half increased more steeply than that from the right udder half throughout experimental Period II. However, the difference in milk yield between the two halves in Group II was about half of that obtained in Group I. Only 11% more milk was obtained in Group III by 3 times milking a day, although the difference in the yield between the halves was significant. There are significant differences in both milk yield and milk yield ratio between Group I and Group II. Since average daily milk yield during Period I was not different significantly among Groups I (18.03±5.25 kg), II (17.20±6.42 kg), and III (15.76±3.21 kg), the difference in Period II among groups can be ascribed to the difference of lactation stage at which experiments were carried out. Essentially the same results were obtained by Elliot (*3*). She found that the udder halves which were milked 3 times daily produced, on average, 12% more milk than the halves milked twice daily in cows at the middle stage of lactation at the beginning of the experiments corresponding to Group II in our experiment.

The experimental period (Period II) was followed by a period during which both halves were again milked normally twice daily for 10 days (Period III). In Period III the differences in milk yield and milk yield ratio markedly declined in each group. In animals in Group III there was no significant difference between the two halves, whereas in animals in Groups I and II, the left udder half produced more milk than the right udder half ($p<0.01$). Difference in milk yield between left and right halves in Group I was significantly higher than that of Group II ($p<0.05$). Since milk yield of the udder halves milked 3 times daily was always higher than the other udder halves in animals of Groups I and II throughout the lactating period postexperiment, it is likely that the differences in milk yield between the two halves would relate to a difference in the amount of mammary tissue. Tucker (*15*) used lactating rats in which some of the teats were ligated and reported that the contents of DNA and RNA were correlated with the intensity of the suckling stimulus. Therefore, frequent milking appears to induce an increment of the secretory unit in the mammary gland. From his experimental results, however, it is difficult to distinguish the effect of the hormonal change associated with more frequent suckling from that of the complete removal of milk on the increase in the activity of the gland. In the present study the comparison of the effect of frequency of milking was made between two halves within a cow. Therefore, the results of the present study suggest that the increase in milk yield is definitely due to the removal of milk and not to the additional release of oxytocin or other hormones caused by the increased frequency of milking stimulation.

Numbers of mammary cells continue to increase during early lactation (*16*). This development probably continues until the peak of lactation. Thereafter the rate of losses of the mammary cells exceeds the rate of cell division. Thus the udder at the end of lactation contains substantially fewer cells than at the beginning. In the present study, the effect of frequent milking appears more markedly in the early stage of lactation than in the late stage. It is reasonable to consider, therefore, that frequent milking increases the milk yield by promoting the rate of proliferation and the activity of secretory cells during early lactation and reducing the rate of involution after the peak.

The difference in milk yield during Period III in which both halves were milked twice daily may be due to a difference in the number of cells which was brought about by the milking procedures during Period II. In other words, cells which had proliferated and were activated during experimental Period II might keep their activity during experimental Period III by regular milking. An experiment was carried out to check whether the difference in milk yield during Period III was maintained during the rest of the lactation stage (Shinde, unpublished results). The difference remained until the end of the lactation stage but not until the next lactation.

The effect of frequency of milking on milk production increased progressively during the experimental period (Period II). Therefore, Experiment II was designed to elucidate the effect of milking frequency on milk production over a shorter period than in Experiment I. Experimental procedures were almost the same as Experiment I. Twelve Holstein heifers were at the 6th day, on average, at the start of the experiment and

TABLE VI. Comparative Milk Yields of Left and Right Half of Udder in Dairy Cows in Experiment 1

Group	Experimental periods			
	II		III	
	Difference in daily milk yield (left−right)	Milk yield ratio (left/right)	Difference in daily milk yield (left−right)	Milk yield ratio (left/right)
I	1.04 ± 0.07 kg[a]	1.13 ± 0.08[a]	0.49 ± 0.04 kg[a]	1.04 ± 0.03[a]
II	3.22 ± 0.56[b]	1.39 ± 0.24[b]	1.91 ± 0.11[b]	1.26 ± 0.08[b]
III	2.66 ± 0.22[b]	1.24 ± 0.12[b]	2.10 ± 0.16[b]	1.24 ± 0.05[b]

Values presented are means ± SD. Dissimilar superscripts indicate significant differences ($p < 0.05$). Each group contains 4 animals. Period II lasted 20 days for Group I, 40 days for Group II, and 50 days for Group III.

average daily milk yield during the 5 preexperimental days was 14.65 kg (Period I). During the experimental period (Period II) which lasted for 20, 40, and 50 days in Groups I, II, and III, respectively, the left half of the udder of each cow was milked 3 times a day and the right half was milked twice daily. Period II was followed by a further 10 days during which both halves were again milked twice daily (Period III). The results are shown in Table VI. The milk yields of the udder halves milked 3 times a day were corrected by the pretreatment differences in the yield between the udder halves. The udder halves milked 3 times a day produced more milk than those milked twice a day. The differences in yields between halves were the least in Group I and the highest in Group III, and the difference was significant ($p < 0.01$). On the other hand, in Period III in which both halves were milked twice daily, the differences in milk yield and milk yield ratio declined from high values in Period II in Groups I and II and they were essentially the same in Group III. In animals in Group I, no significant difference was found between halves, but in Groups II and III the milk yield of left udder half was more than that in the right udder half ($p < 0.01$). These results suggested that mammary tissue *per se* was not affected by such a short trial. Therefore, for activating proliferation and retarding involution of the mammary gland, it is necessary to continue milking 3 times daily from the day of parturition for at least 40 days in heifers.

The effect of frequency of milking on milk production increased progressively during the experimental period (Period II) in Experiments I and II. In another experiment during an experimental period which lasted for 150 days, the left half of the udder of each cow was milked 3 times a day and the right half was milked twice daily (Shinde, unpublished results). Both halves were again milked twice daily for the following 30 days. The daily milk yield of the left udder half (experimental udder half) compared to that of the right udder half (control udder half) increased progressively until the end of the experimental period. Total milk yield of the experimental half was 52% more than that of the control half. In the postexperiment period, furthermore, experimental half yield was 54% more than that from the control half. It appears that among the effects of frequency of milking on the mammary gland, the retardation of involution is regarded as of major importance, since with extended periods of milking 3 times daily, greater effects of milking on milk production were obtained. In the present study, the treatments were applied to different halves of the same udder. Therefore, the effects of frequent removal of milk resulting from frequent milking on the mammary gland could not be ascribed to hormonal factors, since these factors are common to all halves. A finding that the rate of milk secretion is constant during milking intervals of normal length (*4*) suggests that the relief of milk accumulation would not carry any benefit for milk secretion. A possible explanation of the increase in milk yield is the action a local effect on the secretory cells of a smaller amount of residual milk and fat left after the

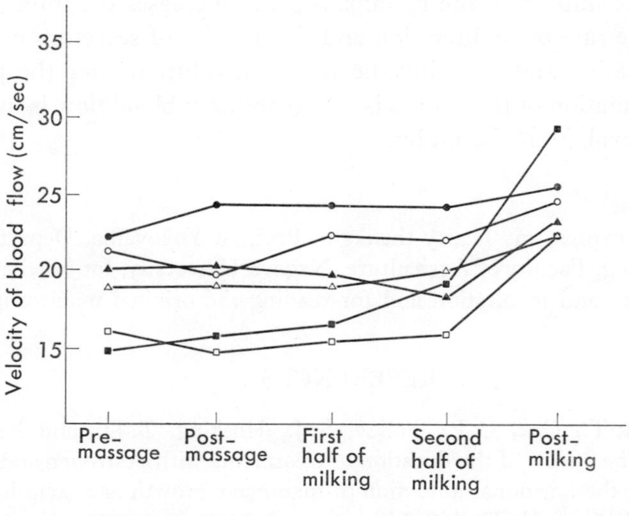

FIG. 3. Effect of milking interval on velocity of mammary blood flow of cows Milking interval (hr): ○ 4, ● 8, △ 12, ▲ 16, □ 20, ■ 24.

shorter-length intervals. It is to be expected that the levels of residual milk and fat when milking is done twice daily will be greater than when milking is thrice daily. But Elliott (*3*) was unable to demonstrate that differences in residual milk levels of this order would influence milk yield sufficiently to account for the milking fequency effect. An alternative explanation (*8*) that an increase in the mammary blood flow resulting from milk removal deserves consideration. Therefore, an attempt was made to assess the velocity of blood flow in a milk vein of the cow. Six Holstein cows at various lactation stages were used. The blood flow was measured after milking intervals of 4–24 hr by the use of an ultrasonic method. The results are illustrated in Fig. 3. The results suggest that milk accumulation has an inhibitory effect on mammary blood flow. At long milking intervals, mammary blood flow is markedly reduced. The decreased rate of milk secretion might also be explained by such biochemical factors as: (a) lesser amounts of hormones reaching the mammary gland, or (b) lesser amounts of milk precursors reaching the mammary gland.

SUMMARY

The present review is concerned with effect of milk removal on lactation in goats and cows using the half-udder technique. It appears that the removal of milk from the mammary gland increases the milk yield by promoting the rate of proliferation and the activity of secretory cells during early lactation and reducing the rate of involution after the peak. A possible explanation of the results is that mammary blood flow is increased by milk removal from the udder.

Acknowledgment

I wish to express my hearty thanks to Prof. A. Yokoyama, Department of Animal Breeding, Faculty of Agriculture, Nagoya University, for excellent intellectual guidance and inspiration and for reading the original manuscript.

REFERENCES

1. Cowie, A. T., Cox, C. P., Folley, S. J., Hosking, Z. D., and Naito, M. (1965). The effects of the duration of treatments with oestrogen and progesterone on the hormonal induction of mammary growth and lactation in the goat. *J. Endocrinol.* **32**, 129–139.
2. Elliott, G. M. (1959). The effect on milk yield of the length of milking inter-

vals used in twice a day milking and three times a day milking and incomplete milking. *Dairy Sci. Abstr.* **21**, 481–490.
3. Elliott, G. M. (1961). The effect on milk yield of three times a day milking and of increasing the level of residual milk. *J. Dairy Res.* **28**, 209–219.
4. Elliott, G. M., Dodd, F. H., and Brumby, P. J. (1960). Variations in the rate of milk secretion in milking intervals of 2–24 hours. *J. Dairy Res.* **27**, 293–308.
5. Gorman, G. M. and Swanson, E. W. (1968). Effects of oxytocin administered during the dry period on the succeeding lactation. *J. Dairy Sci.* **51**, 60–66.
6. Hartmann, P. E. (1973). Changes in the composition and yield of the mammary secretion of cows during the initiation of lactation. *J. Endocrinol.* **59**, 231–247.
7. Kuhn, N. J. (1971). Control of lactogenesis and lactose biosynthesis. In *Lactation*, ed. Falconer, I. R., pp. 161–176. London: Butterworths.
8. Mao, W. and Caruolo, E. V. (1973). Effect of lactose content and milking interval on mammary blood flow. *J. Dairy Sci.* **56**, 729–732.
9. Rowland, S. J., Roy, J.H.B., Sears, H. A., and Thompson, S. Y. (1953). The effect of prepartum milking on the composition of the prepartum and postpartum secretions of cow. *J. Dairy Res.* **20**, 16–23.
10. Schmidt, G. H. (1971). *Biology of Lactation*, pp. 149–162. San Francisco: W. H. Freeman & Co.
11. Shinde, Y. (1971). Effects of prepartum milking on milk secretion of the cow before and after parturition. *Japan. J. Zootech. Sci.* **42**, 501–508.
12. Smith, A., Wheelock, J. V., and Dodd, F. H. (1967). The effect of milking throughout pregnancy on milk secretion in the succeeding lactation. *J. Dairy Res.* **34**, 145–150.
13. Swanson, E. W. (1965). Comparing continuous milking with sixty-day dry periods in successive lactation. *J. Dairy Sci.* **48**, 1205–1209.
14. Swanson, E. W. and Claycomb, J. F. (1968). Oxytocin in dry period inhibits lactation. *J. Dairy Sci.* **51**, 955.
15. Tucker, H. A. (1966). Regulation of mammary nucleic acid content by various suckling intensities. *Am. J. Physiol.* **210**, 1209–1214.
16. Tucker, H. A. (1969). Factors affecting mammary gland cell numbers. *J. Dairy Sci.* **52**, 720–729.
17. Tucker, H. A. (1974). *Lactation*, vol. 1, ed. Larson, B. L. and Smith, V. R., pp. 296–317. New York, London: Academic Press.
18. Wheelock, J. V. and Dodd, F. H. (1969). Non-nutritional factors affecting milk yield in dairy cattle. *J. Dairy Res.* **36**, 479–493.
19. Yokoyama, A. and Ôta, K. (1965). The effect of anaesthesia on milk yield and maintenance of lactation in the goat and rat. *J. Endocrinol.* **33**, 341–351.
20. Yokoyama, A., Shinde, Y., and Ôta, K. (1969). Endocrine control of

changes in lactose content of the mammary gland in rats shortly before and after parturition. In *Lactogenesis*, ed. Reynolds, M. and Folley, S. J., pp. 65–71. Philadelphia: Univ. Pennsylvania Press.

21. Zaks, M. G. (1962). The relationships between milk removal and synthesis. In *The Motor Apparatus of the Mammary Gland*, ed. Cowie, A. T., pp. 141–173. Edinburgh, London: Oliver & Boyd.

II – 10

PHYSIOLOGICAL SIGNIFICANCE OF VARIATION IN THE ELECTROLYTE CONCENTRATION IN COW'S MILK

Masaharu OSHIMA

National Institute of Animal Industry, Chiba, Japan

The major electrolytes in cow's milk are potassium, chloride and sodium and their concentrations are approximately 9 times, 1/3 and 1/10 the concentrations in the blood plasma, respectively.

As milk contains several varieties of substances, a great many reports of biochemical and dairy chemical studies on milk have been published. However, studies on electrolytes, especially on monovalent ions in milk, are relatively few and it is only very recently that a physiological scheme to account for the ionic composition of milk and ion transport in the mammary gland was proposed by Linzell and Peaker (*3*, *4*, *12*).

The scheme proposed by Linzell and Peaker on the basis of physiological evidence indicates that, as far as sodium and potassium are concerned, concentrations of both ions in milk depend on active transport by a sodium pump in the basolateral membrane of the alveolar cell. Both the ions of the alveolar lumen in milk and in intracellular fluid are passively equilibrated across the apical membrane. On the other hand, a portion of the monovalent ions are packed into Golgi vacuoles with protein and lactose, and are discharged from the cell through exocytosis.

Once milk is secreted, its ionic composition is maintained in both the alveoli and the ducts. In the alveoli, a leak of ions through a paracellular route is prevented by tight junctions between the cells, and in the ducts, the ionic composition of milk is preserved by the unusual property which might be termed "a blood-milk barrier."

If cows are healthy, the concentrations of milk electrolytes are maintained nearly constant during long periods of lactation except the initial and the later part of the period (*13*, *14*, *22*, *23*), though small day-to-day fluctuations occur (*5*).

In a routine examination of quarter milk samples collected from different cows, we quite often found a considerable difference in the concentration of the electrolytes among samples taken from quarters of an individual udder. It is well known that a rise in the concentration of Na and Cl with a simultaneous fall in K and lactose often occurs in milk taken from quarters affected with mastitis or subclinical mastitis (*5*, *25*).

We separated the abnormal quarter-milk from the normal according to a definition we proposed (*10*), and examined interrelationships between the constituents in each group of quarter-milk. We first found clear quantitative relations between the changes in the concentration of electrolytes, and between the change in electrolytes and the changes of the major organic constituents in the abnormal milk (*11*). Secondly, we found clear relationships between the concentration of electrolytes and the content of lactose, protein and fat in normal milk collected from different cows (*6*, *7*).

Those interrelationships found between the concentrations of various constituents in both abnormal and normal milk seemed to indicate that the changes in the concentrations occurred in relation with the constancy of the osmotic pressure of milk, as though not only the electrolytes and lactose but also protein and fat were undeniable osmolar components.

1. Variation in the Electrolytes in Milk due to Non-physiological Causes

The chemical composition of milk taken from each quarter of an individual cow udder is supposedly the same from a physiological point of view. However, this is not true when actually examined. Except for heifers in their first lactation, some differences in chemical composition are commonly observed in the quarter-milk taken from individual cows.

We examined the difference between quarter-milk from the udders of a number of cows, and found that about 1/3 of the cows showed abnormality in some of their quarter-milk (*10*). Such abnormal milk appeared only in one or two quarters in about 90% of these cows and appeared repeatedly in the same quarter or quarters of the cow.

This quarter-milk had higher concentrations of sodium and chloride and lower lactose and potassium than the supposedly normal quarter milk from the same udder, and in addition, the milk yield of the former was usually less than the contra-lateral normal quarter. Therefore, this abnormal milk could be considered to be subclinical mastitic milk.

Cows who have both normal and abnormal quarters in their udders, have distinctive merit for study of the changes in composition of the abnormal milk, since they have an appropriate control within their udder, and because the changes in concentrations of milk constituents of the abnormal milk can be estimated quantitatively by taking the difference between the abnormal and the normal or control quarter milk.

We collected several specimens of quarter-milk by routine sampling of the morning milk of many Holstein cows for years, using a separate quarter-milking machine, and measured the concentrations of Na, K and Cl as the major electrolytes, and the contents of fat, protein and lactose as the major organic components. The latter three components were analysed by the infrared milk analyser Mark II, (Grubb and Parsons & Co., England).

1) The quarter difference value between abnormal and normal quarter-milk

In order to study the change of composition of abnormal quarter-milk, we calculated the difference in the concentrations of various constituents between several samples of abnormal and control quarter-milk, and examined interrelationships between them. We defined quarter-milk whose Na+Cl value or the sum of the concentration of Na and Cl was lowest among the four quarters of an individual udder as the normal or control quarter-milk (*10*). The quarter whose milk had the lowest Na+Cl value, with a Na concentration of not more than about 20 mEq/liter, continues to have the lowest value on subsequent successive samplings and in most of such milk, the California mastitis test was negative, and pH value was the lowest among the quarters.

We called the difference in the concentration of a milk constituent between quarter-milk and the control milk within the same udder a "quarter difference value" following Vanlandingham's example (*21*) and designated it by Qd; the quarter difference for the Na+Cl value was, therefore, Qd (Na+Cl).

On the basis of the results of a statistical survey on the distribution of Qd (Na+Cl) values of 368 quarter-milk samples obtained from 20 Holstein cows in good health, quarter-milk whose Qd (Na+Cl) value was higher than 7.2 mEq/liter was defined as abnormal quarter-milk (*10*). We also examined interrelationships between Qds of various constituents

TABLE I. Relations between the Quarter Difference Values (Qds) in 63 Abnormal Quarter-milk Samples from 12 Cows

Correlation between		Regression equation	Standard error (SE) of regression coefficient	Correlation coefficient
x; Qd(x)	y; Qd(y)			
Cl mEq/liter	Na mEq/liter	$y= 1.353x-1.416$	0.062	0.94
K mEq/liter	Lactose mM/liter	$y= 2.198x-1.594$	0.149	0.88
Na+Cl mEq/liter	K mEq/liter	$y=-0.256x+0.901$	0.016	−0.90
Na+Cl mEq/liter	Lactose mM/liter	$y=-0.687x+3.120$	0.022	−0.97
Na+Cl mEq/liter	L+K mM/liter	$y=-0.942x+3.982$	0.029	−0.97
Na+Cl mEq/liter	Protein %	$y= 0.004x-0.012$	0.0006	0.009
Na+Cl mEq/liter	Fat %	$y= 0.001x-0.008$	0.002	0.061

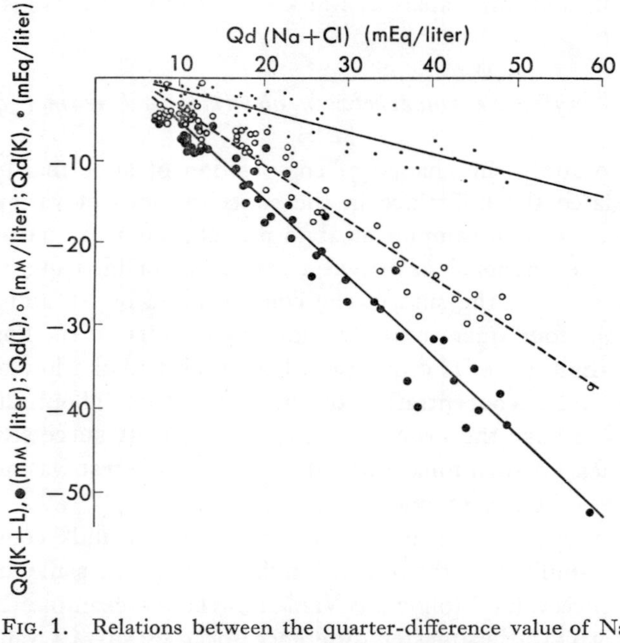

FIG. 1. Relations between the quarter-difference value of Na+Cl, Qd (Na+Cl) (mEq/liter) and of K, Qd (K) and of lactose, Qd (L), and of K plus lactose, Qd (K+L) (mM/liter) in 63 abnormal quarter-milk samples

The straight lines were drawn from the regression equations in Table I.

using 63 abnormal milk samples. The results are shown in Table I and Fig. 1.

Qd (Na) and Qd (Cl) values varied proportionally, and with an increase in them or in Qd (Na+Cl), Qd (K) or Qd of lactose, Qd (L) decreased rectilinearly in abnormal milk. The ratio Qd (Na)/Qd (Cl) of abnormal milk was in the range between 1.2–1.3, and was similar to that of the concentration of Na and Cl in the blood plasma (about 1.36). The ratio Qd (L)/Qd (K) was about 2.0, and was similar to the ratio of the content of lactose to K in normal milk (about 2.3).

2) Qd (Na+Cl) value and admixture theory on abnormal milk

An explanation of the mechanism by which the composition of milk alters in various physiological and non-physiological conditions was proposed many years ago. Barry and Rowland (*1*) found rectilinear relationships between the concentration of Na and K, Na and Cl, K and Cl, and lactose and each of these electrolytes. On the basis of these relationships they explained the change in milk composition by the admixture theory. According to this theory, change in milk composition is caused by the mixing, in varying proportions, of two hypothetical body fluids, one of which is "true milk" which is secreted from mammary alveolar cells, and the other is an iso-osmotic diluent whose composition is similar to blood serum. In milk taken from diseased quarters or mastitic milk, there is little doubt that extracellular fluid enters the milk.

Although the admixture theory of Barry and Rowland explained the mechanism of alteration of composition in abnormal milk, a quantitative estimation of the amount of diluent mixed in individual abnormal milk was impracticable.

The ratio, Qd (Na)/Qd (Cl), in abnormal milk was similar to the ratio of the concentration of Na and Cl in the blood plasma. Therefore, it may also be similar to that of extracellular fluid or exudate of inflammation. On the other hand, the concentration of Na and Cl in bovine blood plasma is 142 and 104 mEq/liter as cited from the literature (*19*). If we postulate that extracellular fluid mixed in the abnormal milk has substantially the same concentrations of Na and Cl as in the blood plasma, its Na+Cl value is about 246 (142+104) mEq/liter.

We can calculate, then, what amount of blood plasma or extracellular fluid will correspond to the Qd (Na+Cl) value of abnormal milk. Thus, we can estimate quantitatively the amount of diluent mixed in each sample of abnormal quarter-milk from its Qd (Na+Cl) value. Further, when some amounts of extracellular fluid were mixed with normal quarter-milk, the concentration of lactose decreased by dilution. If the concentration of lactose in the original or the control milk and the amount of extracellular fluid or Qd (Na+Cl) value of abnormal milk were known, the decreased lactose concentration resulted from mixing can be calculated. And then, if the lactose concentration in abnormal milk calculated as above showed good agreement with that actually measured, it would lend a quantitative confirmation to the admixture theory.

We chose 10 abnormal quarter-milk samples with different Qd (Na+Cl) values from the 63 samples in Fig. 1, and both the calculated and the measured concentrations of lactose were compared. The results are shown in Table II. The ratios of the two lactose concentrations for these samples were about 1.0, and thus the admixture theory was quantitatively confirmed.

It is unnecessary to postulate two hypothetical body fluids for the admixture theory. One of the body fluids, "true milk" should be the normal quarter-milk from an udder and the diluent is extracellular fluid. Insofar as the concentrations of Na and Cl in extracellular fluid do not

TABLE II. A Confirmation of the Admixture Theory for Formation of Abnormal Quarter-milk Using the Quarter Difference Value of Na+Cl, Qd(Na+Cl) (mEq/liter)

Sample No.	A (mEq/liter)	B (1/liter)	C (1/liter)	D (mM/liter)	E (mM/liter)	F (mM/liter)	G
1	17.6	0.072	0.928	119.2	110.6	110.7	1.00
2	18.1	0.074	0.926	119.2	110.4	110.1	1.00
3	19.2	0.078	0.922	117.7	108.5	107.5	0.99
4	20.5	0.083	0.917	117.7	107.9	106.6	1.01
5	26.3	0.107	0.893	124.1	110.8	107.7	1.03
6	26.8	0.109	0.891	128.2	114.2	111.8	1.02
7	33.2	0.135	0.865	117.4	101.6	99.3	1.02
8	36.2	0.147	0.853	130.9	111.7	108.4	1.03
9	40.2	0.163	0.837	130.3	109.1	106.3	1.03
10	45.5	0.185	0.815	130.6	106.4	101.4	1.05

A: The quarter difference value of Na+Cl.

B: B=A/246. The amount of extracellular fluid mixed in a unit volume of abnormal quarter-milk. The concentrations of Na and Cl of the fluid are postulated to be the same as in the blood plasma, *i.e.*, Na, 142 and Cl, 104 mEq/liter, and as a sum 246 mEq/liter of Na+Cl.

C: C=1−B. The amount of the true or normal milk in a unit volume of abnormal quarter-milk.

D: The lactose concentration of normal quarter-milk from the same udder (measured).

E: E=C×D. The amount of lactose a unit volume of abnormal quarter-milk (calculated).

F: The lactose concentration of abnormal quarter-milk (measured).

G: Agreement of E with F, G=E/F.

change substantially, changes in composition of abnormal milk can be explained by the mixture of the two fluids.

3) Relationship between Qd (Na+Cl) value and plasma protein content in abnormal milk

Further information is available on the properties of body fluids which mix in abnormal milk. We estimated the difference in the contents of blood plasma proteins, immunoglobulin G (IgG) and serum albumin (BSA) between abnormal and normal milk, using 30 pairs of quarter-milk samples (*9*). Qd (Na+Cl) values of the abnormal milk samples were less than 50 mEq/liter. The plasma proteins in the milk samples were measured by the single radial immunodiffusion method. The quarter differences of both the proteins were designated by Qd (IgG) and by Qd (BSA), respectively, and the relation between Qd (Na+Cl) and these Qd values were examined. The regression equation was as follows:

$$\log [\mathrm{Qd\ (IgG)}] = 0.0182 \times \mathrm{Qd\ (Na+Cl)} + 1.0943,$$

$$\log [\mathrm{Qd\ (BSA)}] = 0.0346 \times \mathrm{Qd\ (Na+Cl)} + 0.2792,$$

$n=30$ each, Qd (IgG), Qd (BSA), mg/dl, Qd (Na+Cl)$<$50 mEq/liter.

With an increase of Qd (Na+Cl) values, both Qd (IgG) and Qd (BSA) values increased exponentially. In abnormal milk with a high Qd (Na+Cl) value, extracellular fluid mixing with milk could have a considerably high plasma protein content.

The ratio, Qd (BSA)/Qd (IgG) in abnormal milk was from 0.3 to 0.5. Those were substantially different from the ratio of the concentrations of both the proteins in the blood plasma (about 1.6) but were not appreciably different from that in normal milk (0.2–0.3). However, with an increase in the Qd (Na+Cl) value, the proportion of BSA within the plasma proteins in abnormal milk increased. These changes in the blood protein in abnormal milk may indicate a change in the permeability of the mammary gland epithelium to the plasma proteins with an increase of Qd (Na+Cl) values.

2. *Variation in Milk Composition and Osmotic Pressure of Milk*

The osmotic pressure of milk is the least variable and most constant among the many factors in milk, because it is in continuous equilibrium with blood osmotic pressure (*15*, *20*, *24*). In the blood plasma, the solutes which mainly determine osmotic pressure are Na and Cl, whose concentrations in the plasma are very high and are always maintained within a very narrow range. On the other hand, the concentrations of Na and Cl in milk are low compared to the blood plasma and their concentrations change considerably in abnormal milk caused by mastitis or other diseases. In such abnormal milk, however, the milk osmotic pressure is stable and is maintained close to that of blood plasma.

1) The Osmolarity of quarter-milk obtained by routine milking

The osmotic concentration of 208 quarter-milk samples, taken from 26 Holstein cows, two times from each quater of each cow at morning milking was as follows. We used Advance Osmometer Model 3D (Advanced Instruments, Inc., Mass., USA) with 2 ml tubes. The mean and standard deviation for all the samples was 279.91 ± 4.526 m Osm/kg. Analysis of variations in the osmotic concentration data was performed according to the method described by Snedecor and Cochran (*18*).

The components of variance for three sources of variation in the osmotic concentration of quarter-milk were 3.795, 5.801, and 11.180 for cows, quarters in cows and days of sampling, respectively.

2) Variation in composition and constancy of osmolarity of milk

Variation in the osmotic pressure of milk from individual cows was small when sampling was done at ordinary milking. In order to confirm the constancy of the osmolarity of milk, we collected 110 milk samples from 19 Holstein cows using the following sampling method:

1. a) Sampling of fore-milk from normal quarters;
   b) of the middle-milk from the same quarters;
   c) of the latter-milk from the same quarters.
2. a) Sampling of normal quarter-milk taken before prolongation of the milking interval;
   b) of milk from the same quarters taken at the first milking, after prolongation of the milking interval for 38 hr;
   c) of milk from the same quarters taken at the third milking or 24 hr after the first milking;
   d) of milk from the same quarters taken at the fifth milking or 48 hr after the first milking.
3. a) Sampling of normal quarter-milk;
   b) of abnormal quarter-milk from the same cows.
4. a) Sampling of abnormal quarter-milk taken before prolongation of the milking interval;

b) of milk from the same quarters taken at the first milking after prolongation of the milking interval for 38 hr;
c) of milk from the same quarters taken 24 hr after the first milking;
d) of milk from the same quarters taken 48 hr after the first milking.

We measured the osmotic concentration of all the milk samples and determined the concentrations of Na, K, Cl, and fat, protein, lactose in each sample.

Although there was considerable variation in milk composition among the samples, variation in osmotic pressure was small and the values were similar to those of milk taken by ordinary milking. The mean and the standard deviation in osmotic concentration of all the samples were 283.8±4.93 mOsm/kg.

According to the relation between the osmotic concentration and the

TABLE III. Percentage of the Concentration of Major Osmole Groups Constituting Milk Osmolarity to the Osmotic Concentration of Milk Collected in Various Sampling Conditions

Conditions of sampling milk	Percentage to osmotic concentration				Osmotic concentration[a] (mOsm/kg)
	Na+Cl	K	Lactose	All-others[b]	
1. Fractions at a milking					
a. Fore part, $n=8$	18.7	15.6	46.7	19.1	279.1±6.17
b. Middle part, $n=8$	17.6	15.4	45.1	22.0	283.0±5.32
c. Latter part, $n=8$	19.2	14.5	42.7	23.5	283.5±3.02
2. Extention of milking interval					
a. Control, $n=12$	17.1	14.8	45.6	22.5	284.4±3.45
b. First milking, $n=12$	24.8	13.9	39.9	21.4	286.7±6.76
c. Third milking, $n=12$	22.5	14.9	40.6	21.9	284.8±2.37
d. Fifth milking, $n=12$	21.3	15.6	43.2	20.0	282.9±4.17
3. Normal and abnormal quarter-milk					
a. Normal, $n=15$	18.6	15.4	43.1	23.0	282.7±4.59
b. Abnormal, $n=15$	25.6	13.3	38.6	22.6	285.3±5.26
4. Abnormal and interval extended					
a. Control, $n=2$	22.0	14.9	43.4	19.8	286.0
b. First milking, $n=2$	40.3	12.8	33.1	13.9	281.5
c. Third milking, $n=2$	38.7	12.7	31.2	17.3	277.5
d. Fifth milking, $n=2$	30.7	14.7	40.4	14.2	281.5

[a] Mean±standard deviation (SD). [b] All-others represents the remainder after subtracting the sum of the concentrations of Na, Cl, K and lactose from the osmotic concentration of milk.

TABLE IV. Variation in the Concentration of Each of the Four Major Osmole Groups Constituting Milk Osmolarity in the Quarter-milk Samples 1.~3. in Table III (n=102)

Osmole	Mean	SD	Coefficient of variation (%)
Na+Cl mEq/liter	59.44	12.68	21.3
K mEq/liter	41.85	3.97	9.5
Lactose mM/liter	120.5	8.59	7.1
All-others[a] mOsm/kg	62.04	8.80	14.2
Osmolarity mOsm/kg	283.8	4.93	1.7

[a] See the note of Table III.

molar concentration of milk constituents, we divided milk constituents into four major osmole groups: Na+Cl, K, lactose, and all others. And we calculated the percentage of the concentration of each osmole group to the osmotic concentration of each milk sample. The average percentage values for milk collected by each sampling method are shown in Table III.

While the contribution of the sum of Na, K, and Cl accounted for about 1/3 of the osmotic concentration of normal milk, in some abnormal milk samples (4. b, c), it accounted for more than half. While the contribution of lactose accounted for about 45% of the osmotic concentration in normal milk, in some abnormal milk (4. c), it was only 31%.

The mean and standard deviation of the molar concentration of each of the four osmole groups and of the osmotic concentration for 102 milk samples 1–3 in Table III, were calculated and are shown in Table IV. Variation in Na+Cl value was the largest and that of the osmotic concentration was the smallest. We then added up the four groups in milk samples in consecutive order beginning with: Na+Cl (1) and K=(2), (2) and lactose=(3), (3) and all others=(4), and calculated the means and the standard deviations for the 4 sums of the 102 milk samples. The results were as follows.

The sum of parts	Mean	Standard deviation	Coefficient of variation (%)
(1) Na+Cl (mEq/liter)	59.44	12.68	21.3
(2) Na+Cl+K (mEq/liter)	101.3	12.9	12.7
(3) Na+Cl+K+lactose (mM/liter)	221.8	7.70	3.5
(4) Na+Cl+K+L+all-others (mOsm/kg)	283.8	4.93	1.7

When we added up the four groups one by one in successive order, variation in each sum reduced one after another and the coefficient of variation of the total sum or the osmotic concentration of milk was reduced to a minimum. Therefore, even though there were considerable variations in composition among the milk, there was only a slight variation in the osmotic pressure of milk.

3) Change in composition of abnormal milk and constancy of osmotic pressure

In abnormal milk, there is always an increase in the concentrations of Na and Cl. Therefore, some dissolved substances must diminish to compensate for the rise in osmotic pressure due to Na and Cl in order to maintain the stability of milk osmotic pressure. Among 110 milk samples the content of fat showed the largest variation; the coefficient of variation was 34.8%. The coefficient for protein was 12.2%. Contribution of these components to the osmotic concentration, however, may be negligible.

The inverse relationship between Qd (Na+Cl) and Qd (K+L) in abnormal milk is shown in Fig. 1. We obtained nearly the same relation between the two Qds in abnormal milk samples 3.b, in Table III (n=15), as described in the preceding section (1, 1)).

Since the ratios of Qd (K+L)/Qd (Na+Cl) in abnormal milk were within the range 0.8–0.9, most of the effect of increases of Na and Cl on osmolarity of milk was counterbalanced by the decreases in K and lactose in abnormal milk. Therefore, constancy of osmotic pressure depends mostly on the quantitative relationships between the concentrations of Na, Cl, K, and lactose in abnormal milk. Nevertheless, some constituents other than K and lactose may be reduced at the same time, because Qd (Na+Cl) values are bigger than Qd (K+L) values. The divalent cations might be reduced with a rise in pH in abnormal milk.

3. Inverse Relationship between Electrolytes and Organic Constituents in Normal Milk from Different Cows

Composition of cow's milk varies with the stage of lactation, age of the animal and environmental factors. On the other hand, milk composition remains fairy stable in individual animals in mid-lactation period if the udder is free from infections (*13*, *14*, *22*, *23*). Rook and Wood (*16*) reported that the K and lactose contents of milk from heifers in mid-lactation and free from mastitis were fairy stable for individual animals, and found a clear inverse relationship between the two components in such milk. It may be inferred that milk with high K content will have a low content of lactose, and *vice versa*, in order that the balance of the osmotic pressure of milk may be preserved.

We collected several quarter-milk samples from Holstein cows in the Institute herd and examined relationships between concentrations of the milk constituents Na, K, Cl, fat, protein, and lactose using only normal milk samples that were almost certainly free from the influence of mastitis. We found clear inverse correlations, not only between K and lactose, but also between K, Na, Cl, and each of the major organic milk constituents (*6*, *7*).

1) *Normal quarter-milk from individual cows*

We chose normal quarter-milk from individual cows from about 2,000 quarter-milk samples taken at the morning milking of 38 Holstein cows by the following procedure.

1. In the first, all milk samples taken from quarters suspected of subclinical mastitis were excluded by taking only quarter-milk with the lowest Na+Cl value (mEq/liter) in the udder.

2. Milk samples from cows not in mid-lactation were excluded by rejecting the samples taken on a day when the cow's daily milk yield was more than 90% or less than 60% of her maximum daily yield in that lactation.

3. The samples from cows in their fifth or greater number of lactation were excluded.

4. The milk samples taken from the same udder within one month were combined, taking the mathematical means of the concentrations of each constituent.

5. From 58 samples thus obtained, two samples were excluded, since their Na content was higher than the upper limits of Na content in normal milk, which was calculated by (mean+2×standard deviation) of Na content of the 58 samples (20.5 mEq/liter).

Thus, a total of 56 samples of normal milk were obtained from 32 lactation periods of 24 cows.

2) *Relationship between concentration of electrolytes and contents of lactose and protein*

We examined first the relationships between the constituents included in solids other than fat in milk because the relation between electrolytes

TABLE V. Concentration of Constituents of the 56 Normal Milk[a] Samples Taken from 32 Lactation Periods of 24 Cows

Constituents	Mean±SD	Range of distribution
Protein %	3.088±0.274	2.43- 3.72
Lactose %	4.376±0.194	3.95- 4.79
K mEq/liter	44.36 ±2.972	38.3 - 51.5
Na mEq/liter	15.45 ±1.675	12.3 - 20.0
Cl mEq/liter	31.48 ±5.845	20.4 - 45.1
Protein+lactose %	7.462±0.397	6.45- 8.33
Na+K+Cl mEq/liter	91.29 ±9.219	75.3 -115.3

[a] Morning milk.

TABLE VI. Correlation Coefficients between the Constituents in the 56 Normal Milk Samples

a)

Correlation between	Protein and lactose (%)	Na and Cl (mEq/liter)	K and Cl (mEq/liter)	Na and K (mEq/liter)
Correlation coefficient	0.413**	0.718***	0.631***	0.317*

b)

Correlation coefficient between	Na (mEq/liter)	K (mEq/liter)	Cl (mEq/liter)	Na+K+Cl (mEq/liter)
Protein %	−0.203	−0.576***	−0.593***	−0.598***
Lactose %	−0.633***	−0.526***	−0.851***	−0.825***
Protein+lactose %	−0.451***	−0.657***	−0.828***	−0.822***

Correlation coefficients are statistically significant, at $p<0.05$ (*), at $p<0.01$ (**), at $p<0.001$ (***).

and fat may be insignificant in relation with the osmotic pressure of milk.

Concentrations of each constituent of normal milk are shown in Table V, correlation coefficients in Table VI, and regression equations between each constituent in Table VII.

The correlation coefficient between protein and lactose contents in normal milk was positive and statistically significant and correlations between the concentration of each electrolyte were all positive. Therefore, when the concentration of one of the electrolytes is relatively high in normal milk, the concentrations of the other two are also high, and *vice versa*.

On the other hand, every correlation between the concentration of any one of the electrolytes and the content of lactose or protein was nega-

TABLE VII. Interrelations between the Concentration of Electrolytes, and between Electrolytes and Lactose, and Protein Content in the 56 Normal Milk Samples

	Relationship between		Regression equation	SE of regression coefficient
	x	y		
(1)	Na mEq/liter	Cl mEq/liter	$y=2.506x -7.243$	0.3305
(2)	Cl mEq/liter	K mEq/liter	$y=0.321x +34.253$	0.0539
(3)	Na+K+Cl mEq/liter	Lactose %	$y=-0.0174x +5.9633$	0.0016
(4)	Na+K+Cl mEq/liter	Protein %	$y=-0.0178x +4.7188$	0.0033
(5)	Na+K+Cl mEq/liter	Protein+lactose %	$y=-0.0352x +10.6821$	0.0034

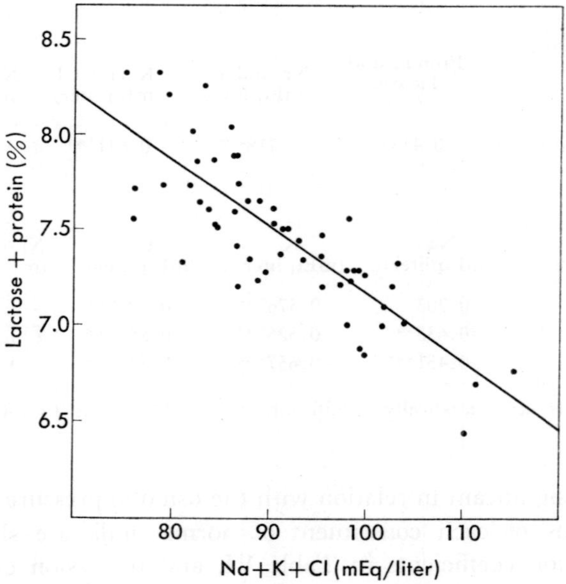

FIG. 2. Inverse relation between Na+K+Cl (mEq/liter) and lactose+protein (%) in the 56 normal milk samples taken during 32 lactation periods of 24 cows The line is: $y=-(0.0352\pm0.0034)\ x+10.6821$, $n=56$.

tive and all were highly significant except the correlation between Na and protein. The correlations between the sum of the electrolytes, Na+K+Cl (mEq/liter) and lactose or protein content (%), and the sum of lactose and protein were, therefore, markedly negative (Table VI). The inverse relation between Na+K+Cl and lactose+protein in normal milk is shown in Fig. 2.

The result of examinations showed that the higher the concentration of electrolytes in normal milk, the less the contents of lactose and protein.

If we now consider two hypothetical normal milk samples, in one of which the electrolyte concentration is relatively high, and in the other relatively low, the contents of protein and lactose in the two milk samples can be estimated using the relevant regression equations shown in Table VII, and further, the difference in the contents of these organic constituents between the two samples can also be calculated.

We postulated first that the Na concentration of milk sample A was 3 mEq/liter higher, and that of the sample B was 3 mEq/liter lower than the mean of Na shown in Table V, therefore, 18.45 mEq/liter for A and 12.45 mEq/liter for B. The concentration of Cl and K in both samples was calculated from Eqs. (1) and (2) in Table VII. The sums of electrolytes, Na+K+Cl were 104.3 mEq/liter or 364 mg/dl for sample A, and 74.8 mEq/liter or 277 mg/dl for sample B, and the difference was 87 mg/dl.

The contents of lactose, protein and the sum of the two in both samples were estimated from Eqs. (3), (4), and (5) in Table VII, and the differences in content, (A−B), were calculated. They were −450, −460 and −910 mg/100 g for lactose, protein and lactose+protein, respectively, against a difference of +87 mg/dl in Na+K+Cl. Thus, it was shown that a small change in the concentration of electrolytes corresponded to considerable changes in the content of lactose and protein or of solids other than fat in normal milk.

3) Inverse relation between electrolytes and fat

Since it seemed that the relationship between the contents of electrolytes and fat would be insignificant, we set aside the examination of the relation between these constituents until later. But when it was examined, an inverse relationship was again found between them.

The normal milk samples used were the same 56 samples as described in the preceding section, except one sample which had a markedly low fat content. The mean and standard deviation of the fat content of the 55 normal milk samples was 2.855±0.507 (%) with a range of 1.78–3.82%.

Correlations and regression equations between the content of fat and other constituents are shown in Table VIII. Every correlation coefficient between the concentration of any one of the electrolytes and the fat

TABLE VIII. Correlations and Regression Equations between Fat and Other Constituents in Normal Milk[a] Taken from 32 Lactation Periods of 24 Cows, $n=55$

Correlation between *x*	Correlation between *y*	Correlation coefficient	Regression equation	SE of regression coefficient	(No.)
Fat %	Protein %	0.756***	$y=0.452x+1.787$	0.0535	(1)
Fat %	Lactose %	0.577***	$y=0.244x+3.666$	0.0473	(2)
Na mEq/liter	Fat %	−0.336*	$y=-0.091x+4.309$	0.0355	(3)
K mEq/liter	Fat %	−0.613***	$y=-0.094x+7.078$	0.0168	(4)
Cl mEq/liter	Fat %	−0.627***	$y=-0.048x+4.424$	0.0085	(5)
Na+K+Cl mEq/liter	Fat %	−0.654***	$y=-0.032x+5.833$	0.0051	(6)
Na+K+Cl mEq/liter	F+P+L %	−0.773***	$y=-0.067x+16.537$	0.0076	(7)

Correlation coefficient are statistically significant, at $p<0.05$ (*), at $p<0.01$ (**), at $p<0.001$ (***).

[a] Morning milk.

content was negative and statistically significant. Accordingly, correlations between Na+K+Cl and fat and the sum of fat+lactose+protein were markedly negative.

Using the previous hypothetical normal milk samples A and B, the differences in the fat content and in the total sum of fat, lactose and protein were calculated in the same way as for the previous example. The fat content and the total sum for sample A whose Na+K+Cl value was 104.3 mEq/liter and B, 78.4 mEq/liter, were estimated from Eqs. (6) and (7) in Table VIII; the fat content of sample A was 2.50% and that of B was 3.32%, and the total sum of fat, lactose and protein in sample A was 9.55% and that of B was 11.28%. Therefore, the difference between the two samples, (A−B), was −820 mg/100 g for the fat content, and −1,730 mg/100 g for the sum of fat, lactose and protein content, against a difference of +87 mg/dl in Na+K+Cl. The difference of −1,730 mg/100 g, consisted of −820, −450 and −460 mg/100 g or the difference of fat, lactose and protein content between the two samples.

Thus, it was shown that a small change in the concentration of electrolytes corresponded to not only big changes in the contents of lactose and protein, but also to a marked change in fat in normal milk. Moreover, the change in the fat content was largest among the major organic constituents.

4) Possibility of ionic regulation of milk synthesis

The inverse relationships between the concentration of electrolytes and the major organic constituents in normal milk were confirmed further by examining 24 normal milk samples collected from 24 cows during 3 months in spring, 1976. We obtained correlations and regressions very similar to those found in the previous normal milk samples (*8*).

A decrease in lactose in milk with a simultaneous rise of Na and Cl in abnormal milk is well known. As mentioned in a previous section, this change seems to be caused by an admixture of extracellular fluid with milk in damaged quarters where an actual breakdown of the mammary epithelium takes place. But, the inverse relation between electrolytes and the content of lactose or other major organic constituents in normal milk would not be attributable to such a process, since the concentrations of electrolytes are positively correlated with each other in normal milk.

We considered osmotic balance as the cause of the inverse relation between the electrolytes and the organic constituents. It may be inferred that normal milk whose electrolytes content is high will have a low content of organic constituents, and *vice versa*, in order that the balance of the osmotic pressure of milk may be preserved.

Linzell and Peaker (*4*) reported that lactose varied and was inversely related to the concentrations of Na, K, and Cl in milk in various species of mammals. As milk in all the animals has very similar osmolarity which is close to the value for plasma, and as lactose and the electrolytes are the predominant osmoles of milk, the inverse relation is what was expected by the authors. In normal milk from different cows, we observed inverse relations not only between the electrolytes and lactose, but also between electrolytes and protein and fat as well.

According to the present conceptions of milk secretion, it is possible to speculate that in cows whose milk has a high electrolyte concentration, the intracellular concentration of the electrolytes of the mammary alveolar cells may be also high, at least in K and Na, since these ions are passively equilibrated across the apical cell membrane. In such an osmotic environment inside the cells, the lactose concentration or other organic constituents may be reduced, especially in the Golgi vesicles where lactose and proteins would be packed together. According to Linzell and Peaker, secretion into a Golgi vesicle is equivalent to secretion into the alveolar lumen (*4*).

On the other hand, the inverse relationship between the electrolytes and fat suggests another possible explanation. Fat droplets of varying size are seen scattered throughout the cytoplasm in lactating mammary cells, and they are discharged from the apical surface of the cell through a process which is independent of secretion of lactose and protein. Therefore, fat seems to be a negligible osmole in milk and inside the alveolar cells. Nevertheless, fat content is inversely related with the concentration of Na, K, and Cl in the normal milk. Moreover, the change in fat content which corresponded to the change in concentrations of electrolytes was largest among similar changes in the major organic constituents in normal milk.

Therefore, the cause of inverse relations between electrolytes and fat, lactose and protein in normal milk is not the osmotic balance between themselves, but rather might be the balance between electrolytes and the precursors of the major organic constituents. And, if the intracellular concentration of electrolytes is determined mainly by the activity of the basolateral membrane of the alveolar cells which transports electrolytes across the membrane, the ion transport activity may have a close relation with the synthetic activity in the mammary alveolar cells.

Recently, the possibility of ionic regulation of lactose and protein synthesis in the mammary cells has emerged through biochemical studies (*2*, *17*). The result of the present study in relations between constituents of normal milk from different cows also indicates the importance of the role of the electrolytes in the mechanism of milk secretion.

SUMMARY

The concentration of sodium, potassium and chloride in cow's milk varies according to physiological and non-physiological causes. The change in the composition of abnormal quarter-milk due to mastitis, compared with normal quarter milk from the same udder, can be explained by an admixture of extracellular fluid with normal milk. The increase in Na and Cl concentrations in abnormal milk indicates quantitatively the amounts of extracellular fluid which mix into the milk. The increase in blood protein, IgG and BSA in abnormal milk bears a quantitative relation with the increase in Na and Cl.

The osmolarity of milk is stable even if milk composition changes considerably. This constancy is, for the most part, due to quantitative interrelations among the concentration of Na, Cl, K, and lactose.

A clear inverse relationship between the concentration of electrolytes and the content of fat, lactose, and protein was found in normal milk from different cows. A small change in the electrolytes corresponds to large changes in the contents of fat, lactose, and protein in normal milk. The relationship seems to suggest that a close relation may exist between the activities of ion transport and biosynthesis in the mammary alveolar cells.

REFERENCES

1. Barry, J. M. and Rowland, S. J. (1953). Variation in the ionic and lactose concentrations in milk. *Biochem. J.* **54**, 575–578.
2. Falconer, I. R. and Rowe, J. M. (1975). Possible mechanism for action of prolactin on mammary cell sodium transport. *Nature* **256**, 327–328.
3. Linzell, J. L. (1972). Mechanism of secretion of the aqueous phase of milk. *J. Dairy Sci.* **55**, 1316–1322.
4. Linzell, J. L. and Peaker, M. (1971). Mechanism of milk secretion. *Physiol. Rev.* **51**, 564–597.
5. Linzell, J. L. and Peaker, M. (1972). Day to day variations in milk composition in the goat and cow as a guide to the detection of subclinical mastitis. *Br. Vet. J.* **128**, 284–300.
6. Oshima, M. and Fuse, H. (1976). Inverse relationship between the concentration of milk electrolytes and contents of lactose and protein observed in the normal milk of individual cows within the same herd. *Japan. J. Zootech. Sci.* **47**, 486–493.
7. Oshima, M. and Fuse, H. (1976). Interrelationships between the concentration of constituents in 'the normal milk' of individual cows, in special reference to the negative correlations found between the electrolytes and the contents of fat, and total solids. *Japan. J. Zootech. Sci.* **47**, 494–499.
8. Oshima, M. and Fuse, H. (1977). Inverse relationship between the electrolyte concentration and the content of fat, protein, and lactose in the normal milks of individual cows from the same herd. *J. Dairy Res.* **44**, 347–350.
9. Oshima, M. and Hodate, H. (1975). Changes in the concentration of serum albumin and immunoglobulin associated with the increase in the concentration of sodium and chloride in the abnormal quarter milk. *Japan. J. Zootech. Sci.* **56**, 81–86.
10. Oshima, M., Fuse, H., and Ishii, T. (1974). Detection of the abnormal quarter milk based upon the quarter difference in the electrolyte concentrations, especially in the Na+Cl value. *Bull. Natl. Inst. Anim. Ind.* **28**, 17–24.
11. Oshima, M., Fuse, H., and Ishii, T. (1974). Interrelations between the increase in sodium and chloride contents and the changes in other constituents in the abnormal quarter milk. *Japan. J. Zootech. Sci.* **45**, 543–550.

12. Peaker, M. (1975). Recent advances in the study of monovalent ion movements across the mammary epithelium: Relation to onset of lactation. *J. Dairy Sci.* **58**, 1042–1047.
13. Rook, J.A.F. (1961). Variation in the chemical composition of the milk of the cow (Parts I and II). *Dairy Sci. Abstr.* **23**, 251–258, 303–308.
14. Rook, J.A.F. and Campling, R. C. (1965). Effect of stage and number of lactation on the yield and composition of cow's milk. *J. Dairy Res.* **32**, 45–55.
15. Rook, J.A.F. and Wheelock, J. V. (1967). The secretion of water-soluble constituents in milk. *J. Dairy Res.* **34**, 273–287.
16. Rook, J.A.F. and Wood, M. (1959). Potassium and lactose in milk in relation to the physiology of milk secretion. *Nature* **184**, 647–648.
17. Silcock, W. R. and Patton, S. (1972). Correlative secretion of protein, lactose and K^+ in milk of the goat. *J. Cell. Physiol.* **79**, 151–154.
18. Snedecor, G. W. and Cochran, W. G. (1967). *Statistical Methods*, 6th ed., pp. 285–288. Ames, Iowa: Iowa University Press.
19. Tasker, J. B. (1971). Fluids, electrolytes, and acid-base balance. In *Clinical Biochemistry of Domestic Animals*, ed. Kaneko, J. J. and Cornelius, C. E., pp. 61–110. New York, London: Academic Press.
20. Tocher, J. F. (1925). *Variations in the Composition of Milk*, pp. 1~195. Edinburgh: His Majesty's Stationary Office.
21. Vanlandingham, A. H., Weakeley, Jr., C. E., Moore, E. N., and Henderson, H. O. (1941). Mastitis. I. The relationship of the development of mastitis to changes in the chlorine, lactose and casein number of milk. *J. Dairy Sci.* **24**, 283–298.
22. Waite, R., White, J.C.D., and Robertson, A. (1956). Variations in the chemical composition of milk with particular reference to the solids-not-fat. I. The effect of stage of lactation, season of year and age of cow. *J. Dairy Res.* **23**, 65–81.
23. Walsh, J. P. and Rook, J.A.F. (1964). Ratio of potassium to lactose in cow's milk and its genetic basis. *Nature* **204**, 353–355.
24. Wheelock, J. V., Rook, J.A.F., and Dodd, F. H. (1965). The relationship in the cow between the osmotic pressure of milk and of blood. *J. Dairy Res.* **32**, 79–88.
25. Wheelock, J. V., Rook, J.A.F., Neave, F. K., and Dodd, F. H. (1966). The effect of bacterial infection of the udder on the yield and composition of cow's milk. *J. Dairy Res.* **33**, 199–215.

SUBJECT INDEX

Acetyl-CoA-carboxylase 258
Adenyl cyclase 252, 259
Adipose 207, 213
Admixture theory
  for change in milk composition 367
Adrenalectomy
  effect on lactational performance 11
  effect on lactogenesis 274, 278, 279
Adrenaline
  effect on milk removal 62
Aggregation
  of epithelial cells 205, 209
Allograft 164
Amygdala 311, 312
  lateral, stimulation of 91
  medial, stimulation of 93
Anterior chamber of the eye 181
Antidiuretic effect 25
Antidiuretic hormone 60
Apical cell membrane 379
Autograft 164
Autoradiography 203

Basal lamina 215
Basement membrane 205
Basolateral membrane
  of alveolar cells 380

Bed nucleus
  of stria terminalis 93
Blood flow 28
  of mammary gland 358
2-Br-α-ergokryptine 73
2-Br-α-ergocryptine methane sulfonate (CB-154) 329
2-Bromo-α-ergocryptine (CB-154) 130
Bromocriptine 73

California mastitis test 365
Casein kinase 256
Cathepsin 257
CB-154 73, 130, 144, 329
Central gray matter 91
Chloride
  in cow's milk 363, 380
Concurrent pregnancy 288–292, 294, 295
Continuous suckling 289, 295
Corticoid 274, 277, 280
Corticosterone 267, 268, 270, 271, 272, 274, 294, 295
Cortisol 8, 10
Cross-circulation experiments 25
Cyclic AMP (cAMP) 11, 12, 252, 253, 259

Dairy cows 76
7,12-Dimethylbenz[a]anthracene (DMBA)-induced mammary tumors 133
DNA
  content in mammary gland 122, 272, 289
  effect of ovariectomy and adrenalectomy 272, 273, 275, 278, 279
  synthesis of 8, 126, 143
Dorsal longitudinal fasciculus 306, 316, 317
Dry period
  of lactation 297, 298

EEG-afterreaction 87
EEG arousal threshold 87
Electrical stimulation
  bed nucleus of stria terminalis 92
  medial amygdala 93
  medial preoptic area 91
Electro-encephalogram(EEG) 87, 89
Electrolytes
  in cow's milk 363, 373, 374, 381
  intracellular concentration of 379, 380
Endoplasmic reticulum 251, 255, 259
Epithelial cell 215
Ergocornine 73, 130, 134
α-Ergokryptine 73
Ergot drugs 111
Ergotamine 77
Estradiol
  effect on mammary growth 184
  implantation into the medial amygdala 93
Estrogen
  effect on mammary tumorigenesis 134
  effect on normal mammary growth 127, 134
  effect on prolactin release 108
  implantation in the amygdala 311, 312
  implantation in the arcuate nucleus 93
  positive feedback sites of 92
Evoked potential 90
Extracellular fluid 367, 380

Fat
  in cow's milk 381
Feto-placentectomy
  effect on lactogenesis 265

Galactopoiesis 44
Genetical predisposition
  on mammary tumorigenesis 136
Gland-free mammary fat pad 175
Golgi body 252, 255, 256
Golgi vesicles 379
Gonadotropin 91, 97
Growth hormone (GH) 26

Heterograft 164
Hippocampus 91
Histocompatibility 165
Human placental lactogen (HPL) 134
Hypophysectomy
  techniques of 49
Hypothalamus 59, 306, 307, 311, 312, 314–318
Hysterectomy
  effect on lactogenesis 275, 278, 279
IgG 332, 369
Immobilization stress 90

Immunoglobulin G 332, 369
Immuno-potentiation
of mammary tumor 138
Immuno-suppression
of mammary tumor 138
Implantation
delayed 288, 291
Induced lactation 45
Initiation of lactation 265
Interscapular brown fat 183
Involution 355–357
Isograft 164

Kinins 27

α-Lactalbumin 266, 332
Lactation 325
hormonal control of 7, 107
induced- 45
initiation of 265
Lactation complex
hormones of 15
Lactation curve 349
Lactational performance 11, 288, 290, 291
Lactational response 349
Lactation stage 354
Lactogenesis
in cow 325, 352
in rat 265
Lactogenic complex 15, 49
β-Lactoglobulin 332
Lactose
content in mammary glands, rat 272, 274
content in mammary glands, mouse 290, 297
content in cow's milk 368, 374, 381
synthesis of 31
synthesis of, goat 332
synthesis of, rat 265, 272
Let-down 59
Life span
mammary parenchyma 195
Lipase 258, 259
Lipogenesis 15
Luteinizing hormone releasing factor (LRF) 114

Magnocellular nuclei 64
Mammary alveolar cells 381
Mammary gland
hormonal control of 129
ion transport of 363, 380
nucleic acids of, mouse 289, 291
nucleic acids of, cow 350
perfused 24
permeability of 369
proliferation of, cow 350, 351, 356
Mammary growth 44, 121
abnormal 128
normal 123, 125, 128, 141,
strain-difference 125
Mammary hyperplastic alveolar nodules (HAN) 130
Mammary tumors 138
pregnancy-dependent 132, 139
Mammary tumor virus (MTV) 126, 136, 137, 142
Mammary tumorigenesis 129, 134, 136, 138, 143
Mastitis 374
subclinical 374
Medial forebrain bundle 306, 307, 315–318
Mesenchyme 217
Mesometrial fat layer 180
Messenger RNA 252, 256, 259
3-Methylcholanthrene 200

Milk
  abnormal 364, 365, 380
  composition of 364
  cow 363
  normal 379, 380
  subclinical mastitic 365
Milk ejection 24
Milk ejection pressure 307
Milk ejection reflex 60, 77, 306
Milk fatty acids 29
Milk proteins
  precursors of 33
Milk removal 347, 351, 352
Milking
  frequency of 353, 355, 356
Milking stimulus 48, 333
Milk synthesis 379
Mini-pigs 75
Multiunit activity (MUA) 91
Myoepithelial cell 215
Myoepithelium 63

Neuroendocrinology 112, 113
Neurohypophysis 306, 307
Neurophysin 26
Neurosecretory cells 64
Neurotransmission 28
Neurotransmitter 113, 114
Nude mice 128

Osmolarity 370
Osmotic balance 379
Osmotic concentration 372
Osmotic pressure 369, 373
Ovariectomy
  effect on lactogenesis 265, 266, 272, 278, 279
Oxytocin 8, 10, 24, 51, 60
  release 305–311, 314, 317

Paradoxical sleep 87
Pararenal fat pad 178
Paraventricular nuclei 307–309
Parenchyma 200
Pathways
  of oxytocin and prolactin release 305, 306, 309–311, 317
  of prolactin release 305, 314, 317
Placental hormone 266, 277, 280
Placental lactogen 125
Placental mammotropins 125
Polysome 255
Potassium
  in cow's milk 363, 380
Pregnancy 287, 292–295
Pregnancy dependent mammary tumors 132, 138, 139
Preoptic area 91
Prepartum milking 352
Progesterone
  effect on lactogenesis 265, 271, 280
  effect on pituitary prolactin content 108
  positive feedback of 92, 328
Prolactin (PRL) 8, 10, 71, 266, 269, 270–280
  binding site of 236, 237, 239–242, 246
  radioimmunoassay of 325
  receptor 231–233, 239, 242–245, 266, 280
  receptor association constant 239 241
  receptor dissociation constant 236, 239–242
  receptor interaction 233, 237, 245
  release of 305, 306, 308–312, 314–318
  secretion of 109
  specific binding of 234, 236, 237, 239, 243, 244

Prolactin inhibiting factor (PIF) 113, 114
Prolactin releasing factor (PRF) 113, 114
Prolonged lactation 145
Protein
  in cow's milk 374, 381
Pseudopregnancy 275, 278, 279

Quarter-milk 364, 365
  abnormal 365, 380
  normal 374, 380

Radioimmunoassay
  of PRL 325
Regeneration 205
Reserpine 109
RNA
  messenger 256
  RNA/DNA, mouse 291
  RNA/DNA, rat 273
  synthesis 8

Secretory cell activity 355
Serum albumin 369
Sex hormone
  feedback mechanisms of 90
Sham-milking 335
Single unit activities of 90
Sodium
  in cow's milk 363, 380
Spinothalamic fibers 310
Spinothalamic system 314, 316, 317
Spinothalamic tract 306
Stress 329
  on prolactin release 329
Stroma 200
Suckling stimulus 59, 305, 312, 315
Supraoptic-hypophysial tract 61
Supraoptic nuclei 307–309
Sympathetic adrenergic nerves 27
Sympathetic discharge 64

Teats 27
Thyroid stimulating hormone releasing hormone (TRH) 113
Thyrotropin (TSH) 325, 336
Triiodothyronine (T3) 325
Trypan blue 172

Vasopressin 61
Vital organs 16
Vital staining 172

Whole mount preparation 121, 124, 131

Xenograft 164